# *Mental Health Consultation in Nursing Homes*

## Clinical Gerontology

GENERAL EDITOR: *Steven H. Zarit*

1. Mental Health Consultation in Nursing Homes

# Mental Health Consultation in Nursing Homes

*Michael A. Smyer*
*Margaret D. Cohn*
*Diane Brannon*

NEW YORK UNIVERSITY PRESS
*New York and London*

First published in paperback in 1990.



**Library of Congress Cataloging-in-Publication Data**

Smyer, Michael A.
Mental health consultation in nursing homes.

(Clinical gerontology ; 1)
Bibliography: p.
Includes index.
1. Nursing home patients—Mental health.
2. Psychiatric consultation. I. Cohn, Margaret D., 1938– . II. Brannon, Diane. III. Title.
IV. Series.
RC451.4.N87S69 1988 618.97'689 88-9982
ISBN 0-8147-7911-5 pbk.

New York University Press books are Smyth-sewn
and printed on permanent and durable acid-free paper.

*This book is dedicated, with affection and respect, to Tex and Alyce Mary Smyer, Hazel McGraw, David A. Decker and his mother, Edith Heffer, Jean and Walter Brannon, and Charlotte Upton.*

# Contents

# Introduction

Nursing homes replaced state mental hospitals as the major receiving site for mentally ill elderly during the 1970s. Estimates vary, but somewhere between 50 and 80 percent of the elderly in nursing homes are believed to have some degree of mental health impairment.[1] Within the nursing home setting, however, there are few organized intervention efforts on a scale comparable to the community mental health system's offerings for community-dwelling elderly.[2] The Institute of Medicine's (1986) recent review of nursing homes summarized the current situation: "(G)reater attention should be paid to mental health aspects of care including appropriate assessment and management techniques for mental and behavioral problems" (p. 381).

This book is designed to provide an introduction to mental-health consultation in nursing homes. It was written with several audiences in mind: administrators in nursing homes, who must provide leadership for their settings in recognizing and responding to recurrent mental health issues; current members of the key mental health disciplines—psychiatry, nursing, social work, and psychology—who are interested in consulting in nursing homes; current staff members of nursing homes who face the day-to-day challenges of providing mental health care in a physical health care facility; faculty members and students in the core mental health disciplines, who are concerned with preparing practitioners to respond to the mental health needs of older adults and their families.

We assume that each portion of the audience is familiar with some of the issues discussed in this book. Few professionals, however, are conversant with the broad range of interdisciplinary topics encompassed by mental health consultation in nursing homes. Therefore, a primary goal of this book is to provide a framework for approaching consultation in this setting.

In chapter 1, we present a conceptualization of nursing homes that contrasts with previous discussions of their detrimental effects: We view nursing homes as communities. In chapter 2, we consider the larger social and economic contexts that affect their functioning, exploring issues such as federal regulations, profit incentives for investors, and staffing patterns. In chapter 3, we discuss the central aspects of mental health consultation, with particular attention to the unique contributions of each mental health discipline.

The first three chapters provide a foundation for considering mental health consultation to key members of the nursing home community: residents, family members, and staff members. In chapters 4, 5, 6, and 7, mental health concerns of individual residents are the focus. In chapter 4, we review the types of mental health problems that occur in nursing homes. In chapter 5, we discuss the process of individual-assessment and specific assessment approaches that are useful. In chapter 6, we present an overview of basic individually oriented treatment approaches. In chapter 7, we focus more closely on treatment efforts aimed at the three most frequent types of problematic resident behaviors: depression, agitation, and disorientation.

In chapters 8 and 9, we turn to the relatives of nursing home residents. We first discuss general patterns of family support throughout later life and then present more specific information on family involvement with nursing home residents, thus dispelling the myth that admission to a nursing home signals the end of family contact and concern. In chapter 9, we consider assessment and treatment approaches for use with family members.

The third major group of nursing home community members are the staff. In chapter 10, we discuss the nature of the caregiving work itself, focusing attention on the largest staff group in nursing homes—nurse's aides and licensed practical nurses (LPNs). In chapter 11, we offer suggestions for mental health–relevant interventions with staff members.

Nursing homes are generally women's worlds where female residents and caregivers far outnumber male counterparts. In contrast, physicians and administrators are more often male, but may be either gender. We also recognize that consultants to this gender-biased system may well be either male or female. Therefore we have attempted to simplify sentence structure by randomly referring to consultants, physicians, and other administrative personnel as *either* he or she rather than he/she, and nursing staff as she.

Writing a book is like making homemade ice cream. At several points in the process, you stop the cranking to inspect the product. Connoisseurs among the group caution patience and renewed work on the mixture. Others, enthusiastic throughout the processes, are eager to have the finished product, no matter how far from perfect. We have benefited from the critical comments and helpful suggestions of several friends and colleagues. We are especially grateful to Steve Zarit for his careful and cogent advice on earlier drafts of the manuscript and to Kitty Moore for her support throughout the project. In addition, Larry Gamm, Ray Horn, Pat Piper, and Jack Spayd read sections of the book and helped improve it. The College of St. Scholastica in Duluth, Minnesota, provided us the opportunity to test the concepts and the manuscript in their graduate seminar on aging and mental health. We appreciate the program's assistance and the students' helpful commentary. Jackie Chapin, Tina Meyers, and Joy Barger provided invaluable secretarial support. Finally, we gratefully acknowledge the helpful support and stimulation of our interdisciplinary professional home, Penn State's College of Health and Human Development.

## NOTES

1. Levine (1981) and Gatz, Smyer, and Lawton (1980) discuss the transformation of the mental-health system and the concomitant change in the nursing home.
2. Glasscote and Biegel (1976) and Lindeman (1985) discuss the contrast between staffing patterns in community mental health and nursing home settings.

*Mental Health Consultation in Nursing Homes*

# 1

# The Nursing Home Community

*Michael A. Smyer*

## INTRODUCTION

Consider the following problems:[1]

1) Cut a cake into eight equal pieces with only three cuts.
2) How are the following numbers arranged?
   0 2 3 6 7 1 9 4 5 8

Solving each problem requires two essential steps: changing our initial expectations of the problem and exploring other possible solutions. For example, most people approach the first problem assuming that a knife is used to cut vertically. When we think about other ways to use it, the answer becomes clear: two vertical cuts and one horizontal cut will give you eight equal pieces from three cuts.

Similarly, most people view the sequence in the second problem as only a set of numbers. After trying out different combinations of addition, subtraction, multiplication, and division most people give up. But some people then shift strategies: They ask another question. If these aren't only numbers, what are they? Asking this question leads to an unexpected solution. Treating the numbers as words, you can eventually get to the solution. These are words in reverse alphabetical order!

Consulting to nursing homes is a lot like trying to solve these problems. An essential first step is examining our expectations about the nursing home setting and the possibilities for treatment there. These expectations structure our assessment of problems and solutions in the setting.

In this chapter, we present three conceptualizations of nursing homes: nursing homes as total institutions, nursing homes as collections of differing realities, and nursing homes as communities. Each view highlights different expectations, problems, and potential solutions. The views are not mutually exclusive, but they do offer contradictory action suggestions.

Throughout this book, we emphasize a view of nursing homes as communities. Therefore, most of this chapter introduces the characteristics of the key community members—residents, residents' family members, and staff members. In doing so, we highlight the importance of these characteristics for mental health consultation. We end the chapter with a suggested view of the nursing home setting that allows all of the community members to identify those tasks that are most appropriate for residents, relatives, and staff members.

## NURSING HOMES AS TOTAL INSTITUTIONS

Where do you work? Is it the same place that you play? The same place that you sleep? For most of us, there are clear divisions among our different activities.

Think about a typical day. Are there activities or times when you are alone, or in the company of relatively few people? How about your schedule? Is it relatively flexible or rigidly scheduled? What about control? Who arranges the schedule for you and your family?

Your answers to these questions help define the type of setting in which you live. For most, daily activities are varied as to where, when, and with whom we do them. Nursing home residents' lives, however, are removed from the world of work, from outside schedules, and from daily contacts. In many cases, the nursing home may function as a "total" institution.

Erving Goffman popularized the term *total institution* to depict a setting that is significantly encompassing.[2] For Goffman, several characteristics are important in describing this kind of setting: first, all aspects of life are conducted in the same place and under a single authority; second, activities occur in the company of others, who are treated alike; third, daily activities are tightly scheduled; and, fourth, activities are controlled under an overall rational plan.

In total institutions, the setting's own schedule, rules, and expectations for behavior come to replace those of other settings. The pervasive influence of such settings varies in how accessible they are to the outside world: the more exchanges between those inside and those outside the institution, the less pervasive the "totality" of the institutional setting. Goffman points out that the separation of the institution's residents from external realities can be most difficult emotionally for one social institution we will refer to in chapters 8 and 9: the resident's family.

## THE MULTIPLE REALITIES OF NURSING HOMES

Another characteristic of total institutions is a basic tension between the resident (the *inmates* is Goffman's term) and the staff. Jay Gubrium[3] has contrasted the perceptions of three groups in the nursing home settings:

"top staff," or administrators; the "floor staff"; and the "patients," or residents.

Gubrium was concerned with how the setting constrains the actions of its key participants. Drawing on his field observations in a nursing home over several months, Gubrium tried to understand how the "work" of everyday life and resident care gets done.

Several themes are important from Gubrium's work: First, the physical setting and role expectations are critical factors in shaping the different views of resident care. Second, the difference between the formal policy and its application is important. Third, informal, unwritten understanding of staff and resident roles, duties, and expectations is very influential in shaping the participants' behavior.

We will return to each of these themes later. For now, however, it is important to emphasize the complexity of the setting and the way in which perceptions shape action in the nursing home.

Gubrium's work, like that of others in the field,[4] emphasizes the differences among the various role players and participants in the nursing home. Although he acknowledges that the floor staff may understand and accommodate the residents' perception and preferences, Gubrium emphasizes the basic tension that arises from differing and conflicting views of the setting.

## THE NURSING HOME AS A COMMUNITY

We view nursing homes as communities, with several different community members. This perspective shifts our attention to the characteristics of community members: administrators and staff, residents, and their family members. Each group brings different talents and expectations to the nursing home—talents and expectations that shape the consultant's task.

The choice of community as a metaphor or theme has several important implications. First, it emphasizes the *shared* interests and concerns of those within the community. For example, Warren's classic discussion of the community in America provides a useful framework for our discussion of the nursing home as a community.[5] He points out that the very label *community* carries with it many meanings:

> The term "community" implies something both psychological and geographical. Psychologically, it implies shared interests, characteristics, or association, as in the expression "community of interest." . . . Geographically, it denotes a specific area where people are clustered. Sociologically, the term combines these two connotations. It relates to the shared interests and be-

havior patterns which people have by virtue of their common locality (Warren, 1963, p. 6).

In addition to outlining the various meanings of *community,* Warren offers a more formal definition of a community:

> *that combination of social units and systems which perform the major social functions having locality relevance.* This is another way of saying that by "community" we mean the organization of social activities to afford people daily local access to those broad areas of activity which are necessary in day-to-day living (p. 9).

Warren outlines five major social functions provided for by communities: production-distribution-consumption; socialization; social control; social participation; and mutual support. These functions range from providing the basic goods and services needed for existence to providing the social friendships and support that give existence meaning. Goffman's work focuses on the total responsibility of the institution for this full range of functions. Our approach acknowledges that totality, but focuses on the analogy between nursing homes and other communities. A major distinction between the two approaches is the "permeability" of the community's boundaries.

Viewing the nursing home as a community suggests that there is an openness among this community and between it and other social groups—a commerce of people, ideas, regulations, services, and so forth. For example, Warren has discussed what he calls the "vertical patterns" of communities, the links between the community's subsystems and systems that are outside of the immediate community. For example, the local bank or grocery store may be part of a larger regional or national chain. Thus, regional and national economic policy may have an indirect impact on the well-being of those community structures. Similarly, several social scientists have identified the major role that federal and state legislation has played in shaping the treatment provided in nursing homes.[6] We will return to this theme in the next chapter.

The metaphor of the nursing home as a community also suggests a third important link for mental health consultants: using mental health consultation and education strategies developed for community settings in institutional settings like nursing homes. In later chapters, we will give examples of how solutions to nursing home problems can be found in approaches already proven effective in community settings.

These themes—the common bonds of community members, the open boundaries of communities, and the applicability of community mental health approaches—provide an underlying optimism for intervention that is missing from the work of Goffman or Gubrium. In later chapters, we will document the basis for this optimism by noting the effectiveness of various treatment approaches—even with severely impaired elderly. For now, however, we will focus on the three primary groups of community members in the nursing home: residents, their families, and the staff members.

## NURSING HOME RESIDENTS

At any one point in time 5 percent of the older population can be found in long-term-care institutions. In 1985, for example, there were 1.3 million elderly residents in nursing homes. The 5 percent figure can be misleading, however, since it represents a "snapshot" of the elderly at any one point in time. If we take a longer view, the lifetime chances of spending time in an institutional setting are approximately 20 percent.[7]

Barry Gurland suggests that three elements are associated with the need for mental health services among older adults with mental health problems: a concomitant medical disorder; problems with caring for themselves; and the absence of an effective social-support network.[8] These elements are also associated with nursing home placement for older adults.

Gurland's three elements provide a useful framework for describing the patient population of nursing homes.[9] Consider, for example, the medical disorders represented in nursing homes settings.

Table 1.1 summarizes information on the disease states of nursing home patients. It is clear that older adults in nursing homes report a variety of both physical and mental health problems.[10]

In terms of self-care capacity, nursing home residents are again likely to be more impaired than community-dwelling elderly. For example, Cohen and his colleagues (1986) found that "the more severe the functional disability, the greater the likelihood of nursing home entry" (p. 790). Johnson and Grant[11] caution, however, that the relationship between functional disability and institutionalization is moderated by the third element of Gurland's framework: an effective social-support system.

## FAMILIES OF NURSING HOME RESIDENTS

The popular image of the process of institutionalization is one of abandonment: a son or daughter "dumps" Mom in the nursing home, abandoning her with little thought given to the care and concern that she has shown for her offspring earlier in life. Information from three sources undercut the myth and provide a more realistic view of family involvement in the institutionalization process: data on the family ties of nursing home resi-

TABLE 1.1: Nursing Home Residents by Selected Health Status, United States, 1977

| *Health Status* | *Residents (%)* |
|---|---|
| *Diseases of the Circulatory System* | |
| Arteriosclerosis | 48 |
| Hypertension | 21 |
| Stroke | 16 |
| Paralysis or palsy, other than arthritis, related to stroke | 6 |
| Heart trouble | 34 |
| *Mental Disorders and Senility Without Psychosis* | |
| Mental illness | 11 |
| Chronic brain syndrome | 25 |
| Senility | 32 |
| Mental retardation | 6 |
| Alcoholism | 3 |
| Drug addiction | — |
| Insomnia | 10 |
| *Other Chronic Conditions or Impairments* | |
| Diseases of the musculoskeletal system and connective tissues: Arthritis and rheumatism | 25 |
| Chronic back/spine problems, excluding stiffness and deformity | 5 |
| Permanent stiffness or deformity of back, arms, legs, or extremities, including feet, toes, hands, or fingers | 14 |
| Missing arms, legs, or extremities, including feet, toes, hands, or fingers | 2 |
| *Diseases of the Nervous System and Sense Organs* | |
| Blindness | 5 |
| Glaucoma | 3 |
| Cataracts | 6 |
| Deafness | 7 |
| Parkinson's disease | 4 |
| Paralysis or palsy, other than arthritis, unrelated to stroke | 4 |
| *Accidents, Poisonings, and Violence* | |
| Hip fracture | 8 |
| Other bone fracture | 4 |
| *Endocrine, Nutritional, and Metabolic Diseases* | |
| Diabetes | 14 |

Source: National Center for Health Statistics (1979).

Note: These disease categories are based on the *Eighth Revision International Classification of Diseases, Adapted for Use in the United States (ICDA)*.

Figures do not add to 100 percent because some residents have more than one reported condition or impairment. Total number of residents is 1,303,100.

*Continued on next page*

TABLE 1.1: *Continued*

| *Health Status* | *Residents (%)* |
|---|---|
| *Neoplasms* | |
| Cancer | 5 |
| *Diseases of the Respiratory System* | |
| Chronic respiratory disease | 7 |
| *Diseases of the Digestive System* | |
| Constipation | 24 |
| *Diseases of the Blood and Blood-forming Organs* | |
| Anemia | 5 |
| *Diseases of the Skin and Subcutaneous Tissue* | |
| Bedsores | 3 |
| *Other Conditions* | |
| Edema | 18 |
| Kidney trouble | 10 |
| *None of These Conditions* | 1 |

dents; information on functional disability among community-dwelling elderly; and patterns of service use prior to admission to the nursing home.

Most elderly living in institutions have living relatives. Approximately 63 percent have at least one living child, and 16 percent have a living spouse. The availability of family members, however, varies with age: fewer family resources are available at advanced ages.[12]

These relatives are also likely to be part of an *effective* social-support network—Gurland's criterion. For example, almost two-thirds of all nursing home residents in the 1977 national survey received daily or weekly visitors, while only 13 percent received no visitors. Relatives were a majority of the nursing-home visitors.

Even before the nursing home placement, however, family members are likely to have provided a wide range of services and support.[13] Johnson and Grant (1985), for example, reviewed information on the functional ability of community-dwelling and institutionalized elderly. They presented the now-familiar relationship of increasing difficulty with activities of daily living with increasing age. More importantly, however, they focused on the ratio of those with activities-of-daily-living (ADL) difficulties in the community and those within the nursing home setting (see table 1.2). They concluded that two and a half times as many functionally dependent people live in the community as in nursing homes between ages sixty-five and seventy-four.

This ratio drops to 1.6 after age eighty-five. Johnson and Grant (1985) speculate that changing family structure combines with increasing disability to alter the family's capacity to keep impaired relatives in community settings. Certainly this impression is consistent with the reports that for every institutionalized individual, there are two other older adults in community settings who are equally impaired.

TABLE 1.2: Persons Having Activities-of-Daily-Living (ADL) Dependency and Persons in Nursing Homes, by Age, United States, 1977

| *Age Group* | (1) *% Having ADL Dependency*[a] | (2) *% Residing in Nursing Homes* | (3) *Ratio Between (1) and (2)* |
|---|---|---|---|
| 45–64 | 1.2 | 0.3 | 4.0 |
| 65–74 | 3.5 | 1.4 | 2.5 |
| 75–84 | 11.3 | 6.4 | 1.8 |
| 85 + | 35.1 | 21.6 | 1.6 |

Source: Health Care Financing Administration (1981).
[a]These include all persons who reside either in a nursing home or in the community and who are dependent in one or more activities of daily living (ADL).

Another indication of the important role of family caregivers comes from a recent report of the types of problems encountered by family members and older relatives prior to institutionalization. Smallegan (1985) found that approximately 80 percent of her sample of institutionalized elderly required assistance before admission. The caregivers were primarily relatives: Children were the most frequent caregivers, while spouses and other relatives were also important contributors of care. Again, this pattern is consistent with earlier reports of substantial family involvement in meeting the challenges of decline in later life prior to institutionalization.

The following example illustrates the difficulties family members face before turning to nursing home settings.[14]

In the mid-seventies, my mother began to suffer from arthritis of the spine, which made it increasingly difficult for her to get around, but at the time we persuaded her to come to Chicago in 1978, she was still able to shop and cook and clean and take care of her physical needs. In 1978, we enrolled her as an individual member in the Health Maintenance organization I belong to through Loyola. For forty-five dollars a month, she was able to call and bug the doctors endlessly about her complaints, although she was in essentially good health. She took medicines daily to ease the arthritic pain and control the high blood pressure. She was able to administer the medicines herself, and to take care of her daily needs.

During the winter of 1982, the arthritis got worse. She was in more pain, less able to move, and often mentally confused as to the time of day, nonsequential in conversation, and so on. Finally, one day in the summer of 1982, she could/would not get out of bed. The fire department had to break down the door and my mother entered Evanston Hospital for three weeks. In the hospital, my mother received physical therapy and was taught to walk using a wrap-around walker.

The HMO doctor assured us that she would recover her ability to walk unaided through therapy and practice. My wife believed him. But I knew differently. I knew that Mama was making her bid for life as a semi-invalid. And so I went to see my first social worker.

The social worker was employed by the hospital and she gave me three pieces of information:

1) She would visit my mother. She did and my mother refused to speak to her.
2) I was not financially responsible for my mother. This is true, at least until the present administration is successful in changing this concept.
3) My mother could go on welfare when she had five thousand dollars in the bank. This is untrue.

After three weeks of therapy, the hospital informed us via the doctor that it would no longer keep my mother under Medicare. She could remain in the hospital only as a full-paying customer. My wife and I talked to my mother about the possibility of her entering a home. The very mention of the word terrified her. She refused and told us that she preferred to spend her money on at-home care.

For the next year and a half, my mother had a Home Health Aide with her for five hours a day, seven days a week. The aides are supplied by commercial agencies listed in the yellow pages. They cost \$7.50 an hour plus transportation, with time and a half for weekends and holidays. For five hours a day, the average monthly bill was approximately one thousand dollars.

What did we get? In the course of approximately eighteen months, we got forty-eight different women. We went through two different agencies. Thirty-eight of the forty-eight stayed less than five days. Eight stayed between a week and a month. One stayed two months and the last one stayed three. At the beginning I was careful to be there when each new person arrived, show her around, introduce her to my mother, and so on. After the seventh or eighth, I gave up, and from then on, on any given day, I had no idea who was in charge.

Why did this happen?

1) The agencies are set up for short-term care. They employ a great many people who want a part-time job for a brief time. Few of their employees want to work seven days a week. Few of them want to work on Saturday and Sunday. Typically, there would be one person there three or four days a week and several other people the rest of the week.
2) My mother got rid of them. She would be absolutely charming to them for a morning or a day, lavishing praise on them, then send them down for a container of milk and when they got back accuse them of stealing. When the women denied the accusation, my mother called me, the agency, the janitor of the apartment house, my secretary, the security post at Loyola, the police station, the telephone operator, etc., etc., etc. After a few phone calls, she was hyperventilating, getting flushed, muttering incoherently; and the terrified home aides would call the agency, who would immediately instruct them to leave.

What did the home aides do? They shopped, cooked, made two meals, did light housekeeping, assisted my mother in dressing, bathing, and so on, and above all set up her daily medicines. But that is not what you are really paying for. What you are really paying for is:

1) Total reliability. The agencies have someone there every day, including Christmas.
2) Honesty. My mother was totally wrong. They never stole a thing.

What we got was highly reliable, relatively unskilled labor. The women ranged from college students on a spring break to practical nurses my mother's age. I was particularly struck by their need for emotional reinforcement. Many of them took the fact that my mother was not making progress as a sign of personal failure. They became depressed, cried, asked to be relieved, and so on.

Halfway through this experience, it was obvious that 1) my mother was not improving and 2) she was bankrupting herself. And I began to look for advice. I opened the phone book and called the Department on Aging. What I wanted to know was the following:

1) Could my mother receive government assistance to defray the cost of the home aides?
2) Precisely when could I apply for welfare on her behalf?
3) Could she stay in her present apartment and receive welfare?

What happened when we placed my mother in a home?

1) By the time she entered a home, my mother could/would not move much. Within a week of entering, she fell in the bathroom and cut her scalp open. After that, she remained in bed all day but was still able to feed herself and use the bathroom with the assistance of a nurse.
2) Within a month after entering, my mother was taken to a local hospital for a three-week stay for a blood infection. When she returned to the home, she could no longer feed herself or sit on a toilet. She is now catheterized. She lies in bed all day. Three times a day, a couple of nurses haul her into a wheelchair, tie her in with a sheet, and wheel her into a common room where along with fifteen other people she is mass-fed by a nurse.
3) When people are institutionalized, they begin to behave like institutionalized people. My mother dozes most of the time. She was clearly depressed, and the home brought in a geriatric psychiatrist, who started her on an antidepressant, which has picked up her spirits. She is still coherent but in view of her rapid decline within the last six months, I expect that she will lapse into an incoherent state within the next year.

---

In chapter 8, we consider more fully the role of family members in later life. For now, however, it is important to see the nursing home setting from the family's perspective: as the most recent in a series of care options that families have tried. Most often, the nursing home is turned to as a last option only after significant economic and emotional resources have been depleted.

## NURSING HOME STAFF MEMBERS

The third major group of participants in the nursing home community are the staff members.[15] For the consultant unfamiliar with nursing home settings, the diversity of staff members, levels of expertise, and degree of contact with patients may be at first bewildering. In this section, we present several indicators for assessing the staffing of the nursing home industry as a whole. These measures are also useful in gauging the staffing patterns of individual nursing homes.

Three different considerations of staffing patterns will underscore the complexity of the nursing home setting: the sheer number of full-time and part-time staff; the ratio of staff members to patients; and the personal characteristics of the primary caregivers, the nurses aides. Once again, the major source for data regarding nursing home staff is national nursing home surveys.[16]

The staffing pattern in nursing homes is a pyramid, with physicians forming the smallest group, followed by increasing numbers of caregivers with less formal education. Among full-time employees in 1977, 800 were physicians; 22,700 administrators; 43,800 registered nurses; 65,900 licensed practical nurses; and 345,000 nurses aides (see figure 1.1). When placed in ratio form, the disparity between physicians and nurses aides is even clearer: one physician for every 431 aides. A similar pattern emerged in the part-time workers, although the differences between physicians and aides are smaller in the part-time segment of the labor force: 13,900 physicians; 2,900 administrators; 40,700 registered nurses; 31,600 licensed practical nurses; and 117,900 nurses aides (see figure 1.2). Again, in ratio terms, there are approximately eight or nine part-time aides for every part-time physician.

One other pattern is important to note: For physicians, involvement in the setting is likely to be on a part-time basis (13,900 part-time compared to 800 full-time physicians). For the nurses aides, the pattern is just the opposite: more aides work full time than part time. These patterns suggest that mental-health consultants must consider different strategies when working with the various levels of staff—not only because of differences in education and disciplinary background, but also because of differences in the amount of contact with members of the nursing home community.

These figures also suggest that communication among the various levels of staff within the nursing home is especially important. Gubrium, for example, emphasized that those with the most frequent contact with the patients may not be in a position to design or influence care plans.[17]

Another gauge of staffing complexity is the intensity of staffing, usually expressed in terms of the number of staff members per 100 beds or 100 patients. For the industry as a whole, the 1985 National Nursing Home Survey reflected a rate of 48.8 employees per 100 beds. This figure includes all staff members—administrative as well as those involved in direct patient care.

Staffing intensity varies as a function of regulatory requirements (discussed in chapter 2) and several characteristics of the facility, including

**Fig. 1.1**

## Staffing Patterns
### Full-Time Employees (n = 478,200)

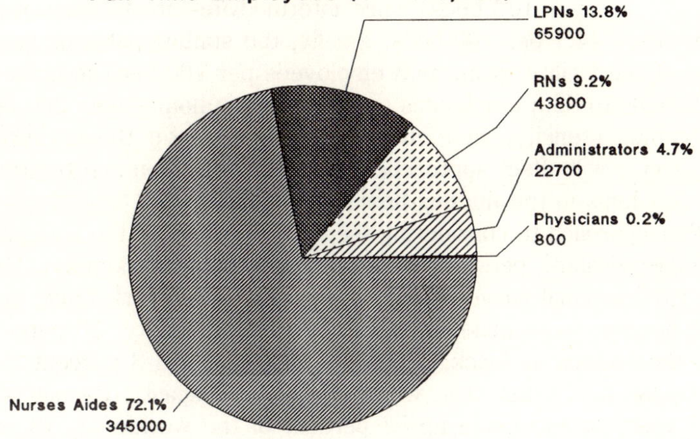


Source: National Center for Health Statistics (1979).

**Fig. 1.2**

## Staffing Patterns
### Part-Time Employees (n = 207,000)

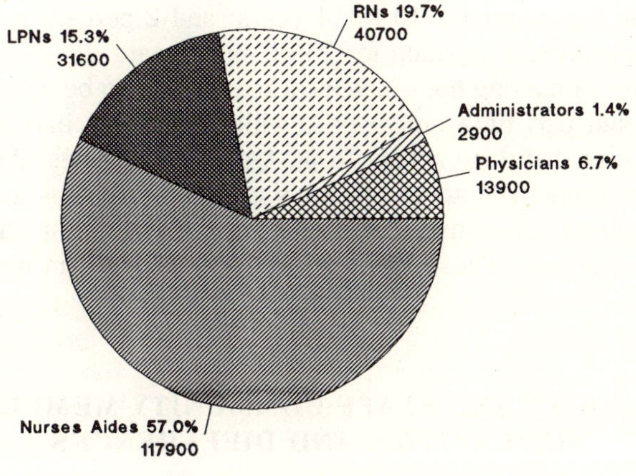


Source: National Center for Health Statistics (1979).

ownership, type of care, and size. Proprietary homes indicated a rate of 46.0 employees per 100 beds, while nonprofit homes reported 54.0 employees per 100 beds. Similarly, skilled-nursing facilities indicated a rate of 55.8 employees per 100 beds, while intermediate-care facilities reported a lower rate—44.1 per 100 beds. Finally, the staffing patterns varied by the size of the facility, from 49.3 employees per 100 beds in homes with 50 to 99 beds to 52.5 employees per 100 beds in homes with 200 beds or more. Staffing intensity, then, offers another indicator of the setting's complexity, which will affect approaches to the identification and treatment of patient problems in the nursing-home community.

Another approach to considering the staff members of the community is through the individual, personal characteristics of the staff members. Drawing on the 1977 national survey data, 94 percent of the work force were female; 6 percent were male. In terms of ethnic diversity, 20 percent described themselves as black, 1 percent Hispanic, and 3 percent from an ethnic background other than white, black, or Hispanic. People younger than 35 years of age made up 53 percent of the workforce, 18 percent were ages 35 to 44, 14 percent were between 45 and 54, and 15 percent were 55 or older. The educational experiences of the caregivers paralleled the professional distribution highlighted earlier: 29 percent of caregivers had less than 12 years of education; 39 percent had 12 years of education; 26 percent had 13 to 14 years of education; 5 percent had 15 to 16 years; and 1 percent of the workforce had 17 or more years of education.

A major concern for the nursing home industry has been staff turnover—particularly at the lowest levels. When asked about longevity in the position, 53 percent of caregivers had been employed in their current position for less than two years; 25 percent for 2 to 4 years; 14 percent for 5 to 9 years; 6 percent for 10 to 14 years; and 2 percent had been employed in their current position for 15 or more years.

In summary, a nursing home's work force is likely to be a complex blend of full-time and part-time employees, with educational backgrounds that range from less than high-school to postgraduate degrees. Their diverse talents and perspectives affect the ways in which problems get identified, treatment options are considered, and effective treatment strategies are eventually employed. These themes will be considered in more detail in chapter 3.

## RESIDENT AND STAFF COMMUNITY MEMBERS: SIMILARITIES AND DIFFERENCES

Thus far, we have sketched the basic dimensions of the major participants in the nursing home community—residents, family members, and caregiving staff. The characteristics of the community's participants are the "building blocks" for mental health consultation.[18] As Swift and Cooper (1986) point out: "Demographic and cultural variables are the consultee characteristics that appear to influence the consultation process most" (p. 373). In this section, the residents' and caregivers' demographic characteristics are contrasted and implications of the contrast are presented.

Figures 1.3 through 1.6 present information on the race, sex, and age of the residents and primary caregivers in nursing homes. A brief review reveals several important contrasts in the nursing home setting. In terms of race or ethnicity, the caregivers are a much more diverse group than the residents. Similarly, in terms of sex distribution, there are clear differences. The caregivers are almost always women (93–98 percent); in contrast, almost 30 percent of the residents are men. Some have noted that nursing homes are places where women often feel comfortable and men often feel out of place. Finally, and not surprisingly, the age distribution of the residents and caregivers shows very little overlap.

These national data provide benchmarks for considering the specific characteristics of an individual facility. They also serve as a reminder that one of the consultant's tasks must be to assess the role of demographic differences in the setting. For example, Knight commented that individual mental health practitioners must be aware of their own cultural and age-related biases when working with older adults.[19] Similarly, consultants should be attuned to the possibility that racial, ethnic, sex-role, and age differences between residents and caregivers may affect the functioning of the nursing home community. (In chapter 3 we will consider the fit between the consultant's characteristics and the settings' characteristics.)

## A CONDITIONAL VIEW OF THE SETTING

A consultant can be very helpful in assessing under what conditions and for which types of patients the nursing home will be effective in producing which types of outcomes. As Litwak asks, "Which groups are best suited to provide which services to older people?" (Litwak, 1985, p. 1).

He provides an important framework for a "conditional" view of the setting.[20] Oftentimes, when mental health problems arise in the nursing home setting, they may occur because family members, staff, or patients are unclear about the roles the nursing home can and should play. Litwak's framework can assist in developing such a "conditional" view. He suggests that the most important element in viewing the nursing home's caregiving is the match between the tasks required and the structure of the caregiving arrangements. For example, he sketches the functioning of several differ-

**Fig. 1.3**

## Race
### Nursing Home Patients and Staff Members

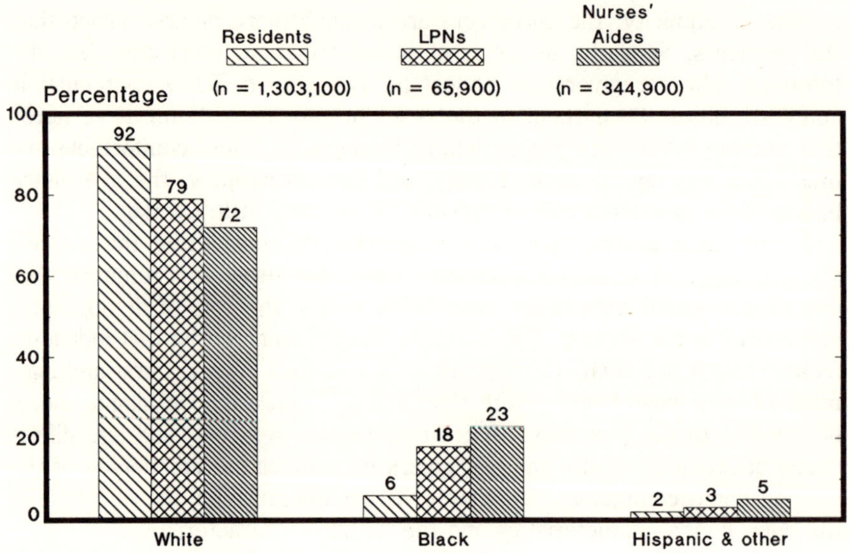


Source: U.S. Dept. of Health, Education, and Welfare (1979).

**Fig. 1.4**

## Sex
### Nursing Home Patients and Staff Members

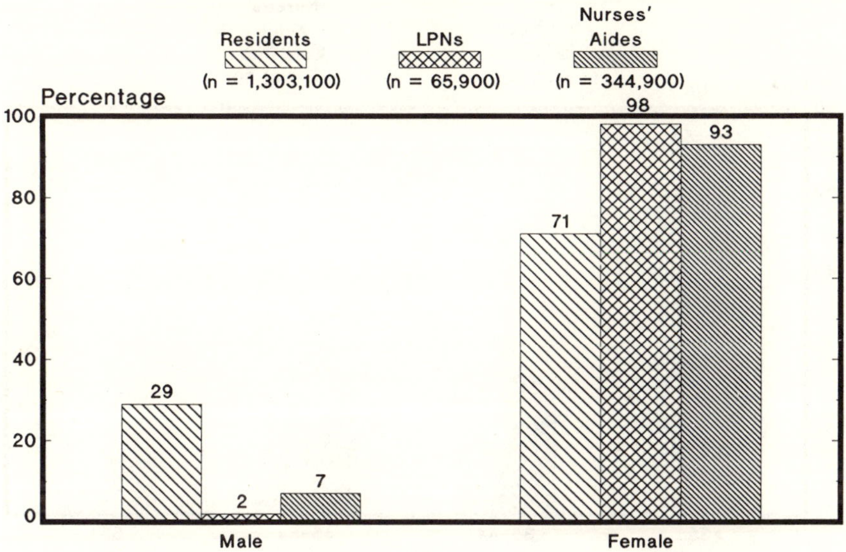


Source: U.S. Dept. of Health, Education, and Welfare (1979).

**Fig. 1.5**

Age
Nursing Home Staff Members

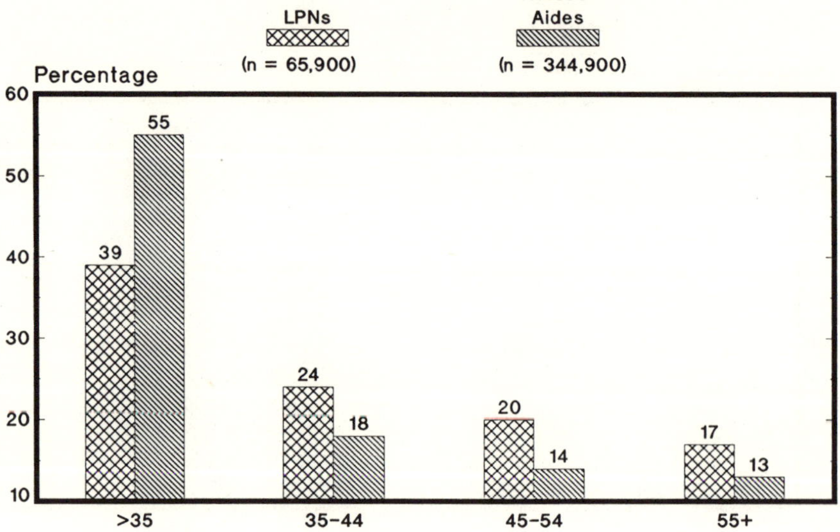


Source: U.S. Dept. of Health, Education, and Welfare (1979).

**Fig. 1.6**

Age

Nursing Home Residents (n = 1,303,100)

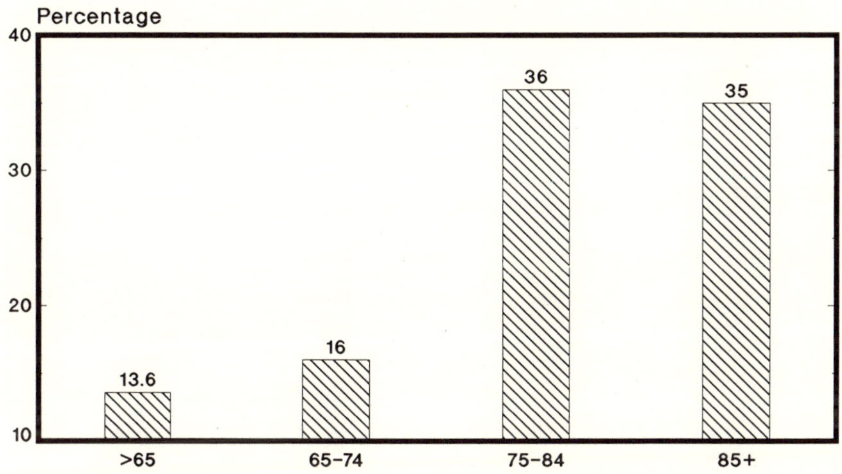


Source: U.S. Dept. of Health, Education, and Welfare (1979).

ent support systems and the types of tasks most appropriate for each (see table 1.3). As noted in the table, some support systems, such as families, are best suited for intense, personal support. Others (such as formal organizations) are best suited for more routine, well-structured tasks. The implications for the members of the nursing home community are clear:

TABLE 1.3: Forms of Differentiation in Primary-Group Structure that have Evolved in Modern Industrial Society

| | SOME TYPICAL TYPES OF PRIMARY GROUPS | | | | |
|---|---|---|---|---|---|
| *Dimensions of Group and Task Structure* | *Marital Dyad* | *Modified Extended Family* | *Friends* | *Neighbors* | *Formal Organization* |
| Face-to-face continual contact of group | Highest | Low | Low | High | Low |
| Long-term commitments | High | Highest | Moderate | Low | Lowest |
| Small size | Smallest | Large | Large | Large | Very Large |
| Affection | High | High | High | Moderate | Lowest |
| Duty to group survival | High | Highest | Moderate | Low | Lowest |
| Common life style (age homogeneity) | High | Low | High | Moderate | Lowest |
| Peer ties | High | High | Highest | High | Low |
| Membership eligibility—everyday socialization | High | High | High | High | Low |
| Division of labor | Low | Low | Low | Low | High |
| *Illustrations of Services That Match Dimensions of Groups in Columns Above* | | | | | |
| | Daily cooking, shopping, housecleaning, laundry | Care for bedridden for 2 to 3 weeks; emotional support in death of spouse | Companions for free-time activities; advice on daily living for widows | Reporting break-ins while out on daily chores; emergency loans of small household items | Major surgery; 24-hour permanent care of older person; selling food; arresting criminals |

Source: Litwak (1985).

> The principle of matching should therefore permit an assessment of (1) which primary-group services will be taken over by the nursing home, (2) which services will be continued to be managed by primary groups, and (3) which will be lost. The ones that will be taken over will be those that can be routinized and economically legitimated by Medicaid. The ones that will continue to be managed by the kin will be those that cannot be routinized or cannot be legitimated by Medicaid and that do not require continual proximity or common life style, or at least require only the most modest time commitments. Those services that will be lost will be nonroutinized services that require continual face-to-face contact and resources (Litwak, 1985, p. 61).

Litwak's work has several implications for mental health professionals concerned with the functioning of nursing home community members. First, it suggests that the consultant should be clear about the tasks that are most appropriate and most likely to be successfully completed by nursing home caregivers. Second, the consultant may have to clarify the changes and losses involved in the transition from a relatively flexible caregiving system to a more routine caregiving setting. For example, individual preferences about breakfast—timing, types of food, and so forth—may have to be given up in order to accommodate the routine of serving two hundred meals in the space of half an hour. Third, the consultant can work with both the caregiving staff and family members to explore ways to maximize the match between caregiving resources and the types of assistance needed. For example, family members may be best suited for providing a sense of personal reaffirmation and connection to both the family's past and its future. In contrast, the staff members may be best at limit setting for the agitated patient. We return to these themes in chapters 8 through 11, where we consider working with families and staff members in more detail.

Finally, Litwak's comments highlight the influence of larger societal structures (such as Medicaid, Medicare, and private insurers) in shaping the caregiving process in nursing homes. We consider the history and current functioning of external influences on the nursing-home setting in chapter 2.

## SUMMARY

Nursing homes are communities with three key sets of participants: residents, family members, and caregiving staff. As in other communities, there are constraints to effective functioning imposed by the characteristics and traditions of the community's residents. Many approaches developed in community mental health settings can be applied within nursing homes. A major task for the mental health consultant is to assess the match between the caregiving demands and the "task structure" provided by the nursing home staff and family members. In some cases, conflicts may arise because of differing personal characteristics among the diverse members of the nursing home community. In many cases, current approaches may at least be influenced by, if not dictated by, funding sources (for example, Medicaid, Medicare, and private insurance) outside of the immediate nursing home community. The effective consultant must develop a conditional view of the setting, assessing under which conditions for which concerns which set of interventions will be most effective.

## NOTES

1. These problems were taken from the Center for Creative Leadership's newsletter.

2. Goffman's work has been summarized in a book, *Asylums* (Garden City, N.Y.: Doubleday, 1961), as well as in several articles (e.g., Goffman, 1968). His sociological perspective has focused on the role structure of settings and the "moral career" of inmates or patients in total institutions.

3. Gubrium (1974) drew upon his participant observation experience to outline the distinctions drawn here. He expanded on these observations to portray the workings of a nursing home in his fuller depiction, *Living and Dying at Murray Manor* (1975).

4. See for instance Gottesman and Bourestom (1974).

5. See Warren (1963) for a fuller discussion of his conceptualization of community functioning.

6. See, for example, Wack and Rodin's (1978) discussion of nursing home legislation and its effects.

7. Kastenbaum and Candy (1973) were among the first to point out the flaws in viewing nursing home admissions cross-sectionally, rather than longitudinally. Others (e.g., Palmore, 1976) have since followed their lead in assessing the lifetime risk of institutionalization. Recent applications of life-table analysis (e.g., McConnel, 1984; Liang and Tu, 1986) have renewed the controversy over the relative risk for institutionalization. Liang and Tu report, however, that an individual born in 1976 could expect to spend 3.34 years in a nursing home. This figure increased to 4.27 years at age eighty-five.

8. Gurland's work (e.g., Gurland, 1980) has focused on assessment issues in the mental and physical health domains. His conceptual contribution to the area of assessment has been significant.

9. Predictors of institutionalization have been studied in detail for some time (e.g., Branch and Jette, 1982; Dunlop, 1976; Greenberg and Ginn, 1979). Recent work by Cohen, Tell, and Wallack (1986) focused on risk factors for institutionalization and their results are consistent with Gurland's framework.

10. The most recent data available on a national sample of nursing home patients come from the 1985 National Nursing Home Survey. Unfortunately, complete reports from that survey are not yet available. Therefore, throughout this volume, we will draw on information from the 1985 survey, when available, and from its predecessor—the 1977 Nursing Home Survey—when the more recent information is unavailable.

11. Johnson and Grant (1985) provide a very informative introduction to the nursing home setting. Their treatment is more policy oriented than our emphasis, but it forms a useful companion volume to our work.

12. These data are drawn from both the 1985 and the 1977 Survey of Institutionalized Persons (1978). Tobin and Kulys (1980) provide a useful discussion of the family arrangements of institutionalized elderly.

13. Many social scientists have commented on the extensive support and service family members provide to impaired older relatives (e.g., Frankfather, Smith, and Caro, 1981; Maddox, 1975; Shanas, 1979; Troll, Miller, and Atchley, 1979). For a fuller discussion of the family's role in long-term-care settings, see chapters 8 and 9.

14. Bloom (1983) provided this compelling example.

15. In chapter 10 we present a fuller description of staffing patterns and the nature of work in nursing homes. Our purpose here is to introduce the types of staff members likely to be found in the setting. Although we recognize that volunteers often play an important role in the nursing home (Crose et al., 1987), our discussion focuses on paid staff members.

16. Haber (1987) summarized the key findings of the national nursing home survey. He also placed the nursing home industry in historical context. The data reported here are consistent with the trends for the 1985 National Nursing Home Survey, although comparably detailed personnel data are not yet available.

17. Gubrium has described the differences among staff members' perception in *Living and Dying at Murray Manor* (1975). His discussion of the gap between the "formal" policy and its informal application is especially helpful.

18. Swift and Cooper (1986) describe the important role that clients' characteristics play in shaping the process and outcome of mental health consultation.

19. Knight's (1986) brief discussion of psychotherapy strategies is useful background reading for mental health consultants working with the elderly. He highlights the role that the individual practitioner's biases can play in affecting treatment goals, process, and outcomes.

20. Litwak (1985) provides a theoretical framework for considering which type of services and which types of care providers are best suited for providing assistance to older adults. These issues are considered in more detail in chapter 8, where we consider the roles of family members, and in chapter 10, where we consider the roles of staff members. Here, however, we emphasize the consultant's role in raising the basic questions for both the institutional caregivers and the family caregivers.

# 2

# The Nursing Home Industry

*Michael A. Smyer and Diane Brannon*

Each morning, more than one and a quarter million Americans awaken in nursing homes. Most of them are very old and very feeble. Most will stay in the nursing home for a long time. For most, it will be the last place they ever live.

*Bruce C. Vladeck, president, United Hospital Fund of New York*

It is obvious that most reimbursement agencies still believe that an individual who at 10:00 a.m. is receiving $400-a-day hospital care can take a 30-minute ambulance ride to a long-term care facility and suddenly need only $40-a-day care.

*R. Siebel, past president of the American College of Health Care Administrators*

## INTRODUCTION

In this chapter we will offer an introduction to the nursing home industry. Our discussion attempts to cover both perspectives represented above—those of the critic and those of the administrator. This material may be familiar to readers who work in or with nursing homes. For others, approaching these issues for the first time we will provide a general review of several important areas.

We begin by briefly sketching the history of nursing home settings and their forerunners in other times and cultures. We contrast the underlying philosophies of philanthropy and the implicit models of human development that each era of institutional care reflected. These comparisons are helpful in placing today's debate and policy considerations in proper historical context.

Next, we focus on nursing home services as an industry. We consider the marketability of nursing home services and their economic health. Along the way, the major costs of nursing homes, income sources, and the general profitability of the industry are considered. We then briefly review the two major issues within the industry: tax status, proprietary or not-for-profit; and ownership, independent or part of a chain. In doing so, we consider whether these distinctions affect the quality of care for nursing home residents and their families. We also focus on the implications of sector differences for mental health consultants.

In the final section, we consider the impact of the changing external environment on the economic well-being and clinical demands of nursing homes. Nursing homes reflect the values and economic priorities of their dominant culture. As these elements change over time, so, too, will the purpose and scope of the nursing home setting.

## CURRENT TRENDS AND HISTORICAL ANTECEDENTS

Recent discussions of catastrophic health insurance for older Americans are reminiscent of a swimmer edging into a cold mountain lake: one toe at a time, the swimmer gets acclimated to the shock. In a similar fashion, debate in Congress and in the popular press has begun to sensitize the public to the potentially expensive costs of an aging society.[1] For example, current proposals to expand Medicare coverage to include pharmaceutical assistance for the elderly acknowledge the importance, and the cost, of prescription medicines in the chronic care of older adults. In 1986, the elderly spent $9 billion on prescription medicines, with $7.3 billion being paid directly by older adults. Unfortunately, the current discussion sidesteps the largest catastrophe in catastrophic health care: the current and future patterns of economic responsibility for long-term care.

Davis (1986) summarized the patterns emerging from the combined effects of increasing numbers of older adults and little projected change in the pattern of chronic disease that accompanies advanced age:

> Future demographic and economic trends will strain the ability of public programs to maintain the current level of assistance, and will further magnify the gaps. Even with the uncertainties of technological change, biomedical research, health-related behavior of the population in future years, it seems safe to predict that the gap between expanding health-care needs and limited economic resources will widen (pp. 234-235).

Several trends provide the foundation for Davis's depiction.

***1) Nursing Home Care Is the Largest Out-of-Pocket Health-Care Expense for Older Adults and Their Families.*** As figures 2.1 and 2.2 indicate, almost 50 percent of out-of-pocket health-related expenses were dedicated to nursing home care. Similarly, older adults and their families paid for approximately half of the costs of nursing home care in 1986 ($19.5 billion out of $38.9 billion).

***2) The Rate of Nursing Home Use Increases with Advancing Age.*** Although at any one point in time, 5 percent of the elderly are residing in nursing homes, the picture changes when the sixty–five–plus age

**Fig. 2.1**

Percentage of Inpatient, Outpatient, and Nursing Home Services Paid Out-of-Pocket

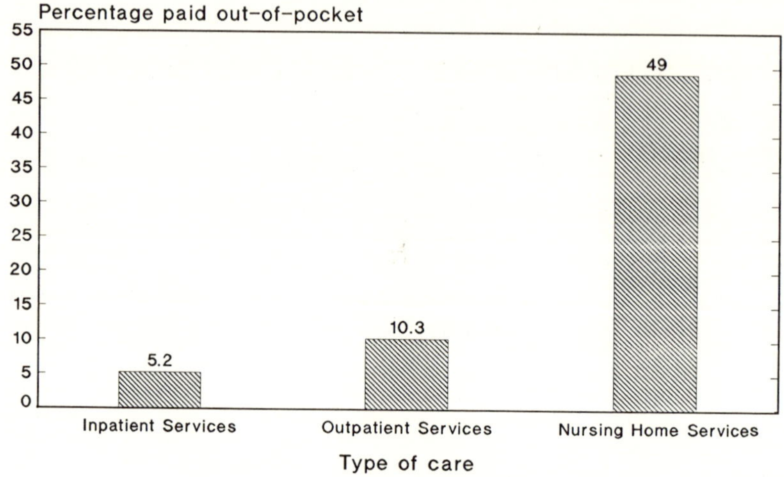


Source: Office of Technology Assessment (1987).

**Fig. 2.2**

1986 Estimated Sources of Payment for Nursing Home Care

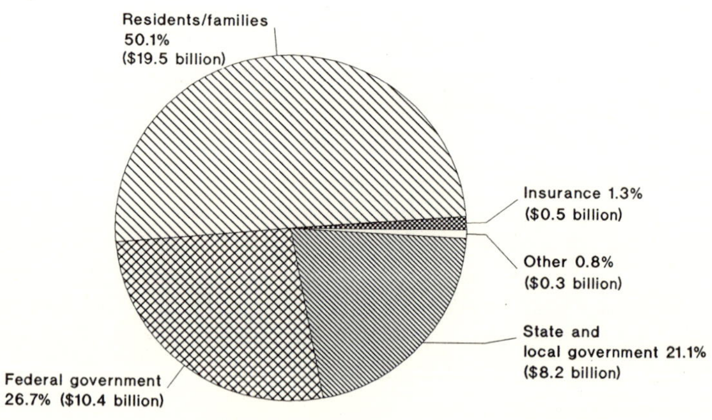


Total: $38.9 billion

Source: Office of Technology Assessment (1987).

group is divided into different segments (see figure 2.3). The rates range from 1 percent of those sixty-five to seventy-four years of age to 22 percent of those eighty-five years old and older.[2]

***3) The Fastest Growing Segment of the Population Is Those Eighty-Five Years of Age or Older.*** As depicted in figures 2.4 and 2.5, this portion of the population is expected to triple in size between 1980 and 2020, and to expand sevenfold between 1980 and 2050.[3] The result will be an "older" group of elderly, with nearly half of the elderly being seventy-five or older by the year 2000.

***4) The Nursing Home Population Will Increase Substantially over the Next Fifty Years.*** The numbers of older adults in nursing homes will increase from approximately 1.4 million to more than 4.6 million by the year 2040, more than tripling during this period (see figure 2.6). In short, from an economic perspective, policy analysts have to be concerned about the current and future patterns of nursing home use. These patterns reflect larger societal assumptions regarding philanthropy and the role of individuals and families in coping with illness and decline in old age.

Today's nursing home settings are the direct descendants, beneficiaries of, and current embodiment of a long history of social debate regarding the role of the state in responding to the needs of dependent populations.[4] Social historians have traced the philosophical and cultural roots of the nursing-home setting's predecessors to almshouses, which were developed within a moral framework that assumed poverty resulted from an individual's own failure. Thus, provision by society carried with it an implicit moral recrimination. By the turn of the twentieth century, however, a shift occurred, with many elderly moving to state mental hospitals, where they might receive better care, at the expense of the state. With the financial difficulties of the 1930s, it was cheaper to subsidize care at home, rather than through construction of new facilities. Cole (1987) summarizes the developments of the last fifty years:

> By 1935, the old myth of healthy self-reliance had been replaced by its opposite—the aged were considered sick, poor, and unable to support themselves.
>
> The growth of a federally supported welfare state accelerated the decline of the almshouse and ultimately transferred to nursing homes the swelling ranks of the elderly in state mental hospitals. The Social Security Act of 1935 banned assistance to inmates of public institutions. Its Old Age Survivors' Insurance and Old Age Assistance provisions greatly expanded the number of people able to purchase boarding home or nursing home care. . . .
>
> By 1960, the nursing home had emerged as the primary long-term-care

**Fig. 2.3**

Number of Nursing Home Residents per 1,000 Population Age 65 and over, by Sex and Age, United States, 1985

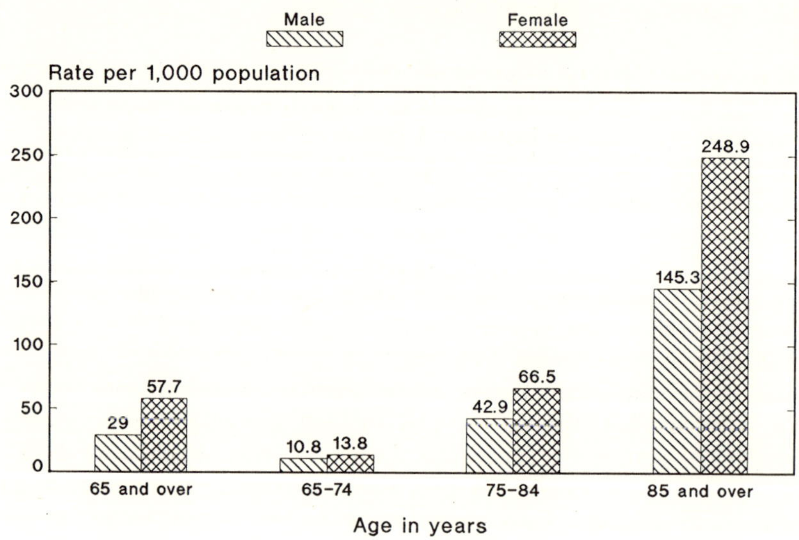


Source: Hing (1987).

**Fig. 2.4**

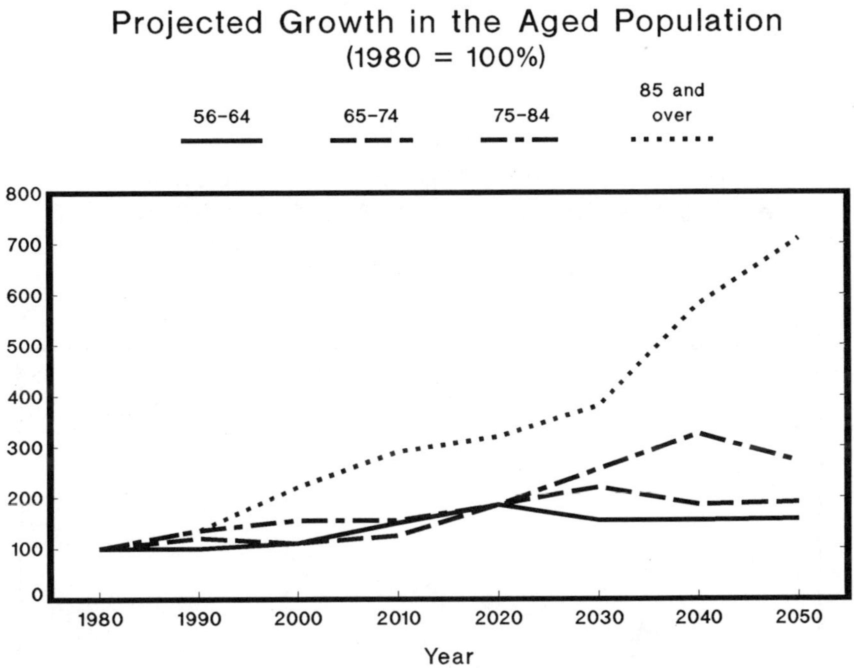


Source: U.S. Senate (1987).

**Fig. 2.5**

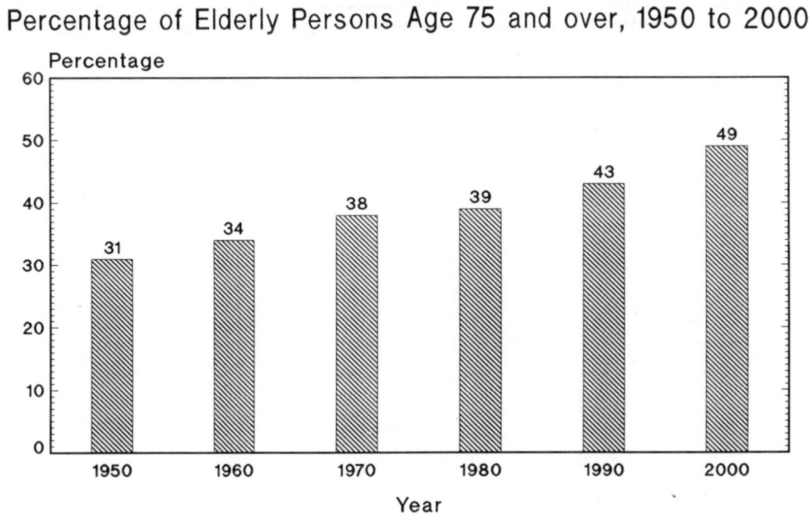


Source: U.S. Senate (1987).

**Fig. 2.6**

Nursing Home Population Projections
Persons Age 65 and over by Age Group, 1980–2040

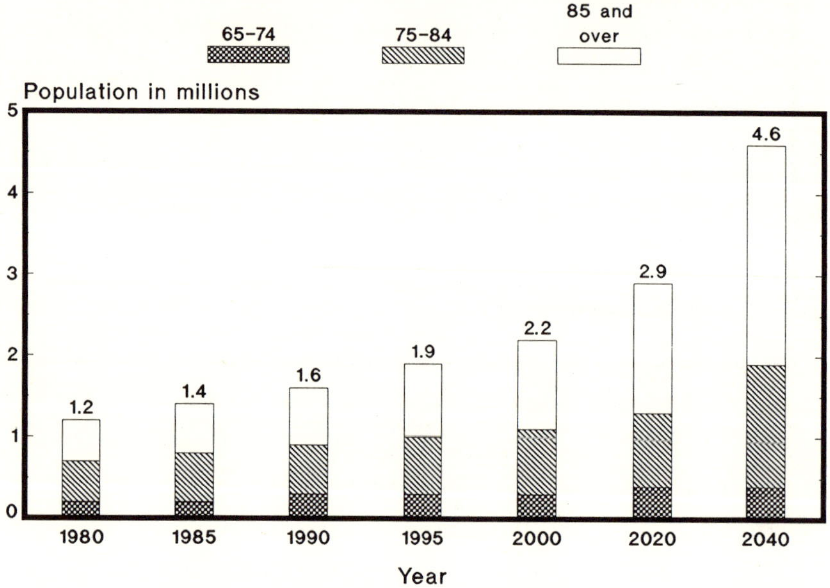


Source: U.S. Senate (1987).

> setting for elderly. . . . The passage of Medicaid and the Supplemental Security Income program accelerated the deinstitutionalization of state mental hospitals, as state executives and legislators came to see that if their patients were placed in privately operated community facilities, the federal government would pick up a substantial share of the costs. . . .
>
> Social Security's restriction of funding to institutions providing health care virtually decimated the boarding home industry. . . . Local and city almshouses either closed their doors or transformed themselves into public nursing homes, continuing to play their traditional role as a place of last resort for the poorest and sickest elderly. Meanwhile, the publicly subsidized proprietary nursing home industry (which receives roughly half of its income from Medicaid) grew at an astonishing rate (p. 14).

As Cole points out, this social and legislative legacy has several effects. Perhaps most importantly, it shapes today's older adults' view of nursing homes and their willingness to consider entering such settings. The history also points out the importance of social structures and social regulation in shaping the nursing-home environment.[5]

The legislative and regulatory climate directly affects the development and functioning of nursing homes. For example, the Medicare and Medicaid legislation of the mid-1960s directly affected older adults' ability to pay for nursing home care. As reflected in figure 2.7, the growth of the nursing home industry accelerated after the initiation of Medicare and Medicaid.

Medicare was enacted in 1965 to insure older adults for the costs of acute illness. Medicaid, in contrast, was developed in 1966 as a joint effort by federal and state governments to provide medical assistance for needy citizens, including older adults with low income.[6] Figures 2.8 and 2.9 indicate the important role that Medicaid plays in providing resources for nursing homes. Two-thirds of the Medicaid budget is dedicated to nursing-home payments; in contrast only 1 percent of the Medicare budget is applied to nursing home care. The irony is that a long stay in a nursing home impoverishes many once-middle-income elderly through the process of "spending down" assets. This creates both a tremendous drain on Medicaid resources and a new class of indigents.

Medicaid is the largest single payer for nursing home services since Medicare pays for only limited use of skilled nursing care. Therefore, Medicaid regulations and their impact have a large effect on the services available in most settings.

While the operational distinctions between skilled nursing and intermediate care have been blurred by variations in practice and reimbursement methods, the two types of certification continue to exist:

> Nursing homes are classified as follows by Social Security's Medicare and Medicaid programs:

**Fig. 2.7**

Number of Nursing Homes,
1963, 1967, 1969, 1971, 1973, 1976, 1980, and 1982

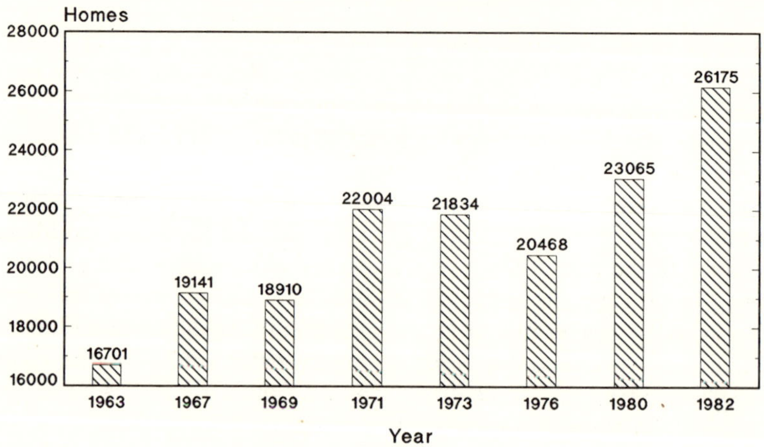


Source: National Center for Health Statistics: Master Facility Inventories, 1963, 1967, 1969, 1971, 1973, 1976, 1980, and 1982.

**Fig. 2.8**

Where the Medicaid Dollar for the Elderly Goes
1984

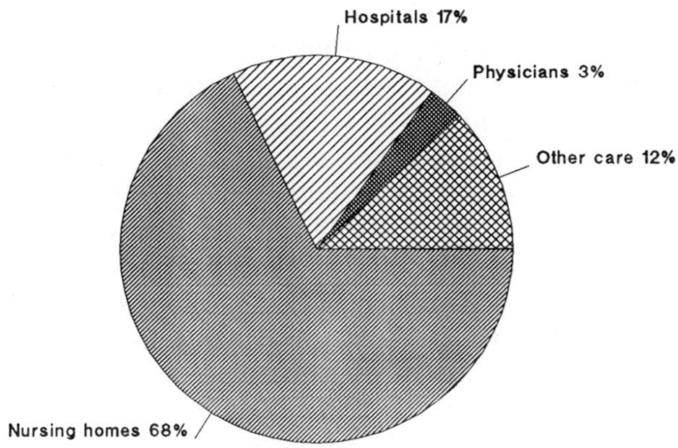


Source: U.S. Senate (1986b).

**Fig. 2.9**

Where the Medicare Dollar for the Elderly Goes
1985

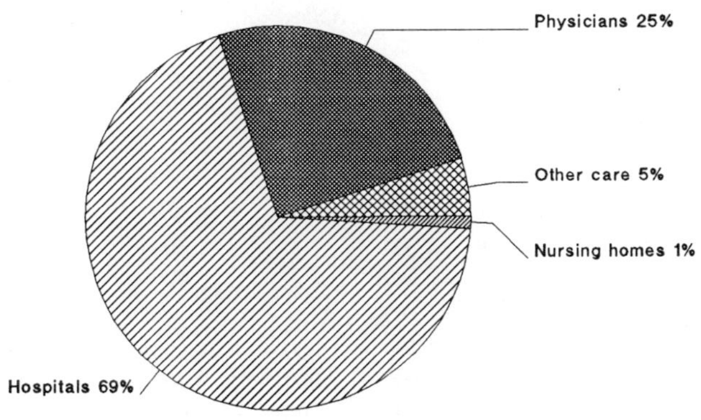


Source: U.S. Senate (1986b).

—Skilled nursing facilities (SNFs) by Medicare (Title XVIII).
—Skilled nursing facilities (SNFs) by Medicaid (Title XIX).
—Intermediate care facilities (ICFs) by Medicaid (Title XIX) (Strahan, 1987, p. 2).

As table 2.1 indicates, more than seventy-five percent of all nursing homes in the 1985 survey were certified as either SNFs or ICFs. Those facilities not certified as either were primarily the independent, proprietary homes. For the mental health consultant, these distinctions among levels of care may be important because they are linked to expectations of services provided, payment sources, and funding streams.

These reimbursement mechanisms and levels have a direct impact on the functioning of nursing home staff members and the likelihood of the setting's interest in mental health consultation. For example, Medicaid coverage is less uniform than Medicare coverage, with twenty-two Medicaid programs recognizing and directly reimbursing independently practicing psychologists for their services. States also vary in which services they cover, with some covering only psychological testing and others reimbursing a wider range of services.

TABLE 2.1: Certification Status of Nursing Homes by Ownership and Affiliation: United States, 1985

| | | CERTIFIED HOMES | | | | |
|---|---|---|---|---|---|---|
| *Ownership and Affiliation* | *Total* | *Total* | *Skilled Nursing Facility Only* | *Skilled Nursing Facility and Intermediate Care Facility* | *Intermediate Care Facility Only* | *Not Certified* |
| Total | 19,100 | 14,400 | 3,500 | 5,700 | 5,300 | 4,700 |
| Ownership | | | | | | |
| Proprietary | 14,300 | 10,500 | 2,800 | 3,900 | 3,800 | 3,800 |
| Voluntary nonprofit | 3,800 | 3,000 | 500 | 1,400 | 1,100 | 700 |
| Government | 1,000 | 900 | 200 | 400 | 300 | 100 |
| Affiliation | | | | | | |
| Chain | 7,900 | 7,400 | 1,300 | 3,200 | 2,900 | 500 |
| Independent | 10,000 | 6,000 | 2,000 | 2,100 | 1,900 | 4,000 |
| Government | 1,000 | 900 | 200 | 400 | 300 | 100 |
| Unknown | 100 | | | | | 100 |

Note: Figures do not add up to totals due to rounding.
Source: Strahan (1987).

Another potential source of reimbursement for mental health consultation may be the long-term-care setting itself. We consider the financial concerns and structure of the nursing home industry in the next section.

## THE MARKETABILITY OF NURSING HOME CARE

The nursing home industry has image problems. Over the years it has been associated in the public's eye with claims of financial and medical fraud, rumored to be linked to organized crime, documented as lacking in competence and requiring greater regulation, and revealed to include administrators and staff who have allowed abuse of frail elders. The goal of individual health behavior and public policy alike is to avoid placement in nursing homes. How, then, has an industry that provides only undesired services survived?

Part of the answer surely lies in the fact that decisions to use nursing home services are often made not by the resident but by the resident's family. The client/consumer discrepancy is evident throughout the health-services sector as physicians and third-party payers play major gate-keeping roles. In the case of nursing homes, however, the client's needs and preferences are further tempered by those of the family.

The clients' physical, mental, and financial dependence make them a relatively weak force in the marketplace. Their caretakers, relatives, or others, as discussed in chapter 8, have limited information and options when they "shop" for nursing homes. Consequently, the nursing-home industry has been able to disregard the potential force of consumer behavior. For example, nursing homes have only recently begun advertising. Pincus (1986) suggests this development has occurred apparently more as a consequence of the professionalization of nursing home management than as a function of concern for the consumer.

Two recent phenomena affect the continued viability of the nursing home industry: the expanding elderly population, as outlined above; and limitations on the use of acute-care facilities imposed by Medicare's prospective payment system. Despite its unattractiveness, then, nursing home care is in demand. Occupancy rates in most areas are in excess of 90 percent. The presence of demand implies not only that there is a need, but also that someone is willing to pay for the needed service. It is to those sources of payment that we now turn.

## THE MAJOR SOURCES OF REVENUE

As indicated in figure 2.2, residents and their families are the largest source of payment for nursing home care. Private pensions, social security, and other sources of resident or family income are used when Medicare does not pay. Medicare and Medicaid are significant sources of income for nursing homes, private health insurance is not a significant revenue source, though there are currently efforts underway to expand this resource.[7]

There are several important factors to understand about the buyers in the nursing home industry. First, the federal government, through Medicare and federal contributions to Medicaid, pays for about one-half of all nursing home care. Consequently, Congress and the Social Security Administration's Health Care Finance Administration (HCFA) are active players in the industry's environment. States administer and contribute to Medicaid programs and are increasingly demanding buyers. Changes in the ceilings on components of what are termed allowable costs by federal or state agencies can have significant impacts on the profitability of the nursing home industry. Since most nursing-home beds are in proprietary facilities, profitability and ability to attract investors are major preconditions to an adequate supply of beds. Policymakers continue to struggle in search of appropriate reimbursement levels that will insure continued investment without raising public expenditures to unacceptable levels.[8]

## THE MAJOR COSTS OF PROVIDING CARE

The major cost centers used to analyze the nursing home industry are listed in table 2.2. In a study of Colorado nursing homes, nursing and nursing aide–service costs were the largest contributors to the operating cost per day of care. They accounted for approximately 44 percent of the total, with room and board second at 35 percent (Shaughnessy et al., 1980).

Significant operating-cost variations have been observed on the basis of location (rural vs. urban), staffing patterns, the extent of rehabilitative therapies offered and case mix (the type and severity of residents' conditions). For-profit facilities operate with lower costs than do nonprofit facilities, in part because of differences in the factors mentioned above (Palmer, 1985).

Since the prospective payment system instituted reductions in Medicare-reimbursed hospital stays, the number of hospital-based skilled-nursing facilities has increased. These facilities have higher costs than free-standing nursing homes with similar locations. Average operating costs for

TABLE 2.2: Cost Categories and Component Cost Centers

| *Cost Category* | *Component Cost Centers* |
|---|---|
| Administrative and general services | Administrative travel and entertainment insurance, other than property<br>Medical records |
| Room-and-board services | Dietary<br>Food<br>Laundry and linen<br>Housekeeping<br>Plant operation and maintenance |
| Nursing and aide services | RNs<br>LPNs<br>Other (aides and orderlies) |
| Therapy services | Occupational therapy<br>Physical therapy<br>Recreational therapy<br>Speech therapy |
| Other ancillary services | Pharmacy<br>Medical supplies<br>Laboratory<br>X-ray<br>Physician care<br>Respiratory care<br>Social services<br>Medical director<br>Utilization review<br>Dental care |
| Personal services | Beauty and barber shop<br>Personal purchases for patients |
| Property | Depreciation<br>Amortization<br>Real-estate taxes<br>Rent<br>Interest<br>Property insurance<br>Other property insurance |
| Other expenses | Income taxes<br>Other nonhealth care nonproperty expenses |

Source: Shaughnessy et al. (1980).

skilled nursing range from around fifty to one hundred dollars per patient per day depending upon the number of rehabilitation therapies, nurse-to-bed ratios and case mix (Sulvetta and Holohan, 1986). Intermediate-care-cost estimates, while somewhat less than skilled care, are difficult to assess since they are determined in response to fifty different state Medicaid reimbursement systems. Increasingly, any significant differences in inputs between ICFs and SNFs have been called into question (Institute of Medicine, 1986) and more refined measures of patient classification for costing out services are in development (see Fries and Cooney, 1985). Even these measures, however, are based on empirical observation of current practice patterns; they do not reflect the potential effects of residents' mental status on staff-resource utilization.

## THE ECONOMIC HEALTH OF THE INDUSTRY

The profitability of the nursing home industry has long been of interest to policymakers and investors alike. Since the passage of Medicare and Medicaid, nursing home owners have allegedly exploited loopholes in reimbursement programs to gain what some have termed unfair profits. For example, the cost-based reimbursement system by which nursing homes were reimbursed enabled facilities to recover the costs of interest in the calculation of the cost of services provided. Consequently, second and third mortgages borrowed from affiliates at high interest rates, became common substitutes for equity. Costs were thereby inflated and investors reaped impressive returns.

After the mid-seventies, as expenditures for nursing home care soared, state Medicaid programs began to confine their definitions of allowable costs. At the same time, Certificate of Need (CON) programs were instituted by the states to control the industry's growth. Some states also imposed quality-of-care standards, which further decreased owners' flexibility. Although these policy adjustments have helped contain the costs of nursing home care, they have also contributed to a shortage of beds available to Medicaid-reimbursed clients.[9]

All of these factors combined to cool investors' interest in nursing homes and slow the industry's growth, as shown in table 2.3. Although there has been a 22 percent increase in the number of nursing homes since the original National Nursing Home Survey in 1973–74, 21 percent of this growth occurred prior to the 1977 survey. A 16 percent increase in the number of beds since 1977 reflects the attention given to expansion of existing facilities during this period of slowed growth in the number of facilities.

Despite the slowed rate of growth in the industry, market analysts continue to view nursing homes as reasonably strong investments. Although nursing home stocks underperformed the Standard and Poors' five-hundred-stock index during the first quarter of 1987, analysts expect improvement. They cite the projected growth in demand resulting from the demographic imperative of an aging population and the strength of the multifacility chains (*Modern Healthcare*, 1987).

## SEGMENTS WITHIN THE INDUSTRY

***The Chains.*** The emergence of the nursing home in the United States has followed a typical path of industrial organization. From simply structured, independently owned and operated facilities, increased complexity and growth opportunities have created a favorable environment for the development of systems of facilities. The nursing home chains as they are known are now changing the composition of the industry. Diminished is the predominant image of the "Mom and Pop" owner-operators, who still control some 60 percent of the homes. Some observers expect that a few chains will operate more than half of the nursing home beds by the end of the decade (LaViolette, 1983). The 1985 National Nursing Home Survey data document this trend (see figure 2.10). Although chains owned 28 percent of the total number of beds in the 1977 survey, that proportion had grown to 41.6 percent by 1985 (Strahan, 1987). Because their average bed size is considerably larger than that of the independently operated facilities, the chains have more actual beds on a national scale than do independent owners. The growth of multifacility systems is a phenomenon of both the for-profit and nonprofit, church-related sectors. The constraints and opportunities associated with chain ownership or affiliation may be confined to financial management or they may be much broader. In a

TABLE 2.3: Number of Homes and Beds and Occupancy Rates for Three Survey Periods

| *Survey Year* | *Number of Homes* | *Number of Beds* | *Occupancy Rate* |
|---|---|---|---|
| 1985 | 19,100 | 1,624,200 | 91.6 |
| 1977 | 18,900 | 1,402,400 | 89.0 |
| 1973–74 | 15,700 | 1,177,300 | 86.5 |

Source: Strahan (1987).

given facility, the consultant should consider the role of the absentee owner in the culture of the nursing-home community.

***The For-Profits.*** The for-profit sector has dominated the nursing home industry since the inception of Medicare and Medicaid. The 1985 survey indicated continuing dominance with almost 75 percent of all homes operating on a for-profit basis (figure 2.11). The continued privatization and corporatization of the industry, which have occurred in recent years, have been decried as major threats to quality of care. While for-profit facilities tend to operate with lower costs than do nonprofits, perhaps by "creaming" the most attractive residents, existing studies do not support the contention that quality of care suffers proportionately.[10] Indeed, the magnitude of these trends toward chain affiliation and proprietary ownership render comparisons with independent nonprofit institutions somewhat moot.

***Quality of Care.*** Recent discussion and policy efforts have focused on improving the quality of care throughout the industry via regulatory reform. In 1986, for example, the Institute of Medicine issued an extensive report with detailed proposals for regulating reform.[11] Current proposals for regulatory reform include increasing the requirements for licensure as a nursing home administrator, increasing and improving the required training provided for nurse's aides, and improving the survey process that provides periodic assessment of the institution's quality of care.

The question of quality of care is complicated by a number of issues, not the least of which is lack of agreement on what constitutes quality. Thorburn and Meiners's study (1986) showed that financial bonuses to facilities for producing improved resident outcomes had no significant effect. Ullman's (1985) analysis of facility data suggested that it is not the high cost, capital-intensive features that affect quality, but the less expensive labor-intensive aspects. Both of these studies suggest the image of an industry in search of effective service-delivery technologies. Neither the ownership nor tax status of a nursing home provides a sound basis for judging the facility's success in achieving effectiveness, however.

## THE CHANGING POLICY CONTEXT

Mental health consultation in nursing homes is affected by two broad dimensions of health-related policy: those regulations and funding decisions that affect who seeks care within the nursing home setting; and those regulations that affect who works in the setting and the types of services they can and must provide.

**Fig. 2.10**

Certification Status of Nursing Homes, United States, 1985
By Affiliation

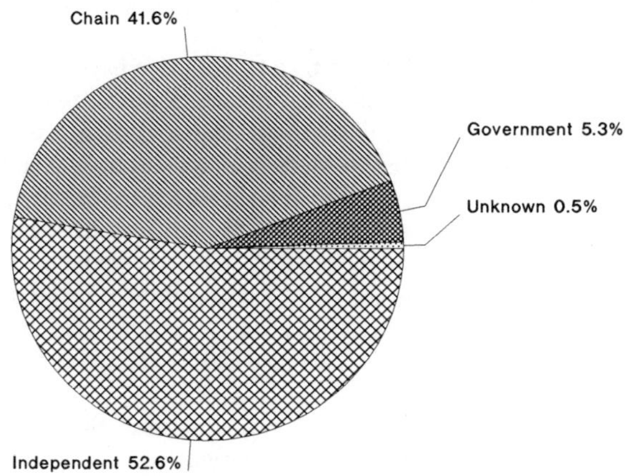


Source: Strahan (1987).

**Fig. 2.11**

Certification Status of Nursing Homes, United States, 1985
By Ownership

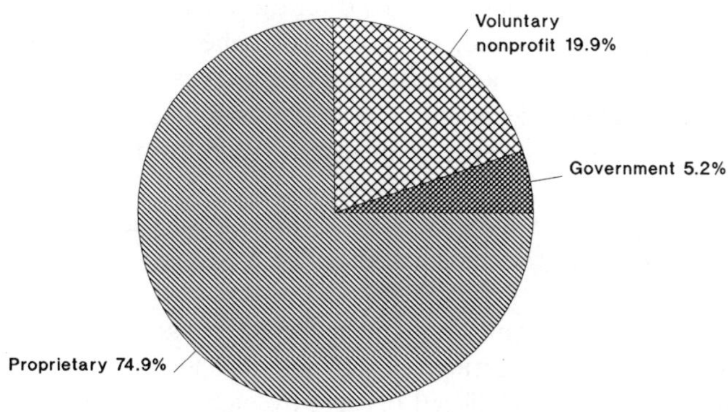


Source: Strahan (1987).

Recent cost-containment developments in Medicare and Medicaid affect who gets referred to nursing homes for care and treatment.[12] In the 1984 fiscal year, the Medicare system adopted a prospective payment system linked to diagnosis-related groups (DRGs). Jones (1984) summarized the approach and anticipated effects of implementing the DRG-based system:

> The new system is based on a target price payment based on the diagnostic category in which each patient is placed. Rates of reimbursement are set prior to the actual admission of a patient. These rates are based on extensive studies of the care provided to Medicare patients by hospitals across the country.
>
> The diagnostic categories which are used to classify patients and determine Medicare payment rates are called diagnostic-related groupings (DRGs). . . . The resulting system contained 23 major diagnostic categories organized by organ systems in the body and causes of diseases. Each category was then divided into diagnostic-related groups. Patients classified within these groups would be similar in services provided and in the lengths of their hospital stays. . . .
>
> As the patient receives care in the hospital, all of the services received are recorded. Once a patient is discharged, his or her utilization of services is reviewed, and he or she is assigned a DRG based on discharge diagnosis. . . .
>
> The government is using fixed prices based on DRGs to estimate Medicare's annual hospital spending. The goal is to place a ceiling on the Medicare budget through prospective pricing based on national DRG rates (p. 20).

The implementation of DRGs has had an important impact on the health-care industry. As pointed out earlier, hospitals have begun to develop and expand hospital-associated nursing home settings. In addition, nursing homes have reported that hospitals are discharging patients earlier and sicker. Lyles (1986), for example, reported on the experience of a group of nursing homes in the Portland, Oregon, area. She found that the initiation of the DRGs system was accompanied by an increase in the employment rate of full-time registered nurses. The homes sampled reported admitting patients with increased severity of illness, increased prevalence of clinical problems, increased use of medical supplies, and shorter lengths of stay. Thus, nursing homes have become a transitional-care setting for patients discharged earlier from hospitals, under DRG-induced cost-containment pressure.

The Medicaid programs in many states have also implemented cost-containment measures. Harrington and her colleagues (1986), for example, reviewed changes in Medicaid policies by eight states from 1978 to 1982. The eight states chosen for study represent one-third of the nation's elderly. They found that states sought to contain costs through several mechanisms: reducing the levels of benefits available; adding restrictions for access to services; increasing the copayment or other costs of services; and restricting the rate of increase in payment for services. Each of these strategies contributed to an overall cost-containment emphasis throughout the states.

Because of their role as major sources of revenue, Medicare and Medicaid can influence the case mix and types of services provided in nursing homes. For example, as pointed out earlier, in twenty-two states, Medicaid regulations do not allow reimbursement for psychological services; this regulatory stance directly affects the feasibility of developing and continuing psychological consultation in the setting. Similar concerns have been raised about the coverage for mental-health services embodied in current Medicare regulations. Uyeda and her colleagues (1986) recently summarized the current situation:

> The acute care orientation of Medicare has meant that many chronic conditions, or conditions requiring long-term care, are not easily accommodated by the program. Mental health services that are now recognized as important for the elderly are minimally covered because they often do not meet the acute criteria or because of questions of efficacy. . . .
>
> In our judgment, the current Medicare coverage for the treatment of mental and nervous disorders reflects the understanding of these conditions, and the prevailing attitudes regarding insurance coverage for them, when Medicare was adopted in 1965. . . .
>
> To the politically naive, it may seem ironic that the same Congress that assured that the provision of mental health services through the discretionary program embodied in the Community Mental Health Center Act was to be functionally oriented and interdisciplinary-based also refused to provide insurance coverage for these same services under Medicare, and apparently included mental health coverage only as an afterthought (pp. 94–98).

Uyeda and her colleagues are somewhat optimistic that Medicare officials will begin to see the preventive, health-promotional contributions that a variety of mental health disciplines can make to the health and well-being of impaired elderly, in both community and institutional settings.

Regardless of the accuracy of these forecasts, however, it is clear that Medicare and Medicaid help set the standard of expectation and payment for services within the nursing-home setting. Thus, the availability of and demand for mental-health consultation in nursing homes will vary as a function of the regulatory climate and the value attributed to such services.

In addition to affecting the access to the setting and the services provided, federal and state regulations also affect those who work within the setting. For example, a common theme of the current legislative debate is a concern for quality of nursing home care. The recent Institute of Medicine report (1986) highlighted staffing patterns and training as a major contributor to a setting's quality of care. Thus, recent proposals for Medicare regulatory reform have suggested requiring up to eighty hours of preservice training for nurse's aides and upgrading the staffing patterns of nursing homes to include more registered nurses (*Nation's Health*, 1987).

These suggestions will affect the setting's willingness to include mental health issues in staff training and preemployment training. Under the not-so-subtle mandate of required training, there may be opportunities to increase the staff's exposure to mental health technologies (as described in chapters 10 and 11). Mental health training programs will likely build upon more general job-training programs' being currently initiated (Kerschner, 1987). The proposed Medicare regulations may also affect the staffing patterns and, therefore, the mix of staff members with whom a consultant would work.

Similar proposals for "toughening" state Medicaid laws are currently being considered in Congress. Some proposals, for example, would require one hundred hours of preservice training for nurses' aides (*Nation's Health*, 1987). Again, such efforts would directly affect a consultant's potential range of issues, as well as the staff's receptivity to mental health consultation.[13]

To summarize this review of policy developments, the nursing home is affected by larger societal concerns regarding quality of care, cost containment, and the provision of services for growing numbers of older adults. Mental health consultants must be aware of the links among state and national developments and the setting's ability and willingness to benefit from and pay for mental-health consultation.

## SUMMARY

In this chapter, we have reviewed the development of the nursing home setting and the growth of the nursing home industry. A variety of constituencies—including federal and state legislatures, insurance companies, and the industry itself—collaborate to define collectively the types of services normally expected in a nursing home setting and the patterns of reimbursement available for mental health consultation. An individual nursing home's approach to the use of mental-health consultation may be a function of these national-, regional-, and state-level contexts, as well as the setting's own fiscal and philosophical commitments. For mental health consultants who are unfamiliar with the business aspects of nursing home care, we have tried to sketch some of the dominant influences on service decisions. These influences shape the constraints and opportunities for mental health consultation in the nursing home setting.

## NOTES

1. See the special issue of *Daedalus* (Winter 1986) that focused on the aging society. The articles by Avorn (1986), Davis (1986), and Callahan (1986) are particularly helpful introductions to the emerging issues of providing adequate health care in an aging society. Mechanic's (1987) article is also helpful.

2. Hing (1987) recently summarized the results of the 1985 national nursing home survey. The data presented here are drawn from her work.

3. See the U.S. Senate's Special Committee on Aging's report, on Developments in Aging: 1986 (1987, volumes 1 and 3) for a good overview of basic demographic changes and current service and expense patterns associated with the aging of the U.S. population.

4. For a general discussion of the difficult issues associated with the development and implementation of social policy regarding care of dependent populations see Gaylin et al. (1978). While their work does not focus directly on the nursing home setting, the issues they raise regarding dependency and the state's appropriate response are applicable to long-term-care settings. Much of our discussion draws upon their work.

5. The work of Cole (1987), Callahan (1986), and McArthur (1970) place the nursing home setting in historical and philosophical perspective. Again, our discussion owes a great deal to their contributions.

6. See Wack and Rodin (1978) for a lucid discussion of the impact of legislation in shaping the services of nursing homes. See Rabin and Stockton (1987) for a discussion of the basic dimensions of federal and state programs that influence the nursing home setting. Also, Blumenthal et al. (1986) provide a helpful review of options for the future of Medicare.

7. Recent Congressional debate regarding catastrophic health care have begun to raise public awareness of the potentially large costs associated with nursing home care. Recent reports in the press (e.g. Pear, 1987) have suggested the importance of developing options for older adults and their families that encourage them to cover a greater portion of nursing home costs before turning to governmental assistance. Wiener, Ehrenworth, and Spence (1987) provide a summary of the currently available options in private long-term care insurance, including information on premium rates, levels of coverage, and restrictions of the policies.

8. For more in-depth discussion of the interaction between reimbursement approaches and the supply of nursing-home beds, see Baldwin and Bishop (1984), Scanlon (1980), and Vogel (1985).

9. Certificate of Need (CON) regulations had been passed in every state by 1979. Under these regulations, a designated state agency reviews plans for new health facilities and purchases of major equipment. For a fuller discussion of the history of this and other regulatory measures, see Vogel (1985).

10. This issue is treated in greater detail elsewhere. See, for example, Greene and Monahan (1981), Ullman (1985), the U.S. General Accounting Office (1987), and Vladeck (1980).

11. The Institute of Medicine's (1986) report focused national attention on the important role that regulatory reform can play in improving nursing-home care. It set the stage for various legislative proposals subsequently considered in Congress. The report also documented the history of regulations linked to the nursing home setting.

12. For a review of Medicare's Diagnosis-Related Groupings see Jones (1984), a report prepared by staff of the Office of Technology Assessment (1983), and the U.S. General Accounting Office (1986).

13. As this book went to press, Congress passed the Omnibus Budget Reconciliation Act of 1987. Signed by President Reagan on December 22, the act includes several steps to improve the quality of care in nursing homes. The nursing home industry, particularly homes that receive Medicaid funding, must respond to the provisions of the act. Although regulations have not yet been promulgated, many areas of the industry—admissions criteria, resident assessment, staffing patterns, and staff training—will be affected. In the area of training, for example, the act mandates that every nurse's aide must receive at least seventy-five hours of training in nursing skills and residents' rights. Those working in the nursing home setting should familiarize themselves with the act and its assorted regulations, once they are available.

# 3

# Mental Health Consultation: Process, Professions, and Models

*Margaret D. Cohn and Michael A. Smyer*

> I know a consultant when I see one. He's the specialist off the jet plane with the flip chart and the black bag who makes it his business to meddle in our business.
>
> *E. J. Heffer*

## INTRODUCTION

The mental health consultant's business is the focus of this chapter. Complementing the background discussion of the community structure of nursing homes in chapter 1, the external environment and its effects on nursing home care in chapter 2, and the mental health issues described in chapter 4, the work of consulting will be described here as it applies to mental health issues in nursing homes. While chapter 2 may have been familiar territory for those who work in nursing homes, it is mental health practitioners who will find that they are well acquainted with the issues covered in this chapter.

Bloom (1975) discussed the key elements of mental health consultation: a process of indirect service in which the consultant works with a consulter or a group of consulters who provide direct service to clients. The focus of the consultation can span a wide range of mental health concerns. In this chapter, we outline the important aspects of mental health consultation and their relevance for nursing homes.

We begin with a reminder of the many reasons for expanding consultative approaches in the long-term-care setting, and an example of how a consultant can help. This is followed by an overview of the structure and process of consultation presented in sections on the basic structural dimensions of the consultation process and differing professional perspectives on consultation. We then consider consultation concerns of the administrator, the consultant, and the board of directors. Finally, we review the two major perspectives emphasized throughout the rest of this book.

## WHY USE CONSULTATION?

Stockdill (1986) introduced the recent NIMH Handbook of Mental Health Consultation with five major reasons for the continuing significance of mental health consultation.[1] They are particularly relevant for consultation in long-term-care settings. First, mental health consultants represent a range of disciplines, from social work and nursing to psychology and theology. These diverse perspectives are also represented by different participants in the nursing home community who may find common ground and a basis for communication and collaboration when focusing on mental health issues.

Second, all points of intervention, from prevention to crisis or chronic care, are apparent in long-term-care settings and are amenable to consultative approaches.

Third, mental health consultation has proven successful in long-term-care settings.[2] If help is needed (and it is), and something works (as this does), then use it.

Fourth, mental health consultation can span a wide range of concerns. Consultants may address psychological factors in resident care, social factors in group structuring, cultural factors in staff training, spiritual issues in dignifying death, economic issues in family counseling strategies, and environmental factors in facility arrangements. Although no single consultant is likely to be able to address all of the topics, each area affects the mental health status of nursing home community members.

Fifth, and final, consultative approaches are, by design, explorations. As such, they can illuminate mental health problems in a particular facility that have relevance for more extensive study and innovation. Other reasons for working with a consultant will become apparent as specific community issues are discussed in subsequent chapters. Now we turn from why consultants are helpful to how they work.

## HOW CAN A CONSULTANT HELP?

A mental health consultant is particularly helpful when a specific problem arises that is beyond the skill of individual staff members and yet appears to influence the emotional well-being of the members of the nursing home community. Under these circumstances, a short-term case consultation provides fresh insights, skills, and confident support to reenergize and direct the staff.

Mental health consultants can also provide programmatic and policy guidance. For example, they can be helpful when staff members require additional skills or insight to work with residents or families. Similarly, consultants can be useful when administrators and staff members want to improve internal communications.

The following case is an example of escalating family-staff conflict in which a case-consultation intervention proved immediately useful. Here a consultant helped identify and restructure interaction patterns that altered the family-staff situation. This strategy, offered by the consultant, was addressed systematically so that the staff could apply it to other situations.

---

Marsha and Sarah alternated days for visiting their mother Georgia F. and made every effort to be at the nursing home for either lunch or dinner to help feed Georgia at these times. Their assistance was appreciated by the nursing assistants. But for several weeks meals were late and some part of the meal did not suit the sisters. At least four times a week they demanded that food be replaced or reheated and were short with and critical of the staff who couldn't "even provide a simple soft meal without spoiling it." Initially the staff apologized and attempted to provide what the sisters requested. But soon they began to avoid that end of the corridor during meals and the family complaints about staff indifference and inadequate basic care went to the nurse in charge and then to the administrators. The nursing assistants involved felt even more harassed and defensive and began seeking any outlet to punish (ignore) Georgia and/or "get those sisters off their backs." Case conferences offered no solutions but were an outlet for staff complaints about insensitive, overbearing relatives.

A mental health nurse practitioner from a nearby university worked with the director of nursing, family caseworker, and all other parties involved to provide a demonstration of conflict resolution–problem solving steps that participants could subsequently use. The consultant structured three meetings: for involved staff members; for staff with the family; and a staff follow-up. Clarification of mutual goals vs. staff and/or family complaints provided concrete behaviors to be sought and identified the benefits of changes. Expressions of approval and appreciation as well as desired changes were solicited. A positive, more trusting cooperation was developed.

Marsha and Sarah continued their vigilance, but found the staff were much more pleasant to deal with when they had complimentary things to say as well as requests to make. The staff approached the sisters with requests for help or with comments about changes they had noted with Georgia more openly after the meetings.

---

Had this consultation process not succeeded in altering the family and staff behavior, the consultant might have referred the sisters to nearby family counseling to alleviate their guilt, overprotectiveness, and anxiety. However, the greatest good for the greatest number was achieved by having a consultant examine and work through existing staff mechanisms and strengthen these links.

## BASIC STRUCTURES IN CONSULTATION

The process of consultation can be viewed in several ways. We begin by outlining the dimensions, or structures, that shape the consultation. We can then explore consultation in terms of its course, or how it unfolds. Subsequently, we will consider the concepts and perspectives that guide this process.

***Dimensions of Consultation.*** As seen in figure 3.1, five elements characterize the consultation process. They frame the questions of who, when, where, and what the consultation is to be about, as well as how it will take place.

The first general question asks, who will participate in this work; who has solicited a consultation and who are the major actors to be involved? For example, although the director of nursing may have requested a consultation, her concerns may be with staff behavior, family interference, or a series of resident incidents. Identification of the appropriate participants clarifies the desired target for change.

The second dimension involves the timing of consultative requests. When is consultation sought? Expectations of the consulter may be understood in terms of the immediacy of the needs presented (crisis situations vs. a more deliberate, considered concern). Administrative patterns, as well as the readiness of the management to initiate preventative therapeutic measures, are evident in the urgency of the initial contact. If, for example, the consultant is contacted because several of the residents are repeatedly abusing their roommates, the need for routine gross motor activities might be presented as a part of the "treatment." However, other resident-safety efforts and behavior-extinguishing procedures would have to be considered first. If management appears crisis oriented, the expanded activity plan may well serve preventative functions, but only secondarily.

The third element shaping consultation is the level, or scope, of the work. On what is the consultation to be focused?. Caplan (1970) specifies two general levels: case and administrative consultation.[3] Case consultation usually works with a specific resident, family, or staff issue, while admin-

**Fig. 3.1**

Dimensions of Consultation

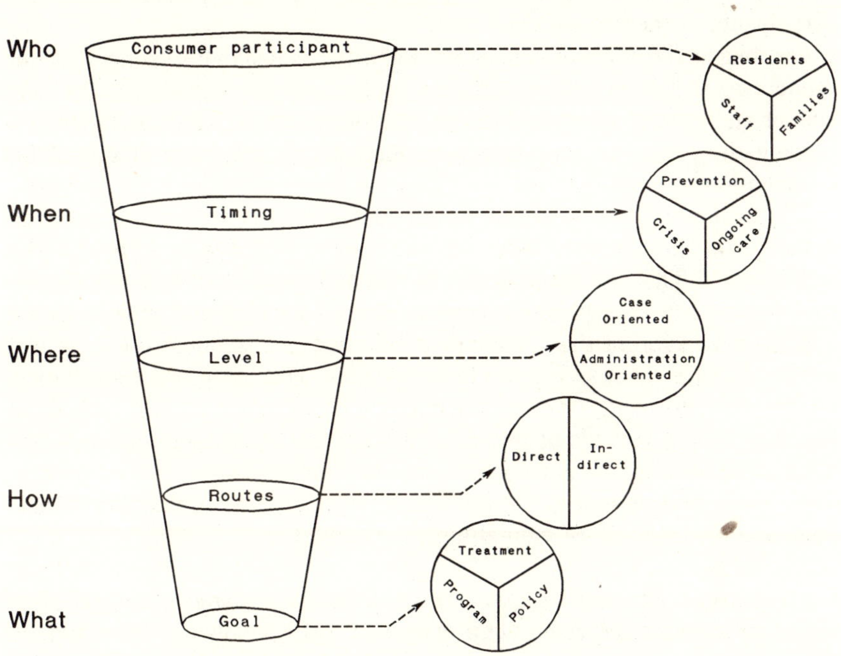

istrative consultations consider the issues of institutional management including policy, protocol, and programs.

The fourth dimension focuses on how to carry out the consultation. We will discuss these aspects in more detail later in the chapter. As an initial categorization of process, however, Caplan (1970) again offers helpful direction. He suggests that consultants use two major modes of action: working directly with the target beneficiary or indirectly through the consulter. For example, consulters may expect, alternatively, that the consultant will provide the intervention or simply design and oversee an intervention that participants in the setting carry out.

Combining the level of consultation and the consultant's mode of action produces a matrix of four consultation prototypes (see table 3.1). The consultant and consulters should develop a consistent set of expectations regarding the form and type of consultation during the early stages of the consultation process.

The final dimension of mental health consultation is the goal, or potential outcome, of the process. What will the consultant leave as a result of his or her work? This can range from a more content resident to a behaviorally specific resident-care plan to recommendations for staff and family policies.

Each dimension of the consultation influences subsequent ones, as well as the ultimate results. When a nursing-home director seeks consultation, he may be unfocused, or even see outcomes that are in conflict with those foreseen by the consultant herself. Through the consultation process, the input of all participants is reviewed and the final focus of intervention clarified. Thus, understanding the process is crucial for understanding the limitations and strengths of mental health consultation.

***Consultation Process.*** Caplan (1970) differentiates among several steps in the consultation process: (1) preparation; (2) relationship development; (3) problem assessment; (4) formulation and delivery of interventions; and (5) follow-up. These categories offer a useful framework for considering major components of mental health consultation.

Preparation for consultation applies to several participants in the consultation process: the consultant, who is presumably an outsider to the nursing home setting; and the members of the nursing-home community—residents, family members, administration, and staff. Each participant in the consultation process has training and experiences that shape his willingness and ability to participate in a mental health consultation. For example, the consultant may have limited knowledge about or experience in the nursing home setting; this gap in training may affect her willingness to seek out consulting experiences in this setting. Similarly, staff members, residents, or family members may have stereotypes of the sorts of issues that are "mental health" issues; a reluctance to label their own concerns as a mental problem may limit the initial acceptance of the consultant or the consultant's suggestions.[4]

Relationship development, Caplan's second step, also applies to several levels of the nursing home community and consultation process. For example, the consultant has to become acquainted with the culture of the nursing home setting, as well as with individual community members. Similarly, community members need to test their assumptions about consult-

TABLE 3.1: Examples of Mental Health Consultation by Route and Level

| *Level* | *Direct-Route Examples* | *Indirect-Route Examples* |
|---|---|---|
| Case Consultation | Psychologist requested to assess and intervene with four very vocal and disruptive residents who persist in cursing at all women visitors. Consultant carries out all procedures. | Social-work consultant confers with on-site caseworker to plan for assessing and working with Essie's alcoholic daughter after several tearful visits have left Essie withdrawn and apathetic. Family interview procedures and counseling strategies are taught or reviewed, but the caseworker carries out all interventions with support from consultant. |
| Administrative | Nurse's aides' job design requested of management or organizational-development consultant for staff in new "wanderers" unit. Consultant initiates all steps from brainstorming to procedural training and evaluation. | In-service educator in the Nursing Department seeks help to provide nursing staff with information and specific skills to help new residents and their families adjust to the nursing home. Class content, suggested teaching strategies, and resources are prepared by consultant, but training and evaluation are carried out by in-service personnel. |

ants against the reality of this consultant. Smith and Corse (1986, p. 257) summarize the delicate nature of the consultant's entry, relationship development, and status in any setting:

> The consultant needs to be in a marginal position, enough inside to understand what's going on and enough outside to be able to bring a fresh vantage point to each critical exchange. . . . The marginality needs to be of two forms. On the one hand the consultant, by definition, is marginal to the system as a whole. This marginality needs to be maintained so that the consultant's independence is not threatened and so that the consultant will continually be able to articulate alternatives insiders overlook. The second type of marginality requires that the consultant not become overidentified with the interests of one or more groups in the system.

The third step of the consultation process, problem assessment, builds upon the earlier steps. The preparation of the consultation participants affects their willingness and ability to identify current problems.[5] Similarly, the consultant's acceptance in the setting affects the kinds of information available for the process of problem assessment. As Smith and Corse (1986) note, there are many ways to gather information as part of the problem assessment. They range from relatively "unobtrusive," unstructured observations to more structured observations, completion of formal questionnaires and review of existing data.[6]

In addition to the dimension of intrusiveness, problem-assessment strategies also vary in the extent to which they involve members of the nursing home community. For example, a consultant may use single interviews with several staff members or a group interview with all the staff. Each strategy both determines and is determined by the preparation of the participants and their relationships.

Caplan's fourth step, formulation and delivery of intervention, requires that some degree of consensus have been reached in the assessment stage. With this as a foundation, the initial goals and strategies for resolving the problem can be outlined and implemented. These may range from case-oriented behavior-management suggestions to broader policy-oriented job-redesign strategies. What unites these diverse activities is their purpose: planned processes of influence and control targeted at individuals and groups.[7]

The fifth step in Caplan's scheme, follow-up, suggests the importance of evaluation and assessment as part of the consultation process. These elements again may vary from formal pre/postassessments that precisely gauge the effects of a specific intervention to less formal, subjective assessments of the efficacy of the intervention.

Caplan's term, *follow-up*, also suggests the dynamic, iterative nature of consultation. The problem assessment, intervention, and outcome are viewed once again—perhaps from the perspective of other nursing home community members, perhaps with a renewed appreciation of the problem's dimensions.

The dynamic nature of mental health consultation is summarized in figure 3.2. Here the consultant approaches the central issues and concerns while sequentially collecting information about varied elements involved. Consecutive reinterpretations eventually produce a manageable intervention that is undertaken and evaluated. This insight into the structure of the consultation process provides a framework for understanding the influence of differing disciplinary perspectives and theoretical models.

## DISCIPLINARY PERSPECTIVES ON CONSULTATION

The task of selecting a mental health consultant for the nursing home setting is influenced by three major elements: the availability of well-trained and effective consultants; a proper "match" between the consultant's expertise and the issue of concern; and the availability of funds to pay for the consultation process.

Thus far, we have not specified the disciplinary training or allegiance of the mental health consultant. To some extent, the four "core" mental health disciplines—nursing, psychiatry, social work, and psychology—share common elements of consultation. Yet each discipline's approach to mental health consultation is distinctive, in part due to its history, tradition, training paradigms, and funding patterns.[8] Consultants and the nursing home staff should be aware of these disciplinary patterns, since they may affect the consultant's skills and effectiveness.

The core disciplines have varied in the emphasis given for consultation training. Schwab (1986) reports, for example, that psychiatry has witnessed a substantial decline in interest in and training for consultant roles. He suggests that despite the contribution of psychiatric pioneers in the mental health consultation field (e.g. Caplan, 1964, 1970), the current trend is a dwindling emphasis on consultation and liaison psychiatry. In contrast, social work, as a field, has continued its historical involvement in consultation activities. Psychology has also focused attention on consultation activities, notably through developments in the subareas of community psychology and industrial-organizational development.

These disciplinary traditions of training and focus may affect the availability, usefulness, and acceptability of consultants for nursing home settings. As indicated earlier, two other elements may structure the choice of a consultant: the differential effectiveness of specific disciplines for ac-

**Fig. 3.2**

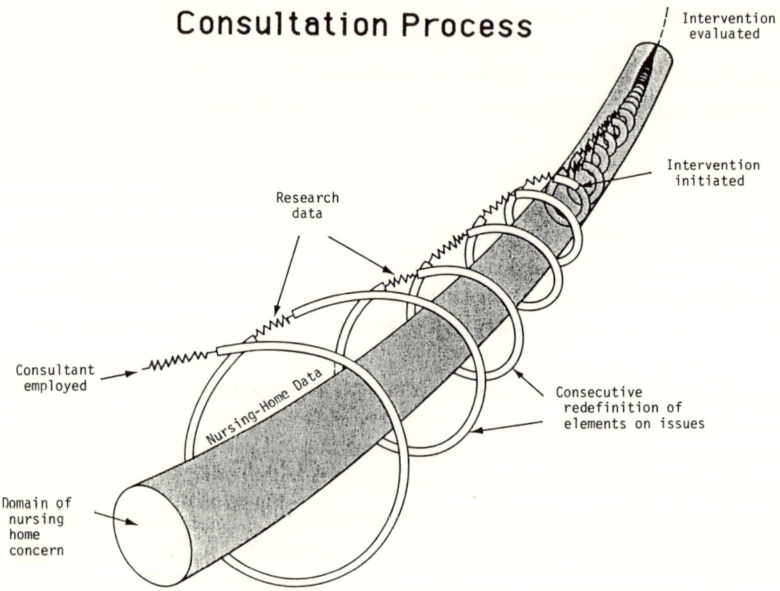


Source:
Adapted from Zeisel (1981).

complishing specific tasks; and the funding mechanisms available to pay for mental health consultation.

As outlined in table 3.2, the disciplines vary in their effectiveness for specific types of consultation. Effectiveness is a function of several elements: the disciplinary orientation of the consulter; status differences and traditions among disciplines and within the nursing home setting; the type of consultant action required (direct or indirect); and the orientation of the consultation (case-oriented vs. administratively oriented).

Although each consultant brings a distinctive set of experiences and training, some generalizations can be made about the types of issues members of each discipline may be best suited for, as well as which disciplines are most acceptable for certain types of problem areas or consulters.[9] For example, psychiatrists may be most effective in consulting with other physicians. Because of training and professional socialization, physicians may respond favorably to another physician as a consultant, in comparison to consultants from other disciplines. With organizational difficulties, the psychiatrist may lack expertise. The bulk of psychiatric training emphasizes case-oriented approaches.

The discipline of nursing, also, has its relative strengths and weaknesses. Like psychiatry, it is a discipline with a clear tradition of training—focusing more heavily on case-oriented issues than organizational or administrative issues. In contrast to psychiatry, however, nursing consultants may find more limited acceptance as consultants to medical or management personnel, because of the heritage of gender-based attributions and the medical tradition of the subsidiary role of nursing to medicine.[10] In short,

TABLE 3.2: Dimensions of Consultant-Consulter Effectiveness

| *Consultant's Discipline* | *Primary Consulter Disciplines* | *Most Effective Consultant Mode of Action* | *Typical Consultation Orientation* |
|---|---|---|---|
| Psychiatry | All, but especially medicine | Direct | Case |
| Nursing | Nursing | Direct/indirect | Case |
| Social Work | Social work | Direct/indirect | Case and administrative |
| Psychology | Medicine/nursing | Direct/indirect | Case and administrative |

status differences may affect the willingness of certain consulters to use the expertise of nursing consultants.

Social work, in contrast to psychiatry and nursing, has a tradition of training expertise in both case-oriented and administratively oriented consultation. Like nursing, however, social work as a discipline has been somewhat limited in its effectiveness in consulting to medical practitioners. Within the profession of social work, however, there is a strong and well-accepted tradition of consultation.

Likewise, psychology has had traditions of training that emphasize a broad range of approaches and strong consultant relationships. In community and industrial psychology, particularly, an emphasis on case-oriented consultation has been linked to broader organizational emphases.[11]

The information in table 3.2 affords the prospective participants only a glimpse of likely consultant strength and fit with consulter needs. Two additional elements affect the choice of a consultant and the conceptualization of the consultation process: the disciplinary background of the nursing home administrator and the inherently interdisciplinary nature of the consultation process.

As indicated in chapter 2, there are no standardized national training or licensure requirements for nursing-home administrators. Therefore, administrators come from a variety of professional and nonprofessional backgrounds, including medicine, nursing, social work, public administration, and other human-service sectors. Thus, although table 3.2 emphasizes the consultant's disciplinary background, it inevitably leaves open the issue of the administrator's disciplinary training. As a primary "gatekeeper" between the nursing home and the outside community, however, the administrator can affect the process and outcome of mental health consultation both indirectly, through support of proposed interventions, and directly, through the selection of the consultant.

Mental health consultation is inherently interdisciplinary.[12] Given the different disciplines working in nursing homes, consultation must be interdisciplinary to be effective. This suggests several cautions for administrators, consultants, and institutional boards in evaluating the prospects for developing a consulting relationship.

## A WORD TO ADMINISTRATORS

Administrators set the terms for consultation. They determine the initial problem areas to be discussed, the range of nursing home community members to be involved, the acceptable scope of change, and, perhaps, the funding sources to be used to pay for consulting services. Administrators must be concerned about the background and training of potential consultants. Two issues are essential in an initial consideration of the fit between the consultant's experience and expertise and the setting's concerns: Will the consultant's training and style fit in well with the facility's culture and staff traditions? Will the consultant's expertise match the perceived tasks? For example, psychologists as consultants may have two types of skills: case-oriented expertise, useful in differential diagnosis of depression and dementia, and/or organizational-consultation skills useful for broader interventions aimed at affecting the working patterns of the nursing-home setting. Thus, it is important not to opt for a member of any discipline without specifying the particular skills needed. Similarly, even if the potential consultant has the necessary skills, the next issue must be the congruence between the facility's culture and the consultant's style and comfort with interdisciplinary collaboration.

## A WORD TO CONSULTANTS

Just as the administrator must examine the match between the consultant's expertise and the facility's concerns, so, too, the consultant should also attend to the match. The consultant is likely to ask similar questions: How open is the setting to outsiders—both administratively and at other levels of staffing? What is the setting's experience in working with outside consultants from similar disciplines and backgrounds? How well does the consultant work with this type of mixture of professional levels and disciplines? Does the consultant have the specific expertise required by the initial consultation request? Will funding be an insurmountable barrier?

## A CONTINUING CONCERN: FUNDING

As outlined in chapter 2, the economic well-being of a nursing home is directly affected by the funding streams of federal programs, notably the Medicaid program. Fees paid by individual families and residents provide the second major source of funds. Each of these sources emphasizes individually oriented, direct-service provision.

These funding emphases can be a major problem for board members who are concerned about identifying resources for indirect-service provision, preventative interventions, or administratively oriented consultations.[13] There are no easy solutions to the funding dilemma. Two strategies seem most feasible, however. When appropriate, case-oriented consultation could be linked to the fee-for-service reimbursement scheme.

Under the Medicaid program, however, there are state-level policy differences in coverage of specific services and specific disciplines. Therefore, both administrators and consultants should explore the potential for third-party reimbursement for case-oriented-consultation services. Similarly, individual residents or their families may provide funding for case-oriented assistance. The cost effectiveness of altering resident behaviors, and altering staff time, must be discussed by the consultant and the administrator.

When administratively oriented consultation is the focus, a different strategy may be necessary. Since the emphasis of such consultation is the improvement of the organization's functioning, the nursing home itself may be the most appropriate source of funding for this activity. Here, however, the initial burden of proof may fall to the consultant: Administratively oriented consultations could potentially affect major cost concerns in the nursing home, such as staff turnover and staff absenteeism. Administrators and board members may be willing to pay for consultation with nursing home funds if that consultation leads to overall savings.[14]

## TWO CONTRASTING AND COMPLEMENTARY APPROACHES TO MENTAL HEALTH CONSULTATION

In this book we emphasize two contrasting and complementary approaches to mental health consultation: behavioral approaches and organizational-development efforts.[15] Vernberg and Reppucci (1986) recently summarized the essential elements of behavioral approaches to mental health consultation:

> The list of principles and practices common to all behavioral consultants is . . . brief: (1) both adaptive and maladaptive behaviors are acquired and maintained through the same learning processes; (2) maladaptive behaviors can be modified through the appropriate application of learning theory; (3) successful interventions should lead to observable changes in behavior; and (4) empirical evaluation of intervention effects is essential (pp. 54–55).

These principles can be applied to all four types of consultation outlined in table 3.1. Later chapters in this book offer illustrations of behavioral approaches to resident issues (chapters 6 and 7), to family functioning in nursing home settings (chapter 9), and to staff issues (chapters 10 and 11).

A second approach to mental health consultation emphasized in this volume is organizational development. Fullan, Miles, and Taylor (1980) summarized the essential elements of organization development (OD):

> . . . a coherent, systematically-planned, sustained effort at system self-study and improvement, focusing explicitly on change in formal and informal procedures, processes, norms or structures, using behavioral science concepts. The goals of OD include improving both the quality of life of individuals as well as organizational functioning and performance (p. 135).

As Keys (1986) pointed out, several aspects of this definition are important to note. First, OD is explicitly focused on the working of the system or institutional setting. Second, the grist for the OD mill are the formal and informal structures of the nursing home. Finally, the outcomes of the OD process can be gauged on both the institutional and individual levels—in our terms we can gauge the health of the nursing home community as a whole, as well as the well-being of specific members of the community. We have already suggested the importance of the institutional context in chapters 1 and 2. In subsequent chapters, we suggest the potentially important role that OD consultation can play in affecting the mental health functioning of different members of the nursing home community, for example, family members (see chapter 9) and staff members (see chapters 10 and 11).

Although we have discussed these two approaches separately, they are often used together. For example, some of our suggestions on OD approaches in chapters 9 and 11 are behaviorally focused. Similarly, behaviorally oriented case consultation inherently requires the cooperation of broader organizational structures.

Our discussion thus far has focused on a single consultant in a nursing home. It is unlikely that a single consultant would have the expertise required to provide the full range of consultations described throughout this book. The task for the consultant and administrator must be to assess the concerns of the setting, the expertise available, and the resources required to achieve the desired outcome—for either the nursing home community as a whole or for special subgroups within the setting.

## SUMMARY

Throughout this chapter, we have described the process of consultation in some detail. Several elements affect the likelihood of successful mental health consultation: the setting's own structure and history; the professional expertise among the staff and potential consultants; the funding streams available for supporting mental health consultation; and the conceptual approaches that guide the consultant and the nursing home in defining problems and seeking solutions. This chapter is designed as a general overview for the specific details of consultation that are considered throughout the rest of the book. In subsequent chapters, we describe mental-health consultation focused on three elements of the nursing home community: residents, their families, and staff members.

## NOTES

1. See James Stockdill's Foreword in the NIMH Handbook of Mental Health Consultation (Stockdill, 1986, pp. v–vi). His five points have been liberally modified in this section to reflect their significance in nursing-home consultation.

2. See Gutheil (1984), Jellineck and Tennstedt (1980), Petry and Gutheil (1979), and Sbordone and Sterman (1983) for example.

3. See Caplan (1964, 1970).

4. See Knight (1986) for a useful discussion of the readiness of different cohorts to seek out mental health treatments.

5. See Maruyama (1983) for a thoughtful discussion of the effects of culture and worldview on problem formation and solution development.

6. In chapters 4, 5, and 9 we discuss problem assessments focusing on individual residents as well as their families.

7. In chapters 6, 7, 9, 10, and 11 we discuss specific intervention strategies. See Birkel, Lerner, and Smyer (in preparation) for a general discussion of the purpose of a wide range of interventions.

8. A detailed discussion of each discipline's particular perspective can be found in Mannino et al. (1986). Specifically, Schwab (1986) focuses on psychiatry; Robinson (1986) and Howard (1986) discuss nursing; Goldmeier and Mannino (1986) detail social work's contribution; and Conoley (1986) summarizes psychology's developments and distinctive contribution. Kelly (1986) provides an integrated discussion of training and traditions across the core disciplines.

9. This discussion draws heavily upon the summaries referred to in note 8. Detailed discussion of each discipline is beyond the scope of this chapter. Interested readers are directed to Birren and Sloane (1980), Busse and Blazer (1980), Santos and VandenBos (1982), and Verwoerdt (1981) for more comprehensive treatments of substantive expertise in core disciplines. In addition, Tobin and his colleagues (1986) provide a thoughtful discussion of the role of pastoral interventions in responding to older adults.

10. Kelly (1986) discusses the relative strengths and weaknesses of the nursing discipline in more detail.

11. See Smyer, Gatz, and Pruchno (1987) for a discussion of the natural links between community psychology and aging.

12. See Levin, Trickett, and Kidder (1986) for a discussion of the obstacles to effective interdisciplinary collaboration.

13. Levin and her colleagues (1986) point out that these concerns are relevant

for the entire field of mental health consultation, not just for the nursing home community.

14. See chapters 10 and 11 for a discussion of administratively oriented mental health consultation strategies focused on staff resources.

15. Our discussion draws from recent reviews by Vernberg and Reppucci (1986) and by Keys (1986).

# 4

# The Mental Health Problems of Nursing Home Residents

*Michael A. Smyer and Adam J. Garfein*

Ya gotta know the Territory.

*"Professor" Harold Hill*
*in Meredith Wilson's* The Music Man

## INTRODUCTION

"Professor" Hill's admonition is a good starting point for consultants beginning to work in nursing home settings. In this chapter, we describe the "territory" of mental health consultation focusing on individual residents. Specifically, we highlight the most frequent mental health problems of nursing home residents. In doing so, we draw on information gathered in three distinct but complementary processes: epidemiological studies; studies based on professional assessments using structured criteria; and surveys of key informants working in nursing homes. Each data approach and its findings is described in a separate section.

The final section of the chapter focuses on the parallels between these national efforts and the consultant's own data-gathering process in beginning a relationship with a nursing home. In approaching a specific setting, many of the questions and data-gathering techniques may be similar, even though the scope of effort may be smaller.[1]

## EPIDEMIOLOGICAL STUDIES

Epidemiology is a changing field. Once focusing on the study of infectious diseases, epidemiology has recently emphasized the study of the distribution and determination of health and disease in humans. Epidemiological efforts now include a broad array of tasks: providing information for planning and policy purposes; evaluating current and projected needs for health care; evaluating new therapies and interventions; and improving basic understanding of the determinants of mental health and illness.[2]

For the nursing home consultant, three subareas of epidemiology are most relevant: the epidemiology of mental illness in general, of mental illness in nursing homes, and of geriatrics. In each domain, the basic process is the same—a study of the distribution of morbidity in time and place, and the factors that influence its distribution.[3] In this section, we focus on epidemiological data relating to mental disorders, moving from community data to institutional data.

Before considering specific results, however, a few definitions are necessary. The results of epidemiological studies are generally expressed as rates of prevalence or incidence of a disorder within a given population. The prevalence rate refers to current numbers of persons who are ill at any given time or during a specified time period. The incidence rate refers to the number of persons who become ill within a specified time period with either first-time illness or recurrent illness. Prevalence studies generally report the percentage of the population with the specific disorder at some specified time. Incidence studies begin by studying a group of individuals who are free of any disorders. The individuals are then followed for a given period of time, and the number who develop a specified disorder are reported as the ratio of new cases over the total number of persons at the beginning of the study.[4] These definitions provide an important background for considering evidence of mental disorders among community-dwelling elderly and institutionalized elderly. We begin with a brief description of the major source of information, the Epidemiologic Catchment Area (ECA) program.

***Epidemiologic Catchment Area (ECA) Program.*** The ECA research program, which is still in progress, was designed to fill the gaps in epidemiological data that existed at the time of the President's Commission on Mental Health (PCMH) (PCMH, 1978a, 1978b). Its main goal has been to obtain prevalence rates of specific mental disorders as defined by DSM-III (*Diagnostic and Statistical Manual of Mental Disorders*)(American Psychiatric Association, 1980)(and *Research Diagnostic Criteria*)(Spitzer, Endicott, and Robins, 1978) rather than prevalence rates of global impairment (Eaton et al., 1981). In addition, the research program is designed to estimate rates of health and mental health services use, to study factors influencing the development and continuance of disorders and to study factors influencing the use of services (Eaton et al., 1984; Regier et al., 1984).[5]

The ECA design includes both community and institutionalized populations, which allows for the identification of treated and untreated mental disorders. When the research is completed each one of the ECA sites will have data on more than three thousand community residents and five hundred institutional residents, for a total of nearly twenty thousand respondents.

Each respondent will be interviewed at least twice by a trained interviewer, with interviews conducted at one-year intervals. Thus, the research employs a short-term longitudinal design with a field-survey data-collection strategy using trained interviewers (Kay and Bergmann, 1980).

The longitudinal format allows each site to calculate incidence, remission, and recurrence rates. Individuals who show no specific disorders at the first interview are followed up at the second interview to determine incidence rates. Those with disorders are followed up to compute remission rates. Finally, individuals with past disorders are followed up to determine recurrence rates (Regier et al., 1984).

The five ECA sites are coterminous with community mental-health center catchment areas and are located at the following universities: Yale University (New Haven, Connecticut), Johns Hopkins University (Baltimore, Maryland), Washington University (St. Louis, Missouri), Duke University (Durham, North Carolina), and UCLA (Los Angeles, California).

Researchers at each of the ECA sites are using the Diagnostic Interview Schedule (DIS) as the case-identification instrument (Robins et al., 1981, 1982). It was selected as the diagnostic instrument because it obtains prevalence rates of specific mental disorders as defined by DSM-III (American Psychiatric Association, 1980) rather than prevalence rates of global impairment. The DIS assesses the presence, duration, and severity of individual symptoms (Regier et al., 1984).

Table 4.1 shows six-month prevalence of DIS/DSM-III disorders for elderly respondents by sex, while table 4.2 provides additional demographic data on impaired DSM-III–diagnosed elders. The data presented are from the New Haven, Connecticut, ECA site, and are based on 2,588 persons age sixty-five or over in an urban community.[6]

Several important findings emerge from these data.[7] First, as Weissman et al. point out, from an epidemiological perspective, the majority of community-dwelling elderly are not experiencing psychiatric distress or severe cognitive impairment. Second, the prevalence rates of psychiatric distress reported for the elderly are somewhat lower than rates reported for younger age groups. Third, the pattern of psychiatric impairment varies with demographic characteristics. Not surprisingly, those demographic factors traditionally associated with risk of psychosocial impairment (for example, widowhood, divorce, poorer education, and older age) are also associated with higher rates of psychiatric impairment. The association between age and cognitive impairment is particularly noteworthy. As Weissman and colleagues note, nearly 17 percent of community-dwelling elderly age eighty-five and older have significant cognitive impairment, yet only about 5 percent of all elderly are institutionalized at any one point in time (as pointed out in chapter 1). Therefore, families and community social-support sys-

TABLE 4.1: Six-Month Prevalence of DIS/DSM-III Disorders for Elderly Respondents by Sex

| *DIS/DSM-III Disorder* | *Male* | *Female* | *Total Respondents* |
|---|---|---|---|
| Any disorder or severe cognitive impairment | 8.9% | 12.1% | 10.8% |
| Any disorder excluding severe cognitive impairment | 5.4 | 7.5 | 6.7 |
| Cognitive impairment | | | |
| Severe | 2.6 | 3.9 | 3.4 |
| Mild | 13.8 | 12.0 | 12.7 |
| Schizophrenia or spectrum | 0.1 | 0.4 | 0.3 |
| Schizophrenia | 0.1 | 0.3 | 0.3 |
| Schizophreniform | 0.0 | 0.0 | 0.0 |
| Affective disorders | | | |
| Major depressive episode | 0.9 | 2.3 | 1.7 |
| Without bereavement | 0.6 | 1.4 | 1.1 |
| Bereavement | 0.3 | 0.9 | 0.6 |
| Bipolar | 0.2 | 0.0 | 0.1 |
| Dysthymia[a] | 1.4 | 3.1 | 2.4 |
| Any affective DX | 1.1 | 2.3 | 1.8 |
| Anxiety disorders | | | |
| Phobia (any below) | 1.8 | 5.3 | 3.9 |
| Agoraphobia[b] | 0.6 | 1.9 | 1.4 |
| Simple phobia[b] | 1.6 | 4.1 | 3.1 |
| Panic | 0.0 | 0.1 | 0.1 |
| Obsessive compulsive | 0.9 | 0.6 | 0.7 |
| Any above anxiety DX | 2.6 | 5.8 | 4.6 |
| Abuse or dependence | | | |
| Alcohol | 1.7 | 0.1 | 0.7 |
| Drug | 0.0 | 0.0 | 0.0 |
| Other | | | |
| Somatization | <0.1 | 0.0 | 0.0 |
| Antisocial | 0.4 | 0.0 | 0.1 |
| Anorexia nervosa | 0.0 | 0.0 | 0.0 |

Note: All respondents age sixty-five or older (n = 2588). Weighted for sample design. Since the numbers of men and women are unequal, column 3 does not equal the sum of columns 1 and 2.

[a]Dysthymia covers a longer period than six months by definition.

[b]Since these categories are not mutually exclusive and there is some overlap, the figures are not added.

Source: Weissman et al. (1985), *Acta Psychiatrica Scandanavica* 71(4): 372. Munksgaard International Publishers, Ltd., Copenhagen, Denmark. Reprinted by permission.

tems must be buffering the effects of cognitive impairment in advanced old age.[8] These community-based data provide an important point of comparison for considering the prevalence rates of psychiatric distress within nursing home settings.

***Prevalence Rates of Psychiatric Distress in Nursing Homes: Early Estimates.*** Early reports (e.g., Goldfarb, 1962; Gottesman, 1977; NIA Task Force, 1980) indicated that between 60 and 90 percent of institu-

TABLE 4.2: Demographic Characteristics for Elderly Respondents by Six-Month Prevalence Rates (%) Cognitive Impairment of DIS/DSM-III Diagnosis

| *Characteristic* | *Cognitive Impairment Severe* | *Any Other DSM-III DX* | *Total* |
|---|---|---|---|
| Sex | | | |
| Male | 2.5% | 5.4% | 7.9% |
| Female | 3.8 | 7.5 | 11.3 |
| Age | | | |
| 65–74 | 1.1 | 7.3 | 8.4 |
| 75–84 | 4.3 | 6.3 | 10.6 |
| 85+ | 16.8 | 3.3 | 20.1 |
| Race[a] | | | |
| Non-Black | 3.1 | 6.8 | 9.9 |
| Black | 5.4 | 4.0 | 9.4 |
| Education | | | |
| 0–8 years | 6.1 | 7.6 | 13.7 |
| 9–12 | 1.3 | 6.9 | 8.2 |
| 13–15 | 0.9 | 2.8 | 3.7 |
| 16+ | 0.2 | 7.5 | 7.7 |
| Marital status | | | |
| Married | 2.0 | 5.7 | 7.7 |
| Widowed | 5.5 | 8.0 | 13.5 |
| Separated/Divorced | 3.6 | 10.0 | 13.6 |
| Single | 1.2 | 5.5 | 6.7 |
| Living Arrangement | | | |
| Alone | 2.7 | 8.2 | 10.9 |
| With spouse/child | 2.4 | 6.0 | 8.4 |
| With Nonrelative | 6.6 | 6.5 | 13.1 |

Note: All respondents age sixty-five or older (n = 2588). Weighted for sample design.

[a]Rates for Hispanic (n = 7) and other races are not presented due to low number (n = 27).

Source: Weissman et al., (1985), *Acta Psychiatrica Scandanavica* 71(4): 373. Munksgaard International Publishers, Ltd., Copenhagen, Denmark. Reprinted by permission.

tionalized elderly were in need of mental health consultation. However, the data base for these estimates was small. Kramer (1986) recently summarized the epidemiological data available prior to the ECA program of research. The major sources of information were the National Center for Health Statistics (NCHS) surveys of nursing homes. Kramer characterized these studies: "The NCHS surveys of nursing homes provide very limited data on the prevalence of mental disorders among nursing home residents" (1986, p. 15). Table 4.3 summarizes the information available from the National Nursing Home Survey (NNHS) of 1977. As indicated in table 4.3, in 1977 approximately 19 percent of nursing home residents had a primary diagnosis of mental disorder or senility without psychosis—almost double the rate reported in the ECA community-based study.

Unfortunately, the NCHS offered little in-depth mental health information, using poorly defined and overly general categories for primary diagnoses at admission. This partially relfected imprecise diagnoses or assessments of residents of nursing homes made upon admission (Sabin, Vitug, and Mark, 1982). Furthermore, many nursing homes have poor record keeping, with little or no past history of residents. Together, the problems of poor record keeping and inadequate assessments limit the precision of such studies (Liptzin, 1986).

***Recent ECA Data for Nursing Homes.*** Early criticisms of the ECA program focused on the lack of reports documenting mental illness among institutional residents (Kermis, 1986). Recently, however, German and her associates at the ECA site in Baltimore have presented data on mental illness among nursing home residents (German, Shapiro, and Kramer, 1986). Their work is important, since it applies the standardized ECA methodology to the nursing-home setting.

The collection of nursing homes in the Baltimore study is unusual since it represents the majority of nursing homes in the area serving the study population. A total of 383 residents were interviewed by one of several methods. Some received a full interview (38.6 percent), including the DIS (Robins et al., 1981, 1982) and Mini-Mental State Examination (MMSE) (Folstein, Folstein, and McHugh, 1975). Approximately 20 percent of the interviews consisted of both patient interviews and proxy interviews, and about 32 percent were proxy interviews only, with less than 9 percent refusals. For the proxy interviews, all information came from someone other than the resident, usually family members who were in frequent contact with the resident.

Residents were categorized by length of stay (less than one year, greater than one year) to examine mental morbidity among different populations at one point in time. This categorization enabled the investigators to compare the mental status of long-term residents to short-term residents, thereby suggesting possible effects of the length of residence in a nursing home. Table 4.4 shows current DIS diagnosis according to length of stay in the nursing home.

Again, several themes are important when reviewing table 4.4. First, the rates of DIS diagnosis and cognitive impairment vary by length of stay

TABLE 4.3: Frequency of Mental Disorders and Senility Without Psychosis Among Nursing Home Residents

| | DIAGNOSIS AT LAST EXAMINATION | |
|---|---|---|
| | *Primary* | *Chronic Condition* |
| | *Number of Residents* | |
| Total | 266,100 | Data not available |
| Mental illness (unspecified)[b] | | 148,300 |
| Chronic brain syndrome | 96,400 | 324,700 |
| Senility (unspecified)[b] | | 416,400 |
| Senile psychosis[a] | 21,200 | |
| Senility without psychosis[a] | 26,600 | |
| Other psychosis[a] | 57,400 | |
| Mental retardation | 42,400 | 79,800 |
| Alcoholism | 6,800 | 36,900 |
| Drug addiction[b] | | * |
| Other mental disorders[a] | 15,300 | |
| Insomnia[b] | | 125,500 |
| | *Percentage of 1,303,100 Residents* | |
| Total | 20.4 | Data not available |
| Mental illness (unspecified)[b] | | 11.4 |
| Chronic brain syndrome | 7.4 | 24.9 |
| Senility (unspecified)[b] | | 32.0 |
| Senile psychosis[a] | 1.6 | |
| Senility without psychosis[a] | 2.0 | |
| Other psychosis[a] | 4.4 | |
| Mental retardation | 3.3 | 6.1 |
| Alcoholism | 0.5 | 2.8 |
| Drug addiction[b] | | * |
| Other mental disorders[a] | 1.2 | |
| Insomnia[b] | | 9.6 |

[a]This diagnostic term was used as a primary diagnosis but not as a chronic condition.
[b]This diagnostic term was used as a diagnosis of a chronic condition but not as a primary diagnosis.
*Diagnosis of insufficient magnitude to record.
Source: National Center for Health Statistics (1979).

in the institutional setting. This should raise at least one question about the initial status of newly admitted residents, as well as the initial impact of the transition to the institutional setting. For the consultant, the data are reminders of the important distinction between recent-onset and long-standing patterns of adaptation—distinctions that are important for both diagnostic and treatment purposes.[9] (See chapters 5 and 6 for more extended discussion of this distinction.) Second, significant levels of psychiatric and cognitive impairment are apparent, within both the short-stay and long-stay nursing home residents. Using the earlier-cited community data for comparative purposes, the prevalence of DIS diagnoses is between approximately 2.5 and 4 times greater in the nursing home setting than in the community setting. Finally, German (1987) indicates that the data are conservative estimates, because of the cautious approach taken in interviewing the sample. The interview team sought to avoid overtaxing particularly confused patients, therefore proxy interviews were used frequently. In those cases, the informants may have been unable to provide full information on the lifetime history of adaptation of the nursing home resident.

Table 4.5 presents information on variation in the reported prevalence of mental disorders as a function of the type of interview approach used. The work of German and her colleagues is important for several reasons.

TABLE 4.4: Current DIS Diagnosis by Length of Stay in Nursing Home

| | LENGTH OF STAY | |
|---|---|---|
| *Current Diagnosis* | *Less Than One Year (174–181)*[a] | *One Year Or More (104–144)*[a] |
| Schizophrenia | 0.6% | 0.7% |
| Affective disorders | 6.8 | 2.1 |
| Phobias | 11.6 | 2.1 |
| Substance abuse or dependence | 0.6 | 0.0 |
| Antisocial personality | 0.7 | 0.0 |
| Other DIS disorders | 3.3 | 0.7 |
| Any DIS diagnosis | 41.1 | 25.3 |
| Cognitive impairment[b] | 24.0 | 21.5 |

[a]These numbers represent the range of individuals for any single diagnosis. Certain diagnoses could not be made because of lack of information. Individuals could have more than one diagnosis, however.

[b]Cognitive impairment here is based on the Mini-Mental State Examination. It does not include chart diagnoses.

Source: German, Shapiro, and Kramer (1986, p. 36). Reprinted by permission.

It documents the significant level of mental impairment among nursing home residents. At the same time, it reflects the difficulty of careful epidemiological investigation in a setting with frail residents. Although the ECA studies used a standardized interview format, they relied upon nonprofessional interviewers. From an epidemiological perspective, this strategy is essential. From a clinical perspective, however, questions arise about the match between research-based diagnostic impressions and those developed by practicing clinicians. The work reviewed in the next section blends clinical and research perspectives.

TABLE 4.5: Mental Status of Patients by Type of Interview and Length of Stay in Nursing Home

| | TYPE OF INTERVIEW | | | | | |
|---|---|---|---|---|---|---|
| | *With Patient Only* | | *Short With Patient, Also With Proxy* | | *With Proxy Only* | |
| | LENGTH OF STAY | | | | | |
| | % | % | % | % | % | % |
| *Current DIS Diagnosis* | *Less Than 1 Year* | *1 or More Years* | *Less Than 1 Year* | *1 or More Years* | *Less Than 1 Year* | *1 or More Years* |
| n | 83 | 63 | 51 | 29 | 58 | 66 |
| Any current DIS diagnosis | 45.8 | 36.5 | 60.8 | 51.7 | 17.2[a] | 3.0[a] |
| Any current DIS diagnosis excluding cognitive impairment | 18.1 | 6.3 | 15.7 | 0.0 | 17.2 | 3.0 |
| Cognitive impairment only | 27.7 | 30.2 | 45.0 | 5.7 | —[a] | —[a] |

[a]Mini-Mental State Examination not administered.
Source: German, Shapiro, and Kramer (1986, p. 37). Reprinted by permission.

## PROFESSIONAL DIAGNOSES OF MENTAL ILLNESS

The epidemiological studies reviewed thus far had two major characteristics: They relied upon trained nonprofessional interviewers, and they involved the use of a structured interview format to limit the effects of the interviewer and to assure comparability across settings. Although these studies improved upon the earlier impressionistic reports of prevalence of mental disorders, they, too, have their limitations. Rovner and his colleagues summarized the current state of research:

> We know of no studies to date on the prevalence of mental illness among random samples of nursing home residents in which psychiatrists systematically examined the residents and made diagnoses of mental disorders according to DSM-III criteria (Rovner et al., 1986, p. 1446).

Rovner's group improved upon previous efforts in two ways: They interviewed a random sample of intermediate-care nursing home patients, and they used a geriatric psychiatrist to interview the sample and make diagnoses using DSM-III criteria.[10] The results of their efforts are summarized in table 4.6.

TABLE 4.6: Prevalence of Psychiatric Disorders in a Random Sample (n = 50) of Nursing Home Residents

| *Disorder or Problem* | *N* | % |
|---|---|---|
| Psychiatric disorder | | |
| Primary degenerative dementia | 28 | 56 |
| With delusions and/or hallucinations | 11 | 22 |
| With depression | 5 | 10 |
| With mania | 1 | 2 |
| Uncomplicated | 11 | 22 |
| Multi-infarct dementia | 9 | 18 |
| With delusions and/or hallucinations | 1 | 2 |
| With depression | 4 | 8 |
| Uncomplicated | 4 | 8 |
| Parkinson's disease, dementia | 2 | 4 |
| Delirium | 3 | 6 |
| Major depression | 3 | 6 |
| Major depression, in remission | 1 | 2 |
| Paraphrenia | 1 | 2 |
| No psychiatric diagnosis | 3 | 6 |

Source: Rovner et al. (1986). Reprinted by permission.

In contrast to the ECA study, the prevalence of psychiatric disorders was 94 percent. The most frequent psychiatric disorder was dementia. Rovner and his colleagues point out that only one of the residents had a history of previous psychiatric hospitalization. Thus, the high prevalence rate is not the result of "transinstitutionalization" from state psychiatric hospitals to nursing homes.

The significant level of psychiatric disorders may reflect the combined effects of the two distinctive aspects of the study: random sampling and use of a geriatric psychiatrist as interviewer. Rovner et al. (1986) argue that their approach provides the most realistic depiction of the prevalence of mental disorders in the nursing-home setting to date. Their logic is compelling.

In addition to psychiatric disorders, Rovner and his colleagues assessed the prevalence of behavioral disorders among their sample of nursing home residents. Again, the results are striking (see table 4.7). Like psychiatric disorders, behavioral problems were also prevalent at a high rate: 76 percent of the residents had at least one maladaptive behavior.

Rovner's group stresses the importance of recognizing the relationship between psychiatric disorders and behavioral disturbance:

TABLE 4.7: Prevalence of Behavior Problems in a Random Sample (n = 50) of Nursing Home Residents

| *Behavioral Problem* | *N* | % |
|---|---|---|
| Difficulty in communication | 20 | 40 |
| Delusions, hallucinations | 19 | 38 |
| Restlessness | 19 | 38 |
| Passive-aggression | 19 | 38 |
| Demands interaction | 18 | 36 |
| Socially objectionable | 18 | 36 |
| Disruptive | 17 | 34 |
| Active aggression | 13 | 26 |
| Verbal aggression | 13 | 26 |
| Wandering | 12 | 24 |
| Noisiness | 12 | 24 |
| Manipulativeness | 11 | 22 |
| Incoherent speech | 10 | 20 |
| Self-destructiveness | 7 | 14 |
| Elation | 1 | 2 |
| Destructiveness to property | 0 | 0 |

Source: Rovner et al. (1986). Reprinted by permission.

> This study is the first we know of in the literature to relate common behavioral problems in nursing homes to specific psychiatric symptoms. Because neuroleptic medications specifically treat delusions and hallucinations, recognition and appropriate treatment with these drugs will likely reduce the behavioral disturbances associated with delusions and hallucinations (Rovner et al., 1986, p. 1448).

While this study is an important one, it is more suggestive than definitive. Drawing a sample from only one home has potential limitations for generalizability. The approach, however, of using geriatric psychiatrists with a random sample of residents offers the possibility of blending epidemiological and clinical perspectives. German and Rovner are now collaborating on a larger study, drawing a sample of five hundred nursing home residents from eight settings. After initial psychiatric diagnoses, these patients will be followed with interviews after two months and after one year (German, 1987). This type of careful collaboration offers the prospect of even better information on the prevalence of psychiatric disturbance among nursing home residents.

In summary, epidemiological and psychiatric inquiry are congruent in documenting significant levels of psychiatric disorders among nursing home residents. Rovner's group also documents significant levels of behavioral disturbance. For those who are not psychiatrically trained, these may be the key indicators of the need for mental health consultation. In the next section, we focus on key informants' views of problem behaviors in the setting.

## PROBLEMATIC BEHAVIORS: VIEWS OF "KEY INFORMANTS"

Thus far, we have reviewed two essential strategies for documenting levels of psychiatric disorders in nursing homes: epidemiological studies and structured diagnostic interviews by professional staff members. A third major strategy for assessing the most problematic behaviors in the setting is to survey "key informants" in the setting.

Seidman (1983) points out the importance of assessing the views of the key "stakeholders" in an intervention setting. In the nursing home, two sets of major stakeholders are administrators and nursing caregivers—aides and LPNs. We have added a third category of key informant, a sample of psychologists with experience in long-term-care settings.

Each group was surveyed to assess its views of the most frequent mental health problem behaviors in the nursing home setting. The administrators and aides were part of a statewide mail survey of nursing homes in

Pennsylvania.[11] The administrators represented a well-experienced group: 54 percent had worked in the long-term-care setting more than five years; 38 percent had worked between one and five years in such a setting; and only 8 percent had served for less than a year in a long-term-care facility. Similarly, the aides represented an experienced work force: 54 percent had worked in long-care for more than five years; 41 percent for between one and five years; and only 5 percent for less than a year.

The psychologists were members of a national network of psychologists in long-term care.[12] The network serves as a forum for communication among psychologists who consult to, are employed within, or conduct research regarding long-term-care settings or other senior living environments. Twenty-three of the twenty-six licensed psychologists agreed to participate in a fifteen-to-twenty-minute telephone interview. Seventeen states and Canada were represented in the group. As with the administrators and aides, the psychologists were a sample of seasoned professionals, with an average of 7.8 years of consultation experience in long-term-care settings.

The three groups were presented a list of mental health problem behaviors and asked to rate the frequency of each behavior as occurring very often, fairly often, sometimes, rarely, or never. The list of behaviors was as follows:

1. Hostile, threatening, or abusive behavior
2. Disoriented behavior
3. Hallucinations and delusions
4. Depression and withdrawal
5. Suicidal behavior
6. Agitation, wandering and screaming
7. Problematic grief reactions
8. Sensory deprivation
9. Inappropriate sexual behavior
10. Drug and alcohol abuse and misuse
11. Lack of family contact

The ratings of the three groups of key informants are presented in figure 4.1.

Figure 4.1 highlights several important points. First, there is consensus among the three groups of key informants that disorientation, depression, and agitation are among the most frequently occurring problem behaviors. Despite this consensus, however, there was also diversity of opinion about the relative frequency of other problem behaviors. This underscores the importance of recognizing different perspectives within the nursing home

**Fig. 4.1**

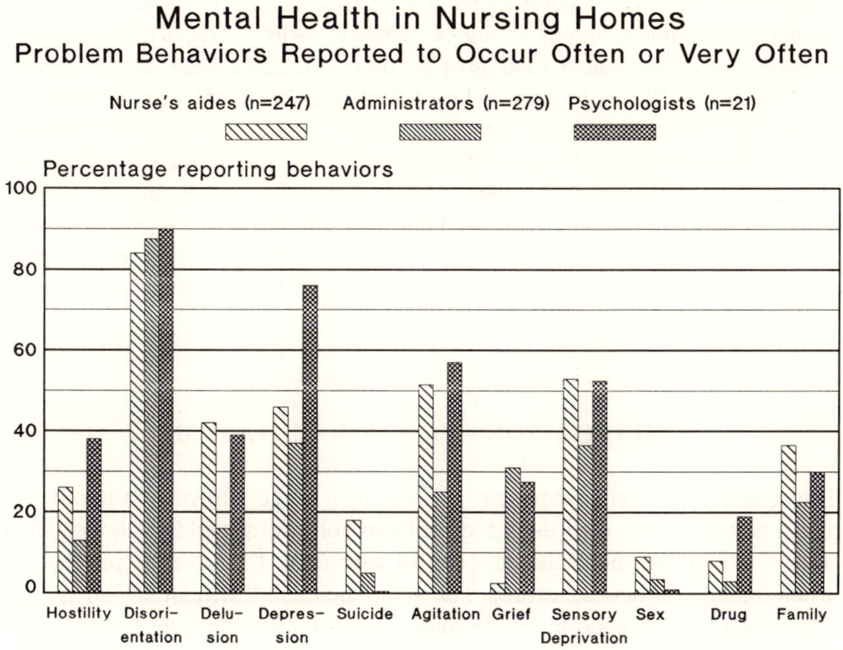
Mental Health in Nursing Homes
Problem Behaviors Reported to Occur Often or Very Often
Nurse's aides (n=247)
Administrators (n=279)
Psychologists (n=21)
Percentage reporting behaviors
100
80
60
40
20
0
Hostility
Disori-entation
Delu-sion
Depres-sion
Suicide
Agitation
Grief
Sensory Deprivation
Sex
Drug
Family

community; often times the consultant is called upon to clarify different assumptions and perceptions about the importance or salience of specific problem behaviors. The differences among the groups may also reflect their exposure to different parts of the nursing home community. For example, a larger percentage of the psychologists rated several problems with higher frequency than the other two groups. This may reflect their consulting experience, which has been focused on particularly problematic patients. Similarly, the aides' higher rating of agitation, when compared to the administrators', may reflect their greater time in contact with the residents.

In summary, three groups of key informants offer another indicator of significant mental health problems in nursing home settings. In addition, their consensus about the prominent role of depression, agitation, and disorientation offer some inidication of likely topics for mental health consultation. It should be emphasized that the key informants focused on behaviors, not psychiatric diagnoses. The importance of this distinction was touched on by Rovner et al. (1986), and will be considered more fully in chapters 6 and 7.

## IMPLICATIONS FOR CONSULTATION

This chapter has two purposes: to introducc basic information about the frequency of mental disorders and problem behaviors, and to help potential consultants think about the process of assessing the level of psychiatric problems in a particular setting. The strategies used with an individual setting parallel those used in establishing norms for the nursing home industry: epidemiological studies, structured professional assessments, and views of key informants in the setting.

To some extent, the particular strategies used to assess the level and type of problem behavior in a particular setting varies upon the characteristics of the setting. Swift and Cooper (1986) summarized the issue well: "The settings in which consultation occurs shape both consultation inputs—the participants and consultation focus—and consultation outcomes" (p. 347).

Consider, for example the following two settings.

---

Devon Manor is a nursing home (with both skilled and intermediate-care beds) attached to a continuing-care retirement community. As part of the community's planning data base, residents have an annual physical examination and complete periodic self-report questionnaires concerning self-care capacity, self-rated mental health, physical health, and social well-being, as well as reporting on physical and mental-health problems. These questionnaire responses are entered into a computerized data base, and are available to reflect changing resident functioning over time.

Centre Manor is also a facility that combines skilled and intermediate care. It is a "county home" with a sizable portion of its residents covered by Medicaid. Although it is a good facility, it relies mainly on chart notes and staffing meetings to identify particular patterns of change that raise concern.

---

Neither setting has a geriatric mental health specialist as a consultant. If called upon to provide mental health consultation to the setting, the consultant should have several sets of questions regarding patterns of adjustment within the nursing home.

1) What is the prevalence of specific types of disorders within the setting?
2) How does that pattern compare to national norms?
3) Are the patterns of adjustment different for recent vs. long-term patients?
4) Is there information available on individual residents' patterns of change over time? On changing patterns and levels of adjustment problems for the facility as a whole over time?
5) What are the views of the key stakeholders regarding the important psychiatric and behavioral problems in the setting?

To answer these questions and to begin to shape an initial treatment strategy, the consultant may want to consider the types of approaches outlined in this chapter. Although the chapter has emphasized epidemiological approaches and research instruments that may be too cumbersome for clinical settings, the underlying strategies may be adapted for nursing homes. For example, structured observational approaches (for example, the Nurse's Observational Scale for Inpatient Evaluation [NOSIE]) could be used by LPNs to document current levels of behavioral problems on specific nursing units and patterns of change following treatment.[13] Similarly, structured psychiatric consultation with targeted samples of patients could be used to assess levels of functioning prior to and following interventions. Finally, administrators' and staff members' views of priority areas for intervention could be assessed, along with their views of change after treatment.

In summary, these approaches can be used to assess the psychiatric and behavioral problems of groups of residents. Prior work suggests that there will be a need for case consultation around psychiatric and behavioral problems in the setting. The approaches outlined here focus on the setting as a whole. In the next chapter, we consider individually oriented assessment procedures.

## NOTES

1. Smith and Corse (1986) provide a helpful introduction to the process of consultation. They emphasize the importance of a variety of data-collection techniques, a theme we will return to later in the chapter. Thus, many of the consultation issues are salient for any institutional or organizational setting, not only nursing homes.

2. Glass (1986) and White (1987) provide informative perspectives on the changing field of epidemiology. Glass, in particular, places current efforts in a broad historical framework.

3. Davies (1985) provides a helpful overview of epidemiology and aging. Blazer (1980) and Kay and Bergmann (1980) discuss the purposes of geriatric epidemiology and they provide in-depth reviews of aging and mental disorders. La Rue and her colleagues (1985) also present a comprehensive review of mental disorders in later life.

4. All epidemiological studies require the identification of two groups of individuals to report morbidity: the population at risk (denominator) and the prevalence or incidence of the given disorder in absolute numbers of persons (numerator). Blazer (1980) and Kay and Bergmann (1980) describe methods for determining the numerator and denominator in epidemiological investigations.

5. The National Institute of Mental Health's Epidemiologic Catchment Area (ECA) program grew out of the 1978 President's Commission on Mental Health (PCMH). In 1978 the PCMH reported on the fields of epidemiology and health services research (President's Commission on Mental Health, 1978a). The PCMH requested that researchers from a variety of mental-health disciplines document the state of their fields and to recommend directions for future advancement. The results of these reports differed widely; the findings lacked uniformity and comparability on the prevalence of mental disorders (Regier et al., 1984). As a result, the PCMH emphasized the need for more precise epidemiological data on mental disorders, and utilization of mental health services by persons with these disorders (President's Commission on Mental Health, 1978b).

6. It is difficult to find a single classification scheme when reviewing studies completed during the last two decades. For example, some investigators use categories like "chronic brain syndrome" to include the diagnosis of senile dementia of the Alzheimer's type. Similarly, others use senility as a catch-all for a variety of types of dementia, including Alzheimer's disease, multi-infarct dementia (dementias related to cerebral-blood-flow complications), and dementias caused by a

mixture of factors. Butler and Lewis (1982) provide a useful discussion of these issues. They note that a major distinction is drawn between mental disorders that have an organic (i.e. physical) cause, and those that are functional in nature (i.e. no known physical cause). In addition, distinctions are drawn between delirium (confusional states caused by potentially reversible causes) and dementia (irreversible brain disorders).

7. Weissman et al. (1985) provide a useful discussion of the ECA project and the Yale-based data on community-dwelling elderly. The summary presented here is designed to alert the reader to the importance of community-based prevalence rates as a point of comparison for considering prevalence rates of institutionalized elderly.

8. We consider the important role of family members' social support in more detail in chapter 8.

9. Kahn (1975) emphasized the importance of distinguishing between two groups of older people with mental disorders: those who are mentally ill and grow old, and those who grow old and become mentally ill. The treatment prospects and approaches are different for each group. We return to these issues in chapters 5, 6, and 7.

10. For the details of the study, see Rovner et al., 1986.

11. For more details of the statewide survey of nursing homes, see Smyer et al., 1985.

12. For more details of the survey of psychologists active in long-term-care settings, see Gatz et al. (in press). For more information regarding the network of psychologists in long-term care, contact the network coordinator: Rita Gugel, Ph.D., P.O. Box 21846, Fort Lauderdale, Florida 33335 (305-763-5030).

13. See Honigfeld and Klett (1965) for a description of the NOSIE.

# 5

# Effective Assessment Approaches

*Michael A. Smyer and Adam J. Garfein*

You can observe a lot by just looking.

*Attributed to Yogi Berra*

## INTRODUCTION

The process of assessment is the starting point for treatment or intervention. Assessment approaches structure our observations, drawing our attention to certain aspects of an individual's behavior, of the environment, or of the family. In this chapter, we present an interdisciplinary perspective on assessment. Our discussion is divided into four major sections. We begin by considering the basic questions that structure assessment efforts with older adults. Next we focus on the participants in the assessment process. In the third section, we consider the most important domains to be assessed. We present information from a recent national survey of key informants who consult in nursing home settings. Finally, we consider problems of assessment in nursing home settings and we provide some suggested solutions.

## BASIC QUESTIONS OF ASSESSMENT

Zarit and his colleagues (1985) identified four core objectives of geriatric assessment: to determine a diagnosis, and find out whether the problems presented by a given individual meet designated criteria for inclusion in a diagnostic category; to assess the broad patterns of behaviors, thoughts, or emotions of the individual in order to provide more complete information about dimensions of current functioning than is encompassed by diagnosis; to evaluate specific variables that can assist in care planning, especially in deciding alternative forms of care; and to measure critical variables for the purpose of evaluating the outcomes of intervention. These suggestions are helpful, since they highlight the broad scope of assessment and its direct link to treatment and evaluation.

Several key questions structure the assessment task for health-care providers working with the elderly (see fig. 5.1).[1] Together, these inquiries embody a differential diagnostic approach to older adults and their problems, providing information to accomplish the objectives Zarit and his colleagues highlighted.

The most general, and in some ways the most difficult, question is often raised by the elderly themselves or by their relatives: Is the presenting problem part of normal aging processes? Is it a pathological pattern of adaptation? Or is it some combination of the two? For example, decline in several biological functions is a natural concomitant of aging in our society. Declining efficiency and effectiveness of heart, kidney, liver, and other major organs and systems have all been documented.[2] Despite this general pattern, however, variability between individuals and within an individual's own various biological systems may make the initial question a difficult one.

An indicator of the problem is the now-familiar story of the seventy-nine-year-old man who visited a doctor complaining of pains in his left leg. After some tests were completed, the physician told the patient that the leg pains were merely the result of the wear and tear of aging. The patient, not to be consoled with this diagnosis, promptly replied; "My right leg is also seventy-nine, why don't I have pains in it?"

In summary, the initial step of the assessment process focuses on differentiating "normal" aging from other patterns. It is important to recognize, however, that even with "normal" age-related changes in functioning, intervention may be essential in helping the older adult accept changes and achieve optimal levels of functioning.

The second phase of the assessment process focuses on the type of problem. Older adults and their families are often aware of the complex interaction of physical and psychological domains in later life.[3] For the assessment professional, the issue is often posed in terms of functional (psychological) bases of problems vs. organic (physical) bases. Not surprisingly, the either/or dichotomy misrepresents the interactive complexity that characterizes the relationships among the biological and psychological elements.[4]

If an organic element is suspected, the focus shifts to examine the expected course of the disorder. Particularly when considering a dementing illness, an important issue is the reversibility of the disorder.[5] With any organic involvement, however, a focus of concern will be the projected trajectory for the older adult's functioning.

The three questions, as outlined above, provide a framework for the specific questions that members of the nursing home community may raise

Fig. 5.1

Basic Questions for Individual Assessment

**Is the problem:**

- **Part of Normal Aging?**
- **An Abnormal Pattern of Adaptation?**
- **A Mixture of the Two?**

**If an abnormal pattern, is it:**

- **A Functional Problem?**
- **An Organic Problem?**
- **A Mixture of the Two?**

**If there is an organic involvement:**

- **Is it a Reversible Process?**
- **Is it an Irreversible Process?**
- **Is it a Mixture of the Two?**

about the functioning of a specific older person. Gatz and her colleagues highlight an additional issue: How severe or disruptive is the problem?[6] They point out the need to get a variety of perspectives on the problem—an issue we explore in the next section.

In summary, geriatric assessment can be thought of as a differential diagnostic process. The task is broader than placing the individual in a specific DSM-III diagnostic category, however. Instead, assessment must be linked to developing and evaluating specific treatment components and approaches. Geriatric assessment is most effective when it capitalizes upon the expertise of many members of the nursing home community. We turn to their contributions in the next section.

## WHO CAN CONTRIBUTE TO THE ASSESSMENT PROCESS?

The broad purposes of assessment sketched earlier suggest that many members of the nursing home community can and should be involved in the assessment process. Following our earlier conceptualization, we focus on the potential contributions of three distinct groups in the settings: residents, their family members, and staff members—both professional and paraprofessional.

The resident can provide an initial perspective on the current set of problems, a starting point for discussion. Several issues are particularly important when gauging the resident's contribution to the assessment process:

1) How reliable is the resident's judgment?
2) From the resident's perspective, is the current problem a recent development or does it represent a long-standing pattern of adaptation?[7]
3) From the resident's perspective, what are the underlying causes of the current problem?[8]
4) From the resident's perspective, what approaches have been helpful thus far? What approaches have been less than useful?[9]
5) From the resident's perspective, what is the most difficult aspect of the current problem?
6) From the resident's perspective, what is the likely outcome of the process?

These questions provide a starting point for assessing the resident's understanding of the underlying problem and expectations regarding treatment and outcomes.

Family members can also provide useful information on the same set of issues. Their perceptions can be useful in three ways: First, as a reliability check on the older adult's reports; second, as another source of information on the older adult's history of adaptation and coping with this sort of problem; and, third, as contributors of important perceptions or aspects that they find to be most problematic in the resident's current functioning.[10]

Finally, staff members can offer valuable information about current resident functioning and changes in the pattern of adaptation within the nursing home setting. The "front-line caregivers" can provide useful observational data on the antecedents, behaviors, and consequences of resident functioning. They can often supplement more formal assessment protocols with behavioral observations before, during, and after treatment attempts.[11]

Professional staff draw upon their expertise and training to provide information in well-structured ways regarding specific domains of resident functioning. For example, nurses can provide information about the effects of differing medication regimens, different treatment techniques, and various physiological states. Other professionals (for example, psychologists, physicians, and so on) add information gathered using various special techniques and protocols.

Assessment should be viewed as a process, not a single occurrence. Assessment procedures should capitalize upon the experience and expertise of the full range of nursing home community members. Their diverse perspectives can help place current resident functioning in the proper perspective. The mental-health consultant can aide in this process in several ways: assuring that input from the various community members is represented in the process; coordinating the range of information; and facilitating the process of discussion and reflection necessary to arrive at a comprehensive view of the patient, the problem, and potential intervention approaches. In the rest of this chapter, we focus on specific domains and methods for gathering the information needed to conduct an effective assessment.

## WHAT SHOULD BE THE DOMAINS AND TECHNIQUES OF ASSESSMENT?

The mental health consultant interested in obtaining comprehensive information on individual resident functioning must determine both the important factors to measure and the specific measurement technology to use.[12] Unfortunately, there is no consensus on either of these topics among practitioners (Institute of Medicine, 1986; Kane and Kane, 1981). In this section, we present a perspective on the most salient domains and most effective approaches.

## DETERMINING DOMAINS TO ASSESS

The specific domains of assessment depend upon the purposes of assessment. There are three major purposes of assessment in the long-term care context: to examine the resident's need for institutionalization; to evaluate the underlying cause of a specific functional problem (for example, disorientation); to estimate the effects of interventions or changes in resident functioning over time.

For example, Gurland (1980) suggests that deterioration in three areas leads to a need for mental-health services and, eventually, to institutionalization: a medical disorder concomitant with psychological difficulties, incapacity in self-care abilities, and lack of an effective social-support system. The salience of these areas is clear in the following case example provided by Rabins and Mace (1986).

---

> Mrs B. was a 68-year-old woman who had been independent all her adult life. For several years her memory had been deteriorating and she was significantly forgetful. She had stopped driving and therefore had no way to shop. Her children had been shopping for her or taking her shopping but her daughter was returning to work and this would no longer be possible. Her family now felt she was unable to live alone any longer. A medical evaluation demonstrated that her health was good and revealed no treatable cause of her thinking impairment. A cognitive assessment found impaired memory and loss of abilities to carry out complex tasks. The family felt that nursing home placement might be best. This was a source of great distress to the patient and she refused to move (p. 507).

---

Gurland's three areas are focal points of discussion in the process of seeking institutionalization, but of course are not the only determinants of care choices.

Similarly, assessment information can be of central importance in developing and monitoring the effects of interventions. The Institute of Medicine's Committee on Nursing Home Regulation stressed the link between adequate assessment procedures and the quality of care provided in nursing homes. It noted that provision of quality care "requires careful assessment of each resident's functional, medical, mental, and psychosocial status upon admission, and reassessment periodically thereafter, with the changes in status noted." (Institute of Medicine, 1986, p. 74)

The institute's discussion reminds us of the importance of comprehensive assessment approaches. Pfeiffer (1975) for example, suggests that more than 80 percent of an individual's functioning could be evaluated by assessing five areas: social resources, economic resources, physical health, mental health, and activities of daily living. Pfeiffer developed a comprehensive assessment instrument, the Older Adults Resources and Services (OARS) multidimensional-functional-assessment questionnaire, around these domains (Fillenbaum and Smyer, 1981). The OARS measure has subsequently been used to provide community-based estimates of service use and effectiveness (for example, USGAO, 1977), evaluations of the comparative effects of different service arrays for impaired elderly (for example, Smyer, 1980), as well as individual-case assessments for initial and subsequent treatment evaluations.

The OARS serves as a useful reminder that several substantive domains and specific measures can be used for all three purposes of assessment in the nursing-home setting: evaluating the need for institutionalization, assessing specific problem areas, and monitoring patient change.

This discussion provides a context for considering the specific domains of assessment. The list below summarizes some of the more common domains of geriatric assessment.[13] It is intended to be illustrative of the range of issues typically covered in geriatric assessment.[14]

*Domains of Geriatric Assessment*

Sociodemographic information
- Age, sex, education, income, marital and family status, religious affiliation, etc.

Cognitive functioning
- Mental status, neuropsychological testing, intelligence testing, memory assessment

Functional ability
- Activities of daily living, instrumental activities of daily living

Nonorganic psychopathology
- Anxiety disorders
- Schizophrenia or paranoid disorders

Affective status
- Depression

Personality

Economic functioning/resources

Social functioning/resources

Behavioral problems
- Disruptive, dangerous, or otherwise problematic behaviors

General mental health

Medical status
    Medical evaluation
    Pharmacological evaluation
Nutritional status
Subjective well-being
    Life satisfaction
Stress or significant life events
Person-environment fit
Productive behaviors

In summary, although the particular assessment questions vary according to the specific questions asked, who is asking them, and the environmental setting they are relevant to, there is some degree of similarity among all approaches. They tend to overlap in areas such as the measurement of functional and cognitive impairment. They represent multidimensional approaches tapping a variety of areas simultaneously to provide the practitioner with vital treatment, rehabilitative, or therapeutic-outcome information.

## DETERMINING APPROPRIATE ASSESSMENT INSTRUMENTS

Once the mental health professional has determined the most appropriate domains to pursue, the next step is to select the corresponding instruments or measurement strategies. One approach to discovering specific assessment instruments that can be used in institutional settings is to turn to key informants in the field: licensed psychologists practicing in long-term-care settings. Gatz and her colleagues (in press) recently surveyed twenty-three psychologists from seventeen states and Canada. The respondents were members of a recently formed network of psychologists active in long-term-care consultation.[15] These practitioners are seasoned professionals, with an average of 7.8 years' consultation experience in long-term-care settings.

In reference to their consultation experiences and familiarity with specific assessment instruments, the licensed psychologists were asked a two-part question: What assessment instruments should be included in a standard "kit" for use by (1) psychologists (for example, themselves) and (2) nonpsychologists (for example, nursing home staff) in all nursing homes?

Their responses were grouped into four assessment categories: cognitive functioning and mental status; personality, psychopathology, and affective status; physical functioning and self-care capacity; and behavioral observations.

## ASSESSMENT INSTRUMENTS FOR PSYCHOLOGISTS

Table 5.1 shows the instruments specifically recommended for use by psychologists. Instruments reported only once were categorized as "other." Thus, the instruments reported by name had to have been mentioned by at least two respondents. References to original sources and research establishing norms for older adults are included in the table.

TABLE 5.1: Essential Assessment Approaches for Psychologists

| ASSESSMENT DOMAINS | | | | | | | |
|---|---|---|---|---|---|---|---|
| *Cognitive Functioning/ Mental Status* | | *Personality and Psychopathology Affective Status* | | *Physical Functioning/ Self-Care Capacity* | | *Behavioral Observations* | |
| Mattis | 3 | GDS | 2 | | | History | 5 |
| MMSE | 2 | BDI | 2 | | | other | 2 |
| Other mental status | 8 | Other depression screening | 1 | | | | |
| WAIS or sub-tests | 6 | MMPI | 3 | | | | |
| | | Rorschach | 3 | | | | |
| WMS | 5 | TAT/SAT | 3 | | | | |
| Bender-Gestalt | 4 | Other personality tests | 1 | | | | |
| Luria-Nebraska | 3 | | | | | | |
| Trail Making | 2 | | | | | | |
| Other neuro-psychological tests | 11 | | | | | | |
| Total tests nominated | 44 | | 15 | | 0 | | 7 |

Note:
Mattis: Mattis Dementia Rating Scale (Mattis, 1976)
MMSE: Mini-Mental State Exam (Folstein et al., 1975)
WAIS: Wechsler Adult Intelligence Scale (Savage and Britton, 1968; Wechsler, 1955)
WMS: Wechsler Memory Scale (Margolis and Scialfa, 1984; Wechsler, 1945)
Luria-Nebraska: Luria Nebraska Neuropsychological Battery (Golden, 1981)
GDS: Geriatric Depression Scale (Yesavage et al., 1983)
BDI: Beck Depression Inventory (Beck et al., 1961)
MMPI: Minnesota Multiphasic Personality Inventory (Hathaway and McKinley, 1951; Pearson, Swenson, and Rome, 1965; Colligan et al., 1984)
Rorschach: Rorschach Test (Rorschach, 1942; Reichlin, 1984)
TAT/SAT: Thematic Apperception Test/Senior Apperception Test (Murray, 1943; Bellak and Bellak, 1973)
Source: Adapted from Gatz et al. (in press). Baltimore, Md.: Williams & Wilkins. Reprinted by permission.

The assessment instruments recommended for use by trained mental health professionals focused heavily upon cognitive functioning, including mental status screening, neuropsychological evaluation, and traditional intelligence testing. In the personality, psychopathology, and affective-status domain, the key informants recommended depression screening, and standard objective and projective personality instruments. There were practically no suggestions for assessing physical functioning and self-care capacity.

Importantly, several of the psychologists indicated difficulty in recommending a standard kit. Six respondents did not suggest a standard battery since they felt that a standard procedure would not be appropriate for all residents.

## ASSESSMENT INSTRUMENTS FOR NONPSYCHOLOGISTS

Since the majority of direct services for the elderly in nursing homes is provided by staff members who are not psychologists, the survey respondents were asked which structured assessment instruments were most appropriate for the staff. Table 5.2 summarizes their suggestions. Three declined to suggest a standard kit.

There was wide agreement that nonpsychologists could use some type of mental-status-screening instrument. Although there were fewer responses, a self-report depression-screening instrument was recommended. The key informants saw a viable role for staff in collecting activities of daily living (ADL) and related data, even though they did not suggest similar measures for use by themselves. In the behavioral domain, many of the psychologists recommended a systematic approach using a behavioral check list.

In summary, the key informants emphasized cognitive measures that could be used by either personnel group. This probably reflects the predominance of cognitive difficulties among nursing-home residents. In the personality, psychopathology, and affective-status arena, psychologists viewed themselves as screening for depression and administering more complex personality batteries or other related methods. Nursing home staff were seen as capable of contributing to the process of screening for depression.

The absence of any functional or self-care capacity measures for mental-health professionals may reflect two elements. First, since many of these measures require ratings by key staff who experience frequent contact with patients, the psychologists may have felt unable to provide these ratings. Second, ADL measures are relatively straightforward and consequently staff can be taught to collect such information accurately and reliably. The latter situation also touches on another important finding from the survey: The licensed psychologists saw a viable role for properly trained mental health paraprofessional assessment "technicians" in the long-term-care setting.

## PROBLEMS OF ASSESSMENT IN THE LONG-TERM-CARE SETTING

Three sets of problems confront the mental health consultant trying to establish a quality program of assessment in nursing homes: difficulties arising from characteristics of impaired elderly; problems arising from the nature of currently available assessment approaches; and, finally, constraints imposed by the nature of the setting and its larger external contexts. We will consider each of these areas briefly.

TABLE 5.2: Essential Assessment Approaches for Nonpsychologists

| ASSESSMENT DOMAINS | | | | | | | |
|---|---|---|---|---|---|---|---|
| *Cognitive Functioning/ Mental Status* | | *Personality and Psychopathology Affective Status* | | *Physical Functioning/ Self-Care Capacity* | | *Behavioral Observations* | |
| MMSE | 7 | GDS | 5 | ADL | 8 | BPRS | 3 |
| MSQ | 3 | Other | | | | Other | 10 |
| SPMSQ | 2 | depression | | | | | |
| Other mental | | screening | 2 | | | | |
| status | 8 | Life | | | | | |
| | | satisfaction | 1 | | | | |
| Total nominations | 20 | | 8 | | 8 | | 13 |

Note:
MMSE: Mini-Mental State Exam (Folstein et al., 1975)
MSQ: Mental Status Questionnaire (Kahn et al., 1960)
SPMSQ: Short Portable Mental Status Questionnaire (Pfeiffer, 1975)
GDS: Geriatric Depression Scale (Yesavage et al., 1983)
ADL: Activities of Daily Living Scale (e.g., Katz et al., 1963)
BPRS: Brief Psychiatric Rating Scale (Overall and Gorham, 1962)
Source: Adapted from Gatz et al. (in press). Baltimore, Md.: Williams & Wilkins. Reprinted by permission.

***Characteristics of Impaired Elderly.*** The variability of cognitive functioning among institutionalized elderly poses a challenge for accurate assessment. Well-functioning or cognitively intact elderly residents may be overly cautious (Pfeiffer, 1980; Schaie and Stone, 1982). If older adults are, indeed, overly cautious, the mental-health professional must be aware of the likelihood that important aspects of their behavior or difficulties may be omitted from responses. Thus, the professional who rushes through assessment procedures, particularly when they are unstructured, risks losing key insights into patient status.

Mentally impaired elderly also pose a challenge. Disoriented or cognitively impaired older adults are likely to take longer to adjust to new challenges or demands placed upon them (for example, the assessment) (Miller, 1980). In addition, cognitive impairment may undermine the patient's reliability and credibility. For instance, most if not all self-reported data are questionable, since the cognitively impaired patient is often unable to recall information accurately (Zarit and Anthony, 1985).

In addition to cognitive impairment, some residents experience difficulty in communication due to impaired hearing or vision or other handicaps or illness (Gurland, 1980; Miller, 1980; Schaie and Stone, 1982). Before beginning the assessment, the mental health practitioner must ensure, for instance, than any sight or hearing loss is corrected or at least remediated to some minimal level of acuity. Providing large-print text or pictures, or thicker, more "tactile" paper are examples of specific techniques that facilitate the assessment of older individuals with sensory loss.

***Characteristics of Measurement Approaches.*** Apart from the characteristics of older adults themselves, the nature of the measurement approaches used with impaired elderly also pose challenges to accurate assessment. Three issues will be highlighted here: the lack of adequate norms for most standardized assessment measures used with the elderly; the inability of most measures to be sufficiently sensitive to change in patient functioning over time; and the difficulty of finding measures that adequately reflect both individual- and group-level functioning.

Many assessment instruments were not developed specifically for use with older clients. Most procedures have been developed in a non-developmental-psychopathology-oriented context (for example, MMPI or the Rorschach) or were based on younger populations such as children or young adults (for example, Wechsler, Army alpha, PMA intelligence tests, Cattel's 16 PF, or the Guilford-Zimmerman) (Schaie and Schaie, 1977; Schaie and Stone, 1982). Therefore, their construct validity may differ significantly between age groups. For example, measures that might have been appropriate or valid with young adults or children may not tap the same experiences or have the same meaning in an older population. Therefore, the mental health consultant must exercise caution when selecting instruments for use with older adults, and when possible, select cohort-appropriate measures with norms for older adults.

When standardized norms are used as a reference for interpreting where an individual falls on a cohort-specific measure, the norms must reflect up-to-date cohort levels (Schaie and Stone, 1982). The implicit assumption is that the individual is measured or diagnosed in reference to normative society-wide levels of functioning. What may have been considered normative or appropriate in earlier historical time periods may now be considered unhealthy or nonnormative; the opposite may also be true. The argument is that age-adjusted norms are inappropriate since they are usually based on cross-sectional data, which risks confounding actual indivdual development with intergenerational differences.[16]

Lezak (1987) recently reviewed the availability of age norms for the ten most commonly used psychological-assessment approaches. Her summary reflects the current state of the field: "Despite decades of awareness of the need for age norms for psychological tests, of the tests in most common use today, few have adequate age norms if any" (p. 12). Unfortunately, even in the desirable instance where standardized cohort-specific norms are available, the assessment consultant must then determine if the norms were derived specifically for application in the institutional setting.

A second problem with many of the assessment strategies available is their implicit and explicit assumption of stability of functioning.[17] If a major purpose of assessment is to reflect differing patterns of change subsequent to intervention, then the measurement approaches must be suitable for repeated measurements. Multiple versions of the measures and information on test-retest reliability are essential, in addition to appropriate age-norms (see Lubin and Rinck, 1986). Again, such information is generally not available for the most frequently used assessment measures.

A third difficulty arises because of the need to use assessment approaches both to identify individual's problems and to characterize the functioning of groups of older adults. Kane and Kane (1981) point out the desirable qualities of group and individual measures. Table 5.3 shows attributes of each approach and brings to light some of their trade-offs. Both approaches require reliable and valid measures. In terms of their differences, individual measures focus on identifying modifiable problems (for example, those able to benefit from treatment) and detecting small but important changes relevant to evaluating treatment outcomes. On the other hand, group procedures emphasize the importance of interrater reliability and the identification of instruments that can provide aggregate data on the target groups of people.

In choosing an assessment strategy, the consultant and staff must focus on the purpose of the assessment, the resources (both staff and time) available for the assessment, and the potential audience for the results. As table 5.3 indicates, there are differing requirements depending upon the focus of the assessment (for example, individual-oriented behavioral monitoring; group data collection using paraprofessional staff; and so on).

***Characteristics of the Setting and Its Contexts.*** Three characteristics of the nursing home and its larger, external environment place constraints on the types of assessment approaches used in nursing homes: lack of adequately trained professional staff; the implicit model of staff functioning often endorsed in the setting; and the absence of payment mechanisms to cover the costs of assessment.

Perhaps the most immediate problem is the lack of trained personnel with expertise in geriatric assessment. The small number of licensed psychologists listed in the Psychologists in Long Term Care Network Directory is one indicator of the dearth. Storandt (1977) put the problem in perspective when she reported the findings of a survey of psychologists.

TABLE 5.3: Attributes Desired in Individual and Group Measures in Long-Term Care

| *Individual* | *Group* |
|---|---|
| Reliability | Reliability |
| Across raters | Across raters |
| Over time | Over time |
| Validity | Validity |
| Minimizing false negatives | Capability of producing useful broad categories of functional ability across whole spectrum of performance |
| Minimizing false positives | Minimizing time and costs of administration |
| Capability of documenting problems amenable to intervention | Minimizing cost of analysis |
| Capability of documenting conditions requiring a service strategy | Portability; minimizing equipment required |
| Capability of documenting small changes in functioning | Reproducibility across geographical and cultural lines |
| Defensible strategy for sampling behaviors measured | Minimizing dependence on professional judgment or implicit criteria |
| | Defensible strategy for sampling from the population |

Source: Adapted from Kane and Kane (1981, p. 6).

At that time, she identified fewer than one hundred clinical psychologists in the entire country who had been trained in one way or another to work with older persons! The impact on practitioners is clear. Santos and VandenBos (1982) reported on a survey by the American Psychological Association that found that only 0.4 percent of psychological practitioners reported spending the majority of their clinical time working with older patients. They estimated that 2.7 percent of all health services delivered by psychologists were provided to the aged. Since psychologists have traditionally played a major role in the development and implementation of assessment procedures, their lack of contact with older adults has a direct effect on the quality of assessment procedures in long-term-care settings.

The model for geriatric care adopted in the majority of nursing homes (that is, the medical model) also contributes to current and future mental health manpower difficulties. As discussed in chapter 3, the medical model approach to long-term care may be inappropriate as the predominant basis for care. Briefly, this model emphasizes "acute rather than chronic care, diagnostic and treatment services rather than social and rehabilitative services, disease rather than health, and medical professionals rather than other health professionals" (Lindeman, 1986).[18]

We need to rethink and if necessary alter or completely replace this model as a basis for care in order to shift both the way care is provided to the elderly and who will provide what types of services. For example, a "conditional" medical model may serve well as a basis for geriatric care in the long-term-care setting. That is, if there is reason to suspect illness or disease, then this approach is warranted. However, in the absence of any presenting problems, some other model for geriatric care may be more appropriate. For example, mental illness case identification might shift from the physician to an assessment "technician," such as a specially trained nurse. Multidisciplinary collaboration in the identification of pathology and subsequent intervention aimed at "curing," remediating, or coping with the problem is congruent with the view of the nursing home as a caring community (see chapters 1 and 3 for a discussion of differing models underlying mental health consultation in nursing homes).

Determining who will oversee the collection of relevant resident information and manage its storage for immediate and future evaluation is a related personnel problem. Regardless of which qualified mental-health professional interprets the data to ascertain the patient's mental health, someone must ultimately bear responsibility for the routine assessment of the entire nursing home population. Recently, it has been suggested that every certified facility employ an appropriately trained certified nurse with the responsibility of assuring that each resident is assessed upon admission and thereafter (Institute of Medicine, 1986). Although the issue of which personnel should fill this void may be debated, there is growing agreement that such standardized and routine collection of data ought to be a part of the nursing home process.

Another barrier to mental health assessment and treatment services in long-term-care settings is related to third-party-reimbursement policies. Medicare and Medicaid are logical funding sources for such services. However, each system provides reimbursement only with considerable restrictions (Blumenthal et al., 1986). Medicaid coverage is less uniform than Medicare coverage, with approximately twenty-two state Medicaid programs recognizing and directly reimbursing independently practicing psychologists for their services. Even among these states, however, there is variation in which services are covered.[19]

Thus, whether or not mental health services are used by the elderly is largely left up to the resident's, family's, or facility's willingness and capability to pay for such services. As a consequence, standardized comprehensive assessments are the exception rather than the rule, and they are more likely to be conducted as a measure of last resort than on a proactive basis (for example, on admission and periodically thereafter whether or not there are any presenting problems).

## FUTURE DIRECTIONS AND RECOMMENDATIONS

Despite the need for improvement in the content and context of assessment in nursing homes, Gatz and her colleagues (Gatz et al., in press) provide a brief set of recommendations for a standardized set of assessment measures. Their suggestions offer a good starting point for the consultant seeking advice on substantive and procedural approaches for assessment in nursing homes.

They stress several of this chapter's themes in making their recommendations: first, there is no clear consensus on a small number of specific measures that should be used in the assessment task; second, there is greater consensus on the content domains that should be represented; finally, there is general agreement that both professional and nonprofessional expertise should be tapped in the assessment process. Table 5.4 summarizes their recommendations.

TABLE 5.4: Recommended Assessment Domains and Measures

| *Domain* | *Measures for Professional Use* | *Measures for Nonprofessional Use* |
|---|---|---|
| Screening Tests | Folstein MMSE | Orientation/memory/ concentration test |
| Differential diagnosis | MSQ<br>Face-Hand Test[a] | |
| Cognitive functioning | WAIS-R subtests<br>WMS subtests | |
| Affective domain | Self-report items<br>GDS, BDI, or CES-D[b]<br>MMPI-a68[c] | Behavioral checklist<br>Behavioral assessment[d] |
| Activities of daily living | Katz et al., 1963 | |
| Behavioral observation | Detailed History | |

[a]See Zarit, Orr, and Zarit, 1985.
[b]See Radloff and Teri, 1986.
[c]See Overall and Gomez-Mont, 1974.
[d]See Hussian, 1986.
Source: Gatz et al. (in press). Baltimore, Md.: Williams & Wilkins. Reprinted by permission.

## NOTES

1. This chapter provides a framework for assessment. Several reviews of the area provide more detailed discussions of specific measurement approaches or specific domains. See, for example, on the topic of clinical gerontological assessment Brink (1986), Edinberg (1985), Gallagher, Thompson, and Levy (1980), Gurland (1980), Knight (1986), Lawton and Storandt (1984), Schaie and Schaie (1977), Schaie and Stone (1982), Zarit (1980), and Zarit, Eiler, and Hassinger (1985). For consideration of assessment of senile dementia, see Gurland (1980), Kahn and Miller (1978), and Miller (1980). For a treatment of neuropsychological assessment, see Albert (1981). For suggestions on cognitive and memory assessment, see Miller (1980) and Poon (1986). In the area of personality assessment, consult Lawton, Whelihan, and Belsky (1980). Finally, in terms of psychopharmacological assessment, Crook, Ferris, and Bartus (1983), are particularly helpful.

2. See Finch and Schneider (1985) for a recent summary of information on the "normal" aging patterns of major systems.

3. Butler and Lewis (1982) provide a useful overview of the interaction of physical and psychological functioning among the elderly.

4. For a useful discussion of the functional disorders of older adults, see Pfeiffer (1968). Busse and Blazer (1980) provide a helpful discussion of the interaction of biological and psychological processes, as does Verwoerdt (1981).

5. See Gilhooly, Zarit, and Birren (1986) and Zarit, Orr, and Zarit (1985) for a fuller discussion of the dementias and their diagnosis and treatment. Cohen (1987) provides a useful overview of the nature of the dementias and their treatment, focusing particular attention on the shift from "cure" to "care" when a progressive

dementia occurs. Cummings and Benson (1983) offer a helpful discussion of the etiology and assessment of dementia.

6. See Gatz et al. (in press) for a discussion of approaches to assessment in nursing homes, with particular attention given to psychological measures.

7. Kahn's (1975) differentiation between early-onset and late-onset mental health problems has important implications for both assessment and intervention approaches. We return to these issues in chapter 6.

8. Schulz (1980) focuses on the role of individual's attributions and self-perceptions in shaping their adaptation to aging. Seligman's work (e.g., Seligman, 1975; Seligman and Elder, 1986) has also been very influential in exploring the role of individuals' perceptions in shaping their adaptation.

9. Danish, D'Augelli, and Hauer (1979) have suggested that individuals often learn from previous coping attempts. They argue that successful coping is optimized when clients are encouraged to see the parallels between earlier successfully met challenges and current problem situations.

10. In chapters 8 and 9, we discuss the family's role in current functioning in more detail. Here, we want to emphasize that family members can also play a central role in assessment focused on the individual patient.

11. Later in the chapter, we offer specific suggestions for approaches to structure the staff's input. Several structured observational scales can be helpful: The Brief Psychiatric Rating Scale (Overall and Gorham, 1962); the Nurse's Observation Scale for Inpatient Evaluation (Honigfeld and Klett, 1965); the MOSES (Helmes, Csapo, and Short, 1987); and the London Psychogeriatric Rating Scale (Hersch et al., 1978).

12. Kane and Kane (1981) provide an extensive review of comprehensive assessment approaches. Williams (1983) also provides a helpful review of the issues involved in comprehensive assessment.

13. Each of the domains listed has been dealt with in detail elsewhere. For a discussion of the general approaches to geriatric assessment, the reader is referred to Zarit, Eiler, and Hassinger (1985).

14. Again, Kane and Kane (1981) and Brink (1986) provide helpful in-depth treatments of specific assessment domains and measures.

15. For information of the Psychologists in Long Term Care Network, contact Dr. Rita Gugel, P.O. Box 21846, Fort Lauderdale, Florida 33335 (305-763-5030).

16. Schaie (1984) provides a helpful discussion of cohort effects and historical time. His comments are particularly relevant for clinicians working with older patients from different cultural or historical periods than his or her own. Knight (1986) also urges caution in acknowledging the effects of cultural and cohort-specific influences.

17. Nesselroade and Ford (1985) discuss strategies for constructing research designs more appropriate for assessing change in individual functioning. Their rationale and their suggested approach may have clinical utility as well.

18. Lindeman (1986) presents an overview of manpower requirements in nursing homes under the medical model and under alternative-care-model assumptions.

19. Jazwiecki and Press (1986) discuss current federal reimbursement policies for the long-term care of the mentally ill and delineate several areas for future cost-of-care research.

# 6

# Individual Interventions for Nursing Home Residents

*Catherine Selth Spayd and Michael A. Smyer*

Probably the most ubiquitous myth in geriatric mental health is that elders cannot be treated effectively with psychotherapy.

*T. L. Brink*

## INTRODUCTION

A sixty-five–year–old, sophisticated resident who was admitted to the nursing home following a hip fracture, Anna May requested therapy due to "difficulties interacting with her daughter." It soon became clear that these difficulties surrounded the daughter's outspoken belief that her mother was "becoming senile." While Anna May did not fully accept her daughter's description, she did have some doubts, stemming from "memory problems" that she was initially reluctant to acknowledge.

Once these doubts surfaced in a therapy session, they were discussed and then clinically assessed by the therapist. An explanation to the resident that her minor memory difficulties were benign, representing a normal aging process and not of clinical significance, served to lessen her worries. She was thus able to gain a new and more helpful perspective on her daughter's attitude, and on the relationship with her daughter in general.

Anna May's case serves as a caution for the therapist working with elderly residents, and elderly people in general: Be attuned to possible developmental changes in clients, openly address and assess them, and, if necessary, alter therapy to compensate for them.[1]

This chapter is designed to give direct-service providers an overview of fundamental principles in effective mental health intervention with elderly nursing home residents.[2] We begin with a survey of factors to be considered in selecting a psychological intervention: in general, with the elderly and specifically with nursing home residents. An overview of common intervention types, with particular consideration of their efficacy with elderly nursing home residents, will conclude the chapter.[3] This chapter serves as both a "refresher" for the psychological consultant and as an introduction to chapter 7, which reviews specific interventions for the disorders of agitation, disorientation, and depression. This chapter also serves as a basic introduction for those who are unfamiliar with individually-oriented mental health interventions.

## SPECIAL CONSIDERATIONS IN GERIATRIC MENTAL HEALTH INTERVENTION

There are a number of specific considerations in evaluating mental health services for elderly clients, and for nursing home residents in particular, which can be noted in table 6.1. Several obstacles to providing quality therapy to geriatric clients have been identified by Knight (1986). The first of these barriers is the questionable attitude, held by a significant proportion of mental health professionals, that the elderly population is not amenable to psychological or behavioral change. Many therapists avoid contact with elderly clients, or work less effectively with them, due simply to inexperience in working with this population, and, as a result, anxiety regarding their treatment.

TABLE 6.1: Common Obstacles in Geriatric Mental Health Treatment and Ways to Overcome Them

| *Obstacle* | *Compensation* |
|---|---|
| 1. Therapist's belief that elderly clients are not amenable to psychological change | 1. Advocating elderly clients' rights to treatment; reeducation of therapist regarding many elderly clients' appropriateness for treatment |
| 2. Normal possible developmental changes of old age (e.g., slowed cognitive processing, benign memory loss, sensory impairments) | 2. Mutual acknowledgement and therapist assessment of such changes or impairments; discussion of the impact of impairments |
| 3. Client's values differ from the therapist's, resulting from differing cohorts | 3. Mutual and nonjudgmental awareness and acceptance of differing values; open communication |
| 4. Client's lack of familiarity with or trust of psychological services; feeling ashamed to be a client | 4. Client education; discussion of client's feelings |
| 5. Therapist's lack of awareness of the "elderly sub-culture" | 5. Therapist's awareness and assessment of differing life-styles; open communication |

Based on Knight (1986).

Another obstacle involves possible developmental changes in old age, most commonly observed as slowed cognitive-processing time, clinical levels of memory loss, and/or the increasing, debilitating influence of physical impairments.

A third potential barrier to mental health intervention with older people is differential cohort effects between the (presumably) younger therapist and the older client. Older individuals obviously have grown up in a different physical and cultural world than their therapists, with different historical experiences and social values. Knight (1986) lists four common areas of cohort differences: moral values, religious orientations, attitudes toward the family, and the greater tendency of older cohorts to express psychological problems by describing them in terms of physical ailments.

We recognize two additional important cohort differences: the present-day elderly cohort's unfamiliarity with psychological treatment, and its view that psychological treatment is an unnecessary expense in a typically tight budget. Zarit (1980) notes that this group generally views mental health intervention as something to be reserved for serious psychological disturbances, and as slightly shameful. If the therapist and/or client assume that values and attitudes regarding these topics are shared, blocks to effective communication are likely.

A fourth possible barrier to effective mental health service provision with the elderly is the existence of basic differences in life-styles between the client and the therapist, what Knight (1986) refers to as "the elderly subculture." With advancing age, a client is increasingly likely to encounter the experiences of retirement, widowhood, health probelms, financial problems, and ageism—the most common among many such concerns. Further, these losses are more often irreversible for an older person, who cannot, for example, as easily replace a lost job or spouse as a younger client can.

The therapist's lack of knowledge or awareness of these concerns can lead to difficulties relating to them as potential therapy issues. Especially if the client also is not consciously aware of the problems or their impact upon his functioning, their influence on his psychological well-being will not be addressed. The importance of understanding the elderly client's social context in therapy thus cannot be underestimated, and is particularly relevant when he resides in a nursing home. Therapists are well served by visiting or observing the client in this environment, and discussing with him its day-to-day functioning, to gain insights into the influences of its physical and social structures.

In spite of this rather gloomy outlook of the prospects of successful psychological intervention with elderly clients, there is good reason to consider offering such treatment. Brink (1979) cites evidence that an elderly person is less likely to experience a "spontaneous" recovery (one without any formal intervention) than is a younger client. He attributes this circumstance to the greater permanence of experienced losses, such as environmental, financial, physical, and social resources. Thus, the case for mental health intervention with an elderly client is strengthened.

Brink (1979) also notes that elderly clients are often more responsible in their commitments to therapy than are younger clients. He therefore estimates that psychotherapy is often *more* effective with elderly clients than younger ones, in opposition to generally held beliefs.

Goodstein (1982) and Knight (1986) note that the elderly client has another advantage over his younger counterpart: he has a greater, richer psychological history from which to draw examples and possible insights. Further, the elderly exhibit an increased tendency to be introspective, very often recognized as a therapeutic benefit. The nursing home resident's treatment team can use this information in its capacity as an advocate for the resident, to promote him as an appropriate therapy candidate to a reluctant professional.

Additionally, the astute therapist must be aware of, and directly address with the client, these potential obstacles to therapy. As noted in the chapter's introductory case study, possible developmental changes can be assessed and therapy modified to address them. In the same light, recognizing the influences of differing values as possible barriers to therapy, and addressing them with the client, can effectively overcome this potential communication problem.

In evaluating possible mental health interventions for nursing home residents, additional considerations may be noted. Knight (1986) suggests that problems of behavior that are disturbing for the resident himself must be differentiated from those that are more, or exclusively, troublesome to staff or other residents. The nursing home environment itself, and the expectation that the residents will be able to live and work together, make this issue an important one to consider. Training staff to take a broad, environmental perspective to behavioral problems is imperative. A more broadly based perspective will help avoid unnecessary interventions. See the case of Faye for an example.

---

Faye was a cognitively impaired resident who frequently approached the nursing station and sifted through the medical records and other nurses' papers. Despite the nurses' attempts to monitor the desk and repeatedly tell Faye she was not allowed behind it, the problem became quite a serious one when some doctor's orders were discovered missing. In initially trying to resolve the problem, staff considered limiting Faye's mobility by placing her in a Geri-chair.

Taking a broader perspective, however, encouraged the treatment team to ask whether Faye was disturbed by her behavior, or whether it was only the nurses who found it so frustrating. Once the team determined that it was more of an environmental concern than one for Faye, other avenues of intervention became apparent. Staff first tried, then rejected as impractical, an idea to better observe and guard the nursing station. They then settled on the successful intervention of providing Faye with her own set of papers at a small desk: she received positive reinforcement in the form of praise when she sat at this desk, and was verbally redirected to it when she approached the nursing station.

---

Another important issue for the nursing home mental health consultant is the medical orientation inherent in the facility. The people most likely to be identified as the endorsers or mediators of psychological treatments provided are the medically trained physicians and nursing staff. Indeed, the attending physician has the ultimate responsibility for such interventions, in writing the doctor's orders for them. Within such a medical orientation, psychological concerns are often relegated to a secondary status behind physical concerns (Hussian, 1981).[4] This lack of recognition of the significant impact of mental health disturbance upon physical functioning exists despite the fact that the emotional or behavioral problems may be the etiology of the physical concern, exacerbate it, or prevent the resident from concentrating energies upon addressing it.

An interdisciplinary-team effort helps to counteract such possible conflicting philosophies of medical and psychological personnel, and to establish cooperative relationships for the efficient provision of mental health services. Hussian proposes the following measures be taken by both professions: establish "mutual respect" by making mutual referrals; yield to each other's areas of expertise; become familiar with each other's language; and (politely) educate each other regarding each one's own areas of knowledge.

An additional suggestion is to be sure to acknowledge to the nursing staff the invaluable ongoing services that they provide to the resident. In doing so, the consultant emphasizes that the staff's day-to-day interactions with, and care for, the resident provide them with important insights into his functioning that must be taken into consideration in mental health planning.

Another issue pertinent to evaluating appropriate interventions with nursing home mental health clients is the impact of institutionalization itself. This process, a kind of "institutionalization syndrome," is defined by Whanger (1980) as the result of the nursing home's likely-rigid routines, the resident's loss of responsibility for decisions regarding personal care, his lack of privacy, the unavailability of prior social support systems, a lack of intellectual stimulation, and staff attitudes of "infantilization." Residents who suffer the effects of institutionalization may experience lowered self-respect, a narrowing of interests and emotional responsiveness, personality erosion, overdependency, automatic behaviors, and a loss of interest in the external world. The mental health professional must be alert to these symptoms in referred clients, and develop psychological interventions that address and counteract the unnecessary sources as well as the symptoms of institutionalization syndrome.

## SELECTING AN APPROPRIATE INTERVENTION

Keeping these considerations about the nursing home mental health client in mind, five procedural steps guide the mental health consultant's selection of an appropriate and effective intervention:[5]

1) Identify the problem in behavioral terms.
2) Determine realistic and mutually agreeable goals for intervention.
3) Identify all available mental health service resources.
4) Assess the available interventions, in light of the individual resident's problem and characteristics.
5) Consider the potential problems with available treatments and the possibility of not intervening.

***Identify the Problem.*** The first, and very necessary, step is clearly identifying the resident's presenting problem in precise behavioral terms. The goal is to describe the observable behaviors associated with the presumed problem, rather than simply to label it. For example, rather than *inferring* that Blanche and Joe are both depressed, it is preferable to *describe* the behavior of each. While Blanche cries for brief intervals one to three times daily, has a decreased appetite, and verbally expresses extreme guilt and a poor self-concept, Joe appears physically agitated, exhibits poor concentration abilities, and speaks of suicide.

The examples of Joe and Blanche demonstrate several advantages of a descriptive approach. Communication among all parties involved in the resident's care is facilitated, because all are in agreement on the specific behaviors of concern, which in this instance are quite different for each "depressed" resident. Measuring the frequency and intensity of the specific behaviors also helps to evaluate their impact upon the resident's functioning. Baseline (preintervention) rates of the behaviors can be established to assess the efficacy of any interventions. Finally, clearly defined, descriptive behaviors allow for simpler, more concise recording of behavioral progress, thereby increasing the staff's accountability in record documentation.

***Determine the Goals.*** Establishing an objective, behavioral definition of the problem also leads directly to the second step in selecting an appropriate intervention: determining the intervention goals. If Joe and Blanche are "depressed," the intervention goal might be "lessen or eliminate depression," a nebulous and unmeasurable achievement. Behaviorally specific goals may be more helpful. For example, Blanche's treatment may focus on decreasing crying spells to an average of once every three days and improving her appetite. Similarly, goals for Joe might be to improve concentration abilities and eliminate suicidal thoughts.

At other times, objectively outlining the specific behaviors of concern may lead to the realization that they are not troublesome enough to warrant any intervention. While a label of "depression" seemingly must be addressed, brief crying spells twice a week in and of themselves probably do not warrant the inevitable intrusiveness of intervening in the resident's life.

The criteria to be established for mental health improvement will therefore necessarily be individualized, depending upon the specific behaviors of concern, as well as the wishes of the individuals involved. The resident's, staff's, and family's desires for change, which often conflict, all affect the goals of treatment. Blanche or the staff may not view her crying as a problem, although her family sees it as problematic during their visits.

The behavior of concern must be viewed in its environmental context, including the possible value judgments being incorporated by the people involved. Does Blanche, for example, see her crying as relatively normal because her roommate also cries? Is her family embarrassed or feeling guilty when they observe her tears?

The resident, or his court-appointed guardian of person, has the final right to decide on intervention. If the resident is mentally incompetent, but no guardian is appointed, the guardianship issue must be pursued as soon as possible.[6] In the interim, the physician-led treatment team has the responsibility to make decisions jointly regarding necessary psychological interventions. Consultation with concerned family members is especially important in these cases. A few nursing homes also use an "ethics committee" to assist in making difficult treatment determinations, and to broaden the base of responsibility for the final decision.[7] In all cases, the decision makers should be provided whatever professional judgment is available, and strongly consider the resident's verbally or behaviorally expressed wishes.

The concept of limited expectations is important in establishing realistic, achievable treatment goals. Particularly with cognitively impaired elderly, improvement will typically be slow and gradual. In other cases, the goal may simply be the delay of further cognitive or behavioral regression. For example, it is unrealistic to expect that Joe will stop all exhibition of agitated behavior one week into a behavioral intervention that ignores this behavior but positively reinforces appropriate behaviors incompatible with agitation. Perhaps a more realistic, critical goal would be to decrease the frequency or intensity of such episodes over a period of several weeks.

Hussian (1981) notes two advantages of subdividing goals into very small steps toward a desired end: it helps to identify the specific behavioral changes needed to achieve each step, and it provides "minigoals" whose achievement will be viewed as successes rather than being overlooked or dismissed as insignificant. Easily achievable first steps can provide initial success and encourage continued resident and staff efforts.

***Identify Resources.*** The third step in selecting an intervention is to identify all available resources for providing mental health care. The treatment team must be aware of community resources, including community mental health centers and private providers, as well as in-house treatments available. The team also needs to consider the creation of new interventions as necessary. For example, encouraging appropriate, nonagitated behavior by a behavioral modeling technique requires other residents or staff to serve as positive role models.

Identifying possible resources includes assessing the competencies of the professional or paraprofessional individual providing the therapy. Indeed, many people believe that the therapist's qualities may be more influential than the therapist's treatment techniques.

Evaluating "resources" may also include considering the resident's capabilities and characteristics, as well as his receptivity toward mental health services.

***Assess Available Treatments.*** The fourth step in intervention selection is assessing the available treatments through a review of current literature with several elements as a focus, such as the particular problem or intervention under consideration, the particular type of client and therapist, and other situational factors.

Keisler (1971) warns of the danger of the "uniformity myth," which assumes that all clients, therapists, and outcomes or goals are homogeneous. The concern is that individual differences and needs may be obscured. A mildly confused resident with depression, for example, may be frustrated with verbal psychotherapy because of an inability to concentrate in long conversations. He may profit more from behavioral interventions to increase his activity level.

Older nursing home residents, or even community-dwelling elderly, however, are not often subjects in intervention research. Therefore, applying the research conclusions to the nursing home population may require leaps in judgment (Weinstein and Khanna, 1986). Such a second-hand application runs the risk that the results may not generalize to a nursing home population.

Information based upon populations or environments that most closely resemble the nursing home situation may have to substitute if nursing home literature is not available. Close environmental approximations are often found in other institutions such as acute-care or mental hospitals and residential communities for well elderly. The elderly population is also often studied within the context of organized day programs, such as senior-citizen centers or adult-day-care settings. Such research must then be critically reviewed, keeping in mind possible differential influences of mental hospitals or residential communities vs. nursing homes, or outpatient vs. residential placements. A discussion of various therapies' appropriateness for nursing home residents is included in later sections of this chapter.

***Consider Not Intervening.*** The fifth and final step in an evaluation of treatment options is to consider the choice of not intervening. Brink (1979) describes Seegal's related notion of the "principle of minimal interference," which has a goal of disturbing established patterns of living as little as possible. Other authors also note that *any* intervention implies interference with the resident's ongoing life (Burnside, 1980; Sundberg, Taplin, and Tyler, 1983).

Thus, those involved in the resident's care, including the resident himself, must carefully evaluate the possible costs as well as benefits of treatment before making a final determination. Blanche may prefer occasional crying spells, for example, to being continually encouraged to "stay active."

One cost of inappropriate or premature intervention is of particular concern for elderly institutionalized residents: it can minimize their ability to solve their problems independently, thereby encouraging emotional dependency and the "helpless patient" role (Spayd, 1987; Sundberg, Taplin, and Tyler, 1983).

## MAJOR TYPES OF MENTAL HEALTH INTERVENTION

Several modes of mental health intervention can be used with both community-dwelling and institutionalized elderly.

***Individual Psychotherapy.*** The most traditional type of psychological intervention is individual psychotherapy, a one-on-one verbal discussion of the client's psychological, emotional, or behavioral concerns, which may be based on one or more of a variety of theoretical foundations. Wattis and Church (1986) argue that individual psychotherapy is the treatment of choice for older people if they are cognitively intact, if they are ready to accept a psychological explanation for their current distress, and if their problems do not directly relate to family pressures, in which case family therapy would be more appropriate. Clients with mild to moderate levels of cognitive impairment may also benefit from simpler formats of individual therapy, if motivated to participate.

Several authors have noted that practically every known form of individual psychotherapy is appropriate with certain elderly clients, due to the diversity of interests, needs, and capabilities within the population, as well as their experiences of basic emotional concerns and interpersonal problems, similar to those of younger clients.[8] However, some common themes in psychotherapy with the elderly have been identified, including those of loss, impending death, grief over the death of loved ones, fears of illness and dependency, and loneliness. Another common set of issues is the multiple life-role changes often experienced, including changing work, family, and activities structures.

Further, Goodstein (1982) notes that many older clients react to therapy in a qualitatively different manner from younger ones, being more directly expressive of their opinions. He believes that this expressiveness is due to their greater life experience, and the fact that they are "survivors," having made it to old age.

Some factors influencing individual therapy that are unique to this age group have also been delineated. Many therapists note that such therapy with the elderly is typically of briefer duration, and focuses more on the resolution of specific, concrete concerns, than does therapy with younger clients.[9] Zarit (1980) proposes that the therapy tends to emphasize such specific, immediate issues because of the prominent influences that losses have on older adults' psychological well-being. They are thus motivated to resolve these current losses, rather than focus upon previous life experiences.

The minimal-interference principle mentioned earlier also suggests that importance of a goal-defined, short-term intervention. In therapies using this principle, the emotionally distressing problem is defined, facts about its occurrence are collected, alternative solutions to the problem are generated, these solutions are evaluated, and the best one is selected and acted upon. The therapist can thus "move quickly, take care of a specific problem, and then get out," so as to disturb the client's on-going functioning as little as possible (Brink, 1979, p. 153).

A second common category of individual therapy used with older clients is supportive therapy, which is less directive and more empathy-based. It has a goal of nonjudgmentally validating a client's emotional experiences—that is, letting him know that someone is truly listening, understanding, and caring. Supportive therapy is particularly appropriate in cases of irreversible loss, terminal illness, and when maintenance of current psychological functioning is the goal of therapy (Brink, 1979; Zarit, 1980).

Certain pragmatic therapeutic techniques have also been identified as important with older clients in individual therapy. Zarit (1980) notes that because many elderly are unfamiliar with the "psychotherapy client role," they tend to equate it to being a medical patient, with that role's emphasis on passivity and "following the doctor's instructions." For this reason, the therapist must be careful to explain the rationale, process, and especially the interactive roles of psychotherapy clearly. This communication includes reaching a consensus regarding the treatment's goals and duration and the types of interventions to be used.

Wattis and Church (1986) suggest that the older client's therapist is more likely to assume an active advocate or educator role, rather than the more traditional, neutral therapist role. This more active role is likely due to the client's expectations, noted above, as well as his frailer physical well-being and subsequent need for physical, as well as psychological, services.

Also, Wattis and Church (1986) advise writing down important didactic information for the client, and avoiding the use of psychological jargon or complex language, due to normal developmental losses in information-processing abilities. Blazer (1982) suggests that the regular scheduling of therapy sessions is particularly important with this population, because sessions thus serve as a source of constancy in the client's changing and unstable world.

Goodstein (1982) suggests that the therapist be attuned to two common errors in treating older clients in individual psychotherapy: The elderly should not be treated as if they had always been old and were only old—the cliché of being young at heart has some real merit. The therapist should also avoid implying that a disturbing situation must be accepted, and cannot be changed or addressed due to the client's advanced age—the cliché of not being able to teach an old dog new tricks does *not* have the same merit!

***Group Psychotherapy.*** A second type of mental health intervention to be considered is group psychotherapy, in which (typically) one or two therapists work with a number of clients. The group size should be small enough for personal involvement and interactions, but large enough for variety and protection of any one individual. Whanger (1980) recommends that for elderly clients, this number be between six and twelve members, while Burnside (1978) suggests that the size be determined by the type of group, its goals, and the mental capacities of the clients involved. Common themes in group psychotherapy are similar to those mentioned above in the discussion of individual therapies, with the topics of death, losses, boredom, and loneliness being prominent.

Numerous advantages for providing group rather than individual therapy with elders have been outlined: greater cost efficiency; combating loneliness and isolation, while increasing a sense of belonging; providing a means of reality contact and testing, thereby decreasing nonreality-based thinking via mutual group criticism; and providing positive role models for adaptive behavior. Other advantages include providing a source of social contacts to increase socialization and verbalization; increasing self-confidence of members by the acts of helping others in the therapy group; and having multiple listeners and the provision of mutual support and encouragement, which Weinstein and Khanna (1986) note is particularly helpful to elderly clients who have experienced a deterioration of their previous social-support systems. Finally, psychotherapy groups discourage a tendency to withdraw emotionally and socially. By their emphasis on external, interactive sources of satisfaction, they can be less anxiety-provoking for hesitant elders, and they are less likely to promote dependency on the therapist than is one-to-one psychotherapy.[10]

Brink (1979), however, also notes two potential drawbacks to elderly group therapy: its inability to address the needs of clients who are already withdrawn, and the possibility of superficial conversation preventing the achievement of psychological insight.

Various forms of group therapy, typically based upon a specific focus, have been suggested as appropriate for use with elderly clients. These formats include socialization groups, inspirational groups based upon testimonials (for example, Alcoholics Anonymous) or religious beliefs, and problem-specific groups such as groups for widowers, the disoriented, those anticipating nursing home discharge, or the physically disabled. Other groups are defined by the techniques employed.[11] Busch's (1984) review of the literature in this area suggests that the four most common therapeutic strategies used in elderly group therapy are social interaction, reality orientation, life review, and remotivation.

Another form of group therapy often used with older adults is family therapy, appropriate when the client and/or his family members experience hostility, anxiety, or guilt regarding nursing home admission, or otherwise to address and resolve family conflicts that are identified as detrimental to the elderly client's psychological functioning.

Some common modifications to more traditional group-therapy approaches are suggested with older clients. Because of older adults' greater potential for disorientation, it is generally agreed that such groups should focus upon realistic material. Burnside (1978) also suggests that the therapists be more directive and active in their role as facilitator, and that they offer more support and encouragement. She justifies this approach because of the special problems facing elderly clients, such as their preoccupations with death and losses.

Such groups also tend to have goals of immediate problem resolution more often than the achievement of psychological insight. Often, they focus on accomplishing a life-review process for members. The therapists' expectations for the pace of group achievements should also be curtailed, keeping in mind the lesser physical energies of most elderly clients.

Pragmatic considerations in developing the structure of group therapy for older adults have also been delineated. Brink (1979), for example, believes that sessions should initially be very brief but frequent, in order to stimulate interactions among members best, without overwhelming or boring them. He advises that the group then should gradually work up to forty minutes in duration. Burnside (1978) stresses the need to be aware of members' possible sensory deficits, and thus to assure the minimal interference of background noise, and good, nonglaring lighting conditions.

She also promotes scheduling groups at opportune times during the day, not in the evening, to take advantage of clients' "maximum functioning" periods of alertness. To avoid embarrassment, physical disabilities need to be openly addressed when physical group activities are initiated. Such impairments can then also be therapeutically discussed by members.

A final caution in the development of therapy groups with nursing-home residents is in order—such groups will be more successful if homogeneous in basic ability level. Client selection is an especially important consideration with residents, due to their highly variable levels of cognitive ability, sensory impairment, and motivation. Zarit (1987) has warned that the tendency to "put a group together" in order to achieve some predetermined number of participants, without regard to such factors, most often results in a nonproductive resident mix, a frustrating circumstance for therapist and residents alike.

***Behavior Therapies.*** A third major type of therapy used with elderly clients is behavior therapy.[12] In a strict sense, such therapy involves determining the external, observable, environmental events that immediately precede or follow a problem behavior, then altering the events to modify the behavior. However, a broader perspective of multiple behavior therapies is currently more often adopted, and refers to a general orientation to address and resolve immediate, concrete, and behaviorally based problems.

In this model, all behavior is considered *lawful;* that is, it is a function of a specific context. It is assumed to have some purposeful function for the individual, whether or not others believe the behavior to be sensible or appropriate. The specific context may be external events observable to others, or "internal" (psychological or physiological) events experienced only by the individual himself. The emphasis is thus educational, rather than intrapsychic, with a goal of behavior, and not personality, change.

Appropriate and common targets for behavioral intervention with the elderly are identified by Patterson (1982). They include: (1) the acquisition or improvement of skills in the areas of activities of daily living (ADLs), social and leisure activity, and intellectual performance; (2) compensation for psychosocial losses via social skills retraining; and (3) the decrement or elimination of a wide variety of inappropriate or excessive behaviors.

The basic format for providing a behavioral therapy follows: The target problem is first "operationally defined"—defined in terms of the operations used to measure it. Joe's agitation, in our beginning "depression" example, might be defined as 'loud verbalizations, exhibited three or more times in one hour, that are observed to be disruptive to others on the unit, as identified by their physical withdrawal from Joe." Such a behavioral description is clearly designed to be measurable.

Next, the treatment goals are established. Goals fall into four categories according to Patterson (1982): to increase the occurrence of an existing adaptive behavior; to establish the occurrence of a new, adaptive behavior; to decrease the occurrence of a maladaptive behavior; and to maintain or generalize the occurrence of a newly learned or existing behavior. Multiple categories may be employed at one time. For example, one may wish to establish a new behavior of pleasant socialization while decreasing the maladaptive behavior of loud, critical statements.

Behavior therapy does not then employ one or more specific techniques, but stresses the selection of an empirically validated procedure—one with demonstrated effectiveness for the specific problem.[13] Common behavioral treatment strategies include self-monitoring and behavioral assessment, didactic instruction and behavioral rehearsal, behavior modification through positive reinforcement and punishment, modeling appropriate behaviors, and contracting. As exemplified in Table 6.2, these strategies can be combined to increase the treatment's effectiveness. Behavioral therapy is often effectively used in conjunction with other appropriate interventions, such as individual psychotherapy or psychotropic medication. After an intervention is individually designed and implemented, ongoing and follow-up assessment is provided to assure its continuing efficacy.

One major advantage of using behavioral therapies with the elderly is that they are cost- and time-effective.[14] This efficiency stems from the goal of short-term resolution of immediate problems; the frequent strategy of rearranging existing environmental and social resources rather than adding

TABLE 6.2: Categories and Examples of Behavioral Techniques

| *Treatment Goal and Example* | COMMON STRATEGIES: *Category* | *Example* |
|---|---|---|
| Establish new adaptive behavior | Reinforcement | Assertive requests are first operationally defined, then are reinforced by prompt nursing compliance; aggressive demands are met with a neutral request to rephrase them. |
| Learn how to request a change in the nurse's approach to care assertively. | (a) Shaping | Levels of less to more assertive requests are defined. Then, the first level of the desired assertive request is reinforced, as above. Gradually, the criteria for reinforcement change, to approximate more and more closely the goal level of assertiveness. |
| | (b) Continuous Reinforcement | Every occurrence of the desired assertive behavior is reinforced. |
| | Modeling | Desired assertive requests are demonstrated for the client by the therapist or other residents. |
| | Behavioral rehearsal | Assertive requests are role played in a therapy setting, before being attempted on the nursing unit. |
| Increase existing adaptive behavior | Reinforcement | Activity attendance is self-reinforced by the resident's preferred behavior of watching TV after each activity. |
| Increase the frequency of participation in the home's activities, from a baseline average of one, to four times weekly to alleviate depressive inactivity. | Intermittent reinforcement | Contingent TV watching is gradually decreased to once per three activities. |
| | Contracting | The resident agrees to a verbal and written contract that outlines her commitment to attend four activities weekly. |

*Continued on next page*

TABLE 6.2: *Continued*

COMMON STRATEGIES:

| *Treatment Goal and Example* | *Category* | *Example* |
|---|---|---|
| Maintain/generalize existing adaptive behavior | Reinforcement | Unit nursing staff reinforce the resident's oriented statements with verbal praise. |
| Generalize oriented responses outside the Reality Orientation classroom | Modify antecedent conditions | Environmental cues, such as prominent clocks and calendars, are placed on the unit, to enhance appropriate responding. |
| Decrease maladaptive behavior | Punishment | The resident donates one pack from his matchbook collection to his roommate per argumentative behavior. |
| Reduce episodes of loud, argumentative behavior with a roommate | Reinforcement of incompatible behaviors | The resident can earn or reclaim a matchbook for each appropriate, assertive behavior. |
| | Self-monitoring | The resident documents each instance of argumentative and assertive behavior in a notebook, to heighten awareness of both behaviors. |

new ones; and the common use of trained paraprofessionals rather than professional staff. Two additional benefits of using paraprofessional staff in the nursing-home setting are that treatments are provided in the resident's natural environment, which serves to increase the generalizability of results, and that all unit staff can be involved, typically serving to increase the staff's morale and sense of competence when the interventions are effective. Additional discussion of the benefits of staff participation is provided in chapter 10.

Other advantages of behavior therapies with older clients are that such approaches avoid (1) a negative, stigmatizing emphasis on age, (2) inferences regarding intrapsychic causes, and (3) psychiatric labels as the explanation of psychological disturbance. Further, such techniques adopt an optimistic attitude that behavior is flexible and changeable at any age. Clients and staff are typically receptive to the techniques for several reasons: the approaches' quick effectiveness, straightforward rationale, lack of therapy jargon; the more universally accepted notion of "education" vs. therapy; and the direct, active therapist role.

Additionally, the techniques can easily be individualized to clients' diverse needs and ability levels, as well as their preferences, thereby maximizing motivation to participate in the therapy by using techniques that are specifically reinforcing to the client. The common behavioral focus upon self-management and self-control over behavior also serves to increase the elderly client's belief in self-efficacy and self-attribution for resultant positive change, thereby limiting any tendency to depend upon others for behavioral control. The techniques can be applied to whatever is identified as the appropriate target of change: the elderly person's behavior itself, or the reactions of significant others, a point emphasized above in the case example of Faye. Finally, the behavioral therapist's commitment to ongoing assessment of the treatment used helps assure that only effective interventions will be conducted.

Hussian (1981) has further asserted that behavior therapy is particularly appropriate for the nursing home population, partly because of the high frequency of problematic behavior amenable to behavioral intervention that is observed in this setting (see chapter 4). Further, staff can exert a much higher degree of control over external life events than can be achieved in an outpatient setting, due to their opportunities for twenty-four–hour observation of the resident and a unified behavioral approach. And, as has been previously mentioned, the use of paraprofessional caregivers is of particular benefit, when such staff can be trained in behavioral therapy concepts and techniques.

Behavioral interventions can often be used concurrently with other therapeutic regimens found in the nursing home, such as physical therapy or nutritional supplementation (see the case of John, below). The objective emphasis of behavioral assessments, including such techniques as accurate observation and record keeping of targeted behaviors, can also be used to monitor the effectiveness of other psychological and medical interventions objectively.

---

Following a hip fracture, John was quite resistant to participating in his physical-therapy program, claiming that he saw no reason to exert the effort, "since he would never walk again anyway." A psychological consultant, after thoroughly researching the case, recommended incorporating positive reinforcement techniques to increase the resident's motivation. After training staff in the program she designed, and acquiring John's agreement and verbal commitment to try the plan for one week, staff instituted the strategy: John was provided significant verbal praise and a coupon each day following his successful completion of (a gradually increasing number of minutes of) the physical-therapy program. Five coupons could be traded in for a special one-to-one lunch outing with John's favorite social worker, the primary reinforcer that John chose.

Once John earned his first lunch outing, he became more enthusiastic about participating in physical therapy and agreed to continue the program. Gradually, as he regained strength in his legs, he identified the intrinsically reinforcing nature of participation in the physical therapy program, and requested extra time in the physical-therapy room, in order to accelerate his recovery. The luncheons were continued throughout this effort, and culminated in a celebration where John walked, with a cane, into the restaurant.

---

Some disadvantages to the use of behavioral techniques in the nursing home setting are recognized. Although the procedures may ultimately teach new skills, thereby alleviating nursing staff of tasks, they initially require more concentrated and time-consuming efforts than do medications or other psychological treatments provided by outside professionals. Such efforts include the required, initial task of data collection, which may seem burdensome and unjustified to the staff.

To address specific concerns regarding data collection, Hussian and Davis (1985) suggest being sure that the forms are simple to read and complete, are always available to the staff, and require the least duplication of effort possible. Further, the consultant must work with the staff in the development of the assessments, to assure that the problem is being identified accurately. It is also beneficial to share with the staff the compilations, summaries, and interpretations of the data they have collected, to demonstrate the vital value of this information. This feedback will recognize and reinforce their efforts and may serve as motivation for participation in future data collection projects.

Hussian and Davis (1985) point out that nursing staff are also often resistant to behavioral approaches because of some common misconceptions regarding behavior therapy, including the beliefs that: behavior modification is equated to psychosurgery or exclusively aversive conditioning; it is demeaning or too demanding for elderly clients; it works only with animals, children, or retarded people; and it is ineffective with chronic mental health problems or cognitively impaired clients. The existence of these misconceptions is not surprising: In a recent survey of the use of behavior modification techniques in nursing homes, Guy and Morice (1985) determined that while 54 percent of the homes responding to the survey reported using such interventions, only 16 percent of these homes had provided staff any formal training in behavioral therapy.

Hussian and Davis (1985) argue that these staff misconceptions and biases can be overcome by the clear education of nursing staff in the rationale and techniques of behavioral therapies. In particular, the myth that cognitively impaired residents cannot benefit from behavioral intervention needs to be addressed. Williamson and Ascione (1983) report in their literature review that many studies noted improvement among "severely memory-impaired" clients, using behavioral techniques.

Hussian and Davis (1985) advise moving slowly to demonstrate the intervention's efficacy, starting with "easier," more likely-to-be successful clients. They also recommend being knowledgeable regarding organic causes of inappropriate situations. Finally, to increase staff cooperation, they suggest assuring administrative support, positively reinforcing the staff for their intervention efforts, and providing them frequent monitoring, modeling of techniques, and support by a professional behavioral consultant.

A final disadvantage to the use of behavioral techniques is that they appear deceptively easy to apply, resulting in frequent misuse. Because the techniques can produce powerful behavioral change, their application outside the direct supervision of a professionally trained behavioral consultant can be quite disruptive to the resident's well-being. One common mistake that is cause for significant alarm is the inappropriate use of punitive techniques, in the following ways: as a first step intervention, without concurrent positive reinforcement of an appropriate behavior, and inconsistently.

Other frequently observed mistakes of self-appointed "behavioralists" include not obtaining a proper operational definition of the target behavior; incomplete, and thus inaccurate, behavioral documentation, leading to incorrect conclusions regarding program effectiveness; inconsistent application of procedures; and designing behavioral programs without consideration of their impact on the resident's overall behavioral functioning.

Specific modifications to general behavioral techniques have been suggested for nursing-home clients. Strategies to use with cognitively impaired residents include using their shortened attention span to advantage, by distracting them from inappropriate behaviors. In contrast to other, more alert and less confused groups, it is sometimes advisable to use concrete, or even primary, reinforcers; food is the obvious example, if its use is coordinated with dietary recommendations. Continuous reinforcement techniques, and using very small steps to shape new behaviors, are also recommended.

For residents with sensory impairments, the use of multiple sensory modalities, with increased intensities, is recommended, to prompt, shape, and reinforce behaviors. And in the nursing home environment, the behavioral consultant must be aware of possible sources of unintentional interference with an intervention, including noncontingent reinforcement offered by unaware staff, family, or visitors, or the influence of new or concurrent medications.

***Psychotropic Medications.*** A final major area of mental health intervention relevant to the elderly nursing home client is the use of psychotropic medications to alleviate psychiatric symptoms or behavioral disturbances. Table 6.3 provides the reader an overview of common types of medications available for psychological intervention. Unless a physician, the mental health professional will obviously not be prescribing such medications; however, he or she needs to be aware of this mode of intervention for three reasons. First, there are circumstances in which the use of psychotropic medications can be of great benefit to the client in distress, offering an efficient and effective means of assistance (see the case example of Helen in chapter 7). Thus, the treatment team, in deciding upon the

TABLE 6.3: Commonly Prescribed Psychotropic Medications and Potential Side Effects

| *Medication Type* | *Generic* | *Brand* | *Possible Side-Effects* |
|---|---|---|---|
| Antidepressants | Amitriptyline<br>Desimpramine<br>Doxepin<br>Imipramine<br>Nortriptyline<br>Protriptyline | Elavil<br>Norpramin<br>Adapin/Sinequin<br>Tofranil<br>Aventyl<br>Vivactil | Anticholonergic psychosis, agitation, sedation, dry mouth, urinary retention, constipation |
| Antipsychotics | Chlorpromazine<br>Fluphenazine<br>Haloperidol<br>Mesoridazine<br>Thioridazine<br>Thiothixene<br>Trifluoperazine | Thorazine<br>Prolixin<br>Haldol<br>Serentil<br>Mellaril<br>Navane<br>Stelazine | Sedation, restlessness, tremor, muscle tics, ridigity, mouth movements, tongue darting, obesity |
| Antianxiety | Clorazepate<br>Chlordiazepoxide<br>Diazepam<br>Hydroxyzine<br>Oxazepam | Tranxene<br>Librium<br>Valium<br>Atarax/Vistaril<br>Serax | Sedation, depression, confusion, anorexia, excitement, psychotic symptoms on abrupt withdrawal |

Source: Adapted from Responsive Care: *Behavioral Interventions with Elderly Persons,* by R. A. Hussian and R. L. Davis, 1985, Champaign, Ill.: Research Press. Adapted by permission.

appropriate intervention, should consider whether or not the use of medications is warranted, using the advice and assistance of qualified medical personnel.

Secondly, the concurrent use of medications, as briefly noted above, can significantly influence an ongoing psychological intervention, such that the relative efficacy of each individual treatment is obscured and thus cannot be adequately assessed. Therefore, the mental health consultant should closely monitor the frequency, intensity, and duration of targeted behaviors and how they correlate with medication changes made by the physician.

Finally, a variety of medications commonly prescribed for the elderly, including psychotropic medications, can produce side effects that mimic psychological symptoms, including hallucinations, delirium, confusion, lethargy, depression, psychotic behavior, agitation, mania, disorientation, paranoia, amnesia, anxiety, and hyperactivity. For these reasons, the mental health professional must always be aware of all psychotropic and other medications prescribed for the resident, and have a working knowledge of their benefits, side effects, effective dosages, and so on. Referring to the Physician's Desk Reference (Angel, 1987) or consultation with a physician or pharmacist can be extremely helpful in acquiring such knowledge.

The elderly are more sensitive to the effects of medication in general (Hicks et al., 1980).[15] This increased sensitivity is due to physiological differences in older adults' (1) rates of drug absorption; (2) distribution of lean to fatty tissue, where certain drugs are selectively stored; (3) sensitivity of target organs including brain receptors; (4) metabolism rates in the liver; and (5) excretion of medications via renal functioning.

Therefore, medication dosages should be kept to a minimum, with medications only being prescribed following laboratory tests of body-system functioning. When these tests are inconclusive, prescriptions should err on the side of caution by assuming an impaired capacity to metabolize or excrete the drug. Knowledge of these basic principles can facilitate both comprehension of medication usage, and useful communication with medical personnel.

## SUMMARY

This chapter has provided an overview of current research and clinical literature on fundamental issues of mental health interventions with geriatric clients. When available, literature specific to nursing home residents was provided. Five basic, procedural steps in selecting an intervention in general were outlined. These steps include identifying the mental health problem in precise, behavioral terms; determining realistic and mutually agreeable goals for the intervention; identifying available mental health resources; assessing the available interventions; and considering the possible benefits and costs of *not* intervening.

Next, specific considerations in selecting an intervention for elderly clients, and then nursing home residents in particular, were discussed. The chapter concluded with basic descriptions, and relevant considerations for geriatric clients and nursing home residents, of four major types of mental health intervention: individual psychotherapy, group psychotherapy, behavioral therapies, and psychotropic medications.

## NOTES

1. The terms *therapist* and *consultant* are used somewhat interchangeably in this chapter, with both assumed to be trained mental health professionals. The term *therapist,* however, is intended to imply the individual providing a direct psychological intervention. The term *consultant* is intended to imply the individual who is providing recommendations to the treatment staff, but who may also provide direct service to the resident. See chapter 3 for a more detailed discussion of the consultant's role in the nursing home. In the same vein, the term *resident* is used to represent all those residing in the nursing home, while the term *client* indicates specifically those elderly individuals, residents and others, who are receiving mental health services.

2. As Goldfried (1982) strongly emphasizes, prior to considering possible interventions for mental health concerns, one must first have an accurate asessment of the individual resident's problem: its operational definition and, when possible, its cause (see chapter 5).

3. Strategies to treat agitation, depression, and disorientation are the focus of chapter 7. Preventative approaches are not within the scope of this chapter, and will not be addressed. However, the interested reader is referred to excellent overviews of this topic by Gaitz and Varner (1980) as well as specific, applicable interventions described by Banziger and Rousch (1983), Beck (1982), Langer and Rodin (1979), Rodin and Langer (1977), and Zevon, Karuza, and Brickman (1982).

4. The current structure of third-party medical-expense reimbursement encourages this tendency to list mental health concerns as secondary, since they are less likely to be covered by reimbursement.

5. These steps are guided by behavioral methods detailed by Craighead, Kazdin, and Mahoney (1981); Goldfried (1982); Hussian (1981); Hussian and Davis (1985); Rosenstein and Swenson (1980); and Sundberg, Taplin, and Tyler (1983).

6. Burnside (1980) and Wattis and Church (1986) discuss the issue of who ultimately elects intervention. The guardianship process must be recognized as a complex legal, social, and ethical process, best handled through formal legal channels such as the home's or family's attorney. See the summer 1987 issue of *Generations* for a comprehensive discussion of the views involved in guardianship.

7. Hussian (1981, pp. 190–197) provides an excellent and detailed description of the procedural and beneficial aspects of ethics committees.

8. See Blazer (1982), Brink (1979), Goodstein (1982), Gotesman (1980), Wattis and Church (1986), and Whanger (1980).

9. See Brink (1979), Gotesman (1980), and Zarit (1980) for further discussion of individual therapy with older adults.

10. See Blazer (1982), Brink (1979), Burnside (1978), Weinstein and Khanna (1986), and Whanger (1980) for greater detail regarding group therapy with older adults.

11. Carman and Nordin (1984) and Johnson (1985) discuss psychodrama; Brink (1979) presents dream analysis and peer therapy; while Burnside (1978) describes creative-expression opportunities in art, music, dance, poetry, and writing.

12. Hussian and Davis (1985) and Patterson (1982) provide sound introductions to behavioral interventions with the aged.

13. Williamson and Ascione (1983) provide a good overview of the general-category areas of behavioral treatments with the elderly, including antecedent stimulus control, contingency management, and package treatments. They also provide a representative literature review of studies in each area.

14. Hussian (1981), Hussian and Davis (1985), Patterson (1982), Rosenstein and Swenson (1980), and Whelihan (1978) discuss the many benefits of behavioral approaches with older adults.

15. Hicks et al. (1980) provide a background in geriatric pharmacology, while Wattis and Church (1986) explain physiological changes of aging that are associated with altered drug responses.

# 7

# Interventions with Agitated, Disoriented, or Depressed Residents

*Catherine Selth Spayd and Michael A. Smyer*

## INTRODUCTION

---

Sue, the home's social worker, reluctantly entered Helen's room. Helen was a fifty-eight–year–old new admission to the nursing home, diagnosed with Alzheimer's disease, and Sue was wondering how she could face another "hopeless case." The woman was lying in bed with her covers drawn up, although it was two o'clock in the afternoon. She did not respond verbally or physically to Sue's introduction or attempts at conversation—at least at first. After a few minutes, however, she turned her eyes toward Sue briefly, then quickly averted her gaze. It was enough of a response to intrigue Sue, who returned every day that week for one-sided conversations with Helen.

Gradually, Helen became more consistent with her eye contact, though she remained silent—silent until the one day she reached out to touch Sue's long hair in the middle of the social worker's words, and said "My daughter used to have long hair like yours." From that simple connection Helen poured forth months' worth of stored up thoughts and emotions—feelings of depression and despair so intense that her withdrawn behaviors were taken as symptoms of Alzheimer's disease.

---

Helen's true story provides an extreme example of the devastating effects of depression. Once her problem was accurately explained, Sue, Helen, the psychological consultant, and the rest of Helen's treatment team faced another significant and challenging task—that of *treating* the resident's depression. This chapter is designed to provide a current overview of available interventions for depression, as well as for two other major mental health concerns identified within the nursing home setting: agitation and disorientation. Its goal is to provide the mental health consultant with pertinent information regarding various treatments' applications and success rates, in order to assist in selecting an appropriate intervention.

## AGITATION

---

The first question the nursing staff on the third floor typically asked when starting a new shift was "Is Harry behaving himself today?" One could usually gauge the peace and calm of the entire shift by that one measure. New aides were warned to "watch out for Harry in room 304—he's a real handful."

No one really forgave Harry for his loud screaming at the nurses or the more confused residents, his restless "pacing" of the halls with his wheelchair, his vulgar language, or his frequent hurtful criticisms and complaints about his care—it certainly seemed as if he had the mental capacity "to know better." Harry was just *agitated* a lot of the time for no good reason.

---

Direct-care nursing staff have identified agitation among the most important mental health problems of elderly nursing home residents (see chapter 4). Little has been written about "agitation" as a geriatric mental health concern, perhaps because it is a set of behavioral symptoms (including aimless wandering, pacing, cursing, screaming, repetitive statements, spitting, and physical aggression), rather than a psychiatric diagnosis.[1] However, some researchers and clinicians have addressed the symptom. *Agitation* is defined by one such group as "inappropriate verbal, vocal, or motor activity that is not explained by needs or confusion per se" (Cohen-Mansfield and Billig, 1986, p. 712).

By this definition, the purposeful walk of a confused individual to look out the window would not be classified as agitated behavior, whereas disruptive, nongoal-directed pacing of the individual would be. It is the *inappropriateness* of the behavior, as defined by the observer, that is the operational definition. Defined in this way, agitation can be exhibited by confused, cognitively impaired residents; by cognitively alert, psychologically stable, but frustrated elderly; as well as by residents with diagnosed psychiatric impairments, such as schizophrenia or depression.

Agitation can occur for a variety of reasons. It may be caused by an acute physical disturbance. It can occur secondarily as the frustrated reaction to a physical condition. It may be one symptom of a psychiatric disorder, or it may be explained as a learned behavior, reinforced in some way.[2] Selecting a psychological intervention for agitation is, therefore, dependent upon the behaviors' causes and the resident's characteristics. For example, cognitively intact agitated residents, with underlying problems of depression or frustration, may benefit from individual or group psychotherapy that addresses these concerns. More often, however, the symptom of agitation itself is treated with the immediate, specific interventions discussed below.

***Pragmatic/Environmental Manipulations.*** If an underlying physical condition is the behavior's cause, this condition must be addressed. Hussian and Davis (1985) add that staff can beneficially respond to mild agitation caused by a medical condition by reducing the environmental stimulation surrounding the resident.

This intervention could take a variety of forms: calming the resident with a soft voice; reducing other sources of noise; minimizing environmental changes such as room location, furniture, clothes, or bed; keeping lighting low and nonglaring; and minimizing visitors, or forewarning them to be attuned to this need for reduced stimulation.

***Psychotropic Medication.*** The most common intervention for agitation appears to be psychopharmacological, with antianxiety medications frequently prescribed, while more extreme cases of agitation are often addressed with antipsychotic medications. In Cohen-Mansfield's (1986) pilot study of one large nursing home, she found that 77 percent of the residents identified as exhibiting agitation received psychotropic medications for their behaviors, with 62 percent of these drugs being antipsychotic medications. It is notable, however, that psychotropic medications can themselves cause agitated symptoms, as outlined in table 6.3. This new agitation can lead to a vicious cycle of prescribing *more* medications, which produce *more* agitation.

***Behavioral Therapy.*** The last major type of psychological intervention that has been suggested for agitation is behavior therapy, including a behavioral analysis of the situations commonly associated with the agitation. The goal is to identify, and then change, the observable circumstances that may be exacerbating or reinforcing the inappropriate behavior.

In Harry's case, for example, careful observation of the environment revealed that several of the third-floor residents consistently left the area as Harry loudly arrived in the dayroom. He was then left the best spot in the room to enjoy his (now private) television. Others laughed at his vulgarities, providing a ready-made audience for his behavior. Initial staff interventions therefore focused on consistently removing these inadvertent but real sources of positive reinforcement, by educating the other residents to "actively ignore" Harry's rantings, through instruction and modeling techniques. Additionally, Harry's appropriate, pleasant verbalizations were positively reinforced by increased staff attention at these times.

Whelihan (1978) similarly descibes a successful case study in which staff responded to the loud, agitated verbalizations of an elderly woman by simply stating, "I can't hear you." They also positively reinforced softer statements with specific verbal praise. Continued agitation resulted in returning the resident to her room for a short period. Redirection to reality-oriented topics was used when she expressed bizarre statements.[3]

Mishara (1978) describes a research program in which he also used the technique of positively reinforcing appropriate behaviors incompatible to the targeted, inappropriate behavior. A structured, unit-wide token reinforcement system was developed for the elderly chronic patients of a mental hospital with diagnoses of chronic brain syndrome. The program was designed to decrease the frequency of "bizarre and unusual behaviors," which resembled our definition of agitation, as well as other behaviors, and to increase an alternative behavior, conversations with other residents. Tokens were earned by the forty subjects for appropriate social behaviors, and could be traded in for a variety of secondary reinforcers such as cigarettes, wine, and snacks. Mishara concludes that, overall, the frequency of bizarre and unusual behaviors was significantly diminished by the conclusion of the six-month study, although conversations did not increase.

Haley (1983) writes of a case study in which he successfully used more sophisticated, behavioral self-management techniques with an agitated, elderly resident who had a diagnosis of chronic schizophrenia. Specifically, this cognitively alert and motivated resident received progressive relaxation training, assertiveness training, and cognitive-behavioral therapy in the form of coping self-statements. The therapy goal was to decrease her angry expressions of annoyance with troublesome residents and other situations, and more appropriately express her needs and desires.

In summary, agitation is a set of inappropriate behaviors that can be caused by a variety of problems. Common treatments include environmental manipulations, psychotropic medication, and behavioral interventions. The consultant's task is to assess the underlying condition adequately and to aid in the development, implementation, and evaluation of the effects of a structured intervention plan. Such a plan might include more than one therapeutic approach.

## DISORIENTATION

---

Everyone in the home knew Ruth, a tiny ninety-three–year–old woman who walked about with a worn and slightly dirty teddy bear under her arm. She insisted that it was her "baby," and she called it by her daughter's name. Ruth repeatedly stated that she "had to get home to take care of the baby and cook supper." Several times per week she was found attempting to leave the facility or even cross the busy highway outside, and would angrily and physically resist staff efforts to return her to the home.

Most of the residents and staff had come to ignore her over a period of time—after all, Ruth was in her own little world, far removed from their nursing home and the present. Because she rarely responded to their attempts at conversation, there appeared to be little point in trying to interact with her, other than to lead her back to the wing and scold her when she wandered off.

---

Ruth provides a classic example of the second major psychological concern identified as problematic for the staff of nursing homes—disorientation. Like agitation, disorientation is also a symptom rather than a psychiatric diagnosis. Unlike agitation, however, there is a consensus about the definition of disorientation. Disorientation is an individual's inability to recall accurately personal information (such as his name or past occupation), past or present physical locations (such as birthplace or current address), and/or temporal marks (such as time, date, or season). These three areas are commonly referred to as the spheres of self, space, and time. In our example, Ruth knows her own name and her daughter's name, as well as her past occupation as housewife. Thus, she appears to remain oriented to self. With disorientation to space and time, however, she is unable to interact socially with others, and is dependent upon the staff for her safety.

Disorientation can be caused by several physical and psychological conditions such as Alzheimer's disease, cerebrovascular accident, overmedication, sensory loss or deprivation, clinical depression, and social disengagement with its subsequent lack of intellectual stimulation (Hogstel, 1979; Schwenk, 1979). Again, identifying the most appropriate psychological intervention depends upon the behavior's cause and the resident's unique characteristics. An underlying depression must be actively addressed, as discussed below, and the symptom of disorientation monitored, to assure it has been resolved. Reversible physical conditions must, obviously, be reversed, and sensory losses compensated for, by devices such as eyeglasses or hearing aids.

However, many other physical causes of disorientation, such as Alzheimer's disease, cannot by remedied at this time. In these cases, the symptom must be viewed as the primary target of intervention, and an appropriate treatment plan developed. When disorientation is the result of a degenerative organic process, treatment goals must be realistic and may often be modest. Maintenance of current levels of orientation or delay of further regression may be the most attainable goal in such cases.

Cohen (1987) has suggested that in cases of a degenerative organic process the task becomes one of *care*, not *cure*. Such care must be active intervention that does not dismiss the possibility of rehabilitative potential, rather than a vague provision of "TLC." Examples of active interventions are presented below.

***Environmental Manipulations.*** Many environmental interventions for disoriented elderly restructure the environment, to carry more of the "cognitive load" according to Fozard (1980). For example, color cues in hallways and resident photos next to doors support recall through *simple* familiarity and habitual, repetitive association.

Researchers and clinicians from several disciplines have developed pragmatic approaches that are summarized below:[4]

*Practical Interventions for Disoriented Residents*

1) Try to keep a predictable routine, in order to eliminate sources of confusion.
2) Leave some lights on, to minimize the "sundowner's syndrome" of increased disorientation at night.
3) Assure that the resident displays some familiar, personal objects in his room, to assist with orientation to self. Identify rooms by name and with the resident's picture, to augment spatial orientation.
4) Avoid changes in the resident's environment (for example, of room, staff, or roommate) when possible. If change is inevitable, inform the resident in advance of the change; have a familiar person accompany him to the new setting, and remind him of new information as necessary.
5) Never approach a resident from behind.
6) Communicate one piece of information at a time and offer only two choices at a time, to minimize sources of confusion.

***Reality Orientation.*** The current psychological treatment of choice for disorientation is Reality Orientation, a technique developed in the mid-1960s.

RO relies upon the premise that continual, repetitive provision of accurate, realistic information in the spheres of self, space, and time, plus consistent correction of disoriented statements and actions, will increase the individual's level of orientation. Many RO specialists further advocate the use of positive reinforcement for appropriate, oriented statements, but specific ways to apply such reinforcement have not been consistently or operationally defined. The orientation information may be presented by an instructor in a group setting, via environmental clues such as an "RO board" of daily orientation facts, and/or during conversations throughout the resident's day, by nursing and other staff.[5]

RO has gained widespread acceptance in nursing homes over the last twenty years, particularly among clinical personnel. Despite its popularity, there are relatively few empirical research studies that support its effectiveness. In Schwenk's (1979) analysis of controlled, therapy-outcome studies on RO, only three of the six studies reviewed supported the efficacy of RO over a no-treatment, control condition or other therapy technique. More recently, however, another review of the literature concluded that RO was more effective in decreasing disorientation than nonspecific treatments.[6]

Traditional RO therapy may be helpful for some disoriented elderly clients, but it is not universally effective. It may be most beneficial for residents with mild levels of disorientation.[7] Further, its main accomplishment may be to increase the residents' knowledge of the basic set of orientation facts that has been formally presented, rather than providing a flexible skill to be applied in varying situations of the natural environment.[8]

***Modified Reality Orientation.*** Several researchers and clinicians have modified traditional RO approaches to improve the technique's efficacy and generalizability. Hussian (1981), for example, incorporated relevant environmental clues in the training, such as teaching residents to look at nurses' name tags to remember their names, and to use available clocks and calendars to reorient themselves to time. These skills were taught using structured positive reinforcement techniques.

Hart and Fleming (1985) also successfully combined traditional RO techniques with structured positive reinforcement for oriented statements. They further included training in listening skills and role-plays of common unit observations, to increase generalization of the oriented behaviors into the subjects' natural environment. However, no generalization to on-unit conversations was observed following treatment.

***Limitations of Reality Orientation.*** Hussian (1981) cautions that under certain conditions RO therapy may not only be ineffective for the client but it may, in fact, be deleterious: if the disorientation serves to deny the rapid progression of a terminal illness; if a very elderly person has been totally disoriented for two or more years, and is responding to internal stimuli as a compensatory mechanism; and if significant panic or anxiety is observed when a resident's disoriented statements or behaviors are corrected.

Removing an elderly person's disoriented but comforting belief that he or she is living in an earlier, perhaps happier time, can be very threatening. Further, being clearly confronted with his degree of memory loss can in itself be very frustrating for a client who has not acknowledged his level of disorientation. Finally, there are instances when the technique is simply ineffective for the resident, and thus does not address the problematic consequences of disorientation, such as wandering or repetitive questioning.[9]

***Behavior Therapy.*** Despite the problems that some clients experience with RO therapy, few alternative treatment modalities to address disorientation can be identified. Even less empirical research has been completed on other psychological interventions for it. However, Patterson and Teigen (1973) reported one case study in which positively reinforcing an elderly, psychotic woman's oriented conversation served to increase her frequency of oriented responses. Another study by Langer and Rodin (1979) confirms the effectiveness of positively reinforcing oriented responses.[10]

***Validation Therapy.*** Feil's Validation Therapy technique has also been successfully used by some clinicians with severely disoriented clients.[11] In this approach, the elderly client's disoriented statements or behaviors are not corrected, nor are they confirmed. The staff member instead encourages the person to discuss the focal topic of his disorientation by asking nonthreatening questions. The goal is to validate the emotions incorporated in the disoriented belief, in order to alleviate the distress to some extent, and indirectly diminish the disorientation.

In Ruth's case, for example, Reality Orientation–based attempts to inform her gently but firmly that her daughter was not an infant, but had in fact died several years ago, resulted in agitation and significant emotional distress. Because the information was also not retained over time, the treatment team decided to discontinue use of RO to correct the disoriented belief. Instead, when Ruth began to address her stuffed bear as her daughter, the staff encouraged her to talk about her daughter's childhood, asking questions such as how Ruth had dressed her, or about her favorite toys. This approach was not only successful in avoiding agitated behaviors and redirecting Ruth from her attempts to leave the facility, but it also provided some basis for appropriate conversations with the resident.

In summary, disorientation can result from a variety of physical, psychological, and social causes. After appropriate assessment, intervention strategies should be chosen to maximize functioning and offer caregiving staff effective approaches to inappropriate behavior. Common effective treatments include modified versions of Reality Orientation, environmental restructuring, behavior therapies, and Validation Therapy.

## DEPRESSION

This chapter's first case example, that of Helen, the new admission who was initially misdiagnosed as having Alzheimer's disease, provides an illustration of the potentially devastating nature of depression. According to Gallagher and Thompson (1983), depression is the most common psychiatric problem experienced by the elderly.

For a formal diagnosis of a "major depressive episode" an adult must exhibit a dysphoric (sad) mood, and at least four of the following symptoms nearly every day for two or more weeks: changes in appetite, changes in sleep patterns, psychomotor agitation or retardation, loss of interest in usual activities or decreased sexual drive, loss of energy, feelings of worthlessness or excessive guilt, concentration or other thinking difficulties, and/or recurrent suicidal thoughts. Further, these symptoms cannot be caused or complicated by another psychiatric impairment.[12] Clients exhibiting either fewer symptoms or milder intensities of these symptoms may also be in significant emotional distress, while not formally diagnosable as clinically depressed.

However, many elderly people exhibit some of these symptoms, such as decreases in energy levels and sexual interest, as part of the normal aging process; other symptoms, such as appetite and sleep disturbances, are associated with physical diseases, also more prevalent with increasing age. Thus, more reliable indications of depression in the elderly include observable changes in their emotional and/or cognitive status, such as the symptoms of a sad or hopeless mood, psychomotor agitation or depression, apathy, social withdrawal, and concentration, memory, and attention difficulties.[13] In "pseudodementia," like Helen's, the primary symptom is cognitive dysfunction, or nonresponsiveness, which appears similar to dysfunction.

Biological causes are major contributors to the development of depression in the elderly. Salzman and Shader (1978) point out that common illnesses that can produce depressive symptoms include hypokalemia (decreased potassium), anemia, hypothyroidism, and other endocrine disturbances, Parkinson's disease and other neurological disturbances, urinary-tract diseases, and cardiopulmonary insufficiency. Conversely, Lehmann (1982) notes that somatic symptoms in the elderly caused by depression are often mistaken as indications of a physical illness.

Additionally, some medications, including digitalis, antihypertensives, antiparkinsonian medicines, corticosteroids, anticancer medicines, and various psychotropic medications can cause depressive symptoms. Some researchers also believe that neurochemical changes in the brain cause the depression of some elderly (Lehmann, 1982). These presumed, internal causes of depression are often labelled "endogenous."

Psychosocial or environmental stressors can cause "exogenous" or "reactive" depression in the elderly.[14] As noted in chapter 6, elderly individuals increasingly experience the likelihood of disruptive life changes, typically losses, in the realms of finances, the deaths of family members and friends, social interactions, recreational skills, attractiveness, physical infirmities, and previous life roles. Weinstein and Khanna (1986) present one theory of depression in the elderly: these losses result in a self-perceived decrease in mastery or control over the environment, which produces even more feelings of frustration.

Institutionalization is proposed by many as a prime source of loss of environmental control, and thus a likely cause of depression in the elderly. However, Zemore and Eames (1979) argue that there is not adequate scientific evidence for this notion. In their research, which compared institutionalized elderly with those on a waiting list to enter a nursing home, they found no differences in subjects' levels of depression.[15] Activity theorists also promote the concept that loss of social roles and interest in activities, termed "disengagement," is a significant contributor to depression in the elderly; others, however, defend disengagement as an adaptive defense for coping with the changes accompanying advancing age.[16]

More psychological treatments are available for late-life depression, and more therapy-outcome research has been conducted on depression in the elderly, than for the other two mental health concerns under discussion here. A comprehensive presentation of this field of research is beyond the scope of this chapter. However, because the consultant has a wide choice of appropriate interventions to consider, representative studies, incorporating nursing home populations as subjects when available, are provided to exemplify the various treatment types.

### *Individual Psychotherapy.*[17]

*Supportive Psychotherapy.* According to Goodstein (1982), the goal of supportive therapy is to assist a resident with good underlying coping skills through a situational crisis or stressor. Such support is typically achieved through validation, reassurance, and clarification of the resident's emotions and thoughts, and the establishment of a trusting therapeutic relationship, with the therapist assuming a more directive role.

*Insight-Oriented/Psychodynamic Psychotherapy.* Conversely, the goal of traditional insight-oriented (or "psychodynamic") psychotherapy is to change an underlying personality structure. This change is accomplished by a long-term therapy of intensive discussions, which serve to identify and explore the functions of previously unconscious and maladaptive defense mechanisms.[18] Once this insight is achieved, the client theoretically will experience a "catharsis" in which his emotional distress is expressed and addressed, and will gain a basic understanding of his problems and how to resolve them.

Modifications to traditional insight-oriented therapy have been proposed for elderly depressed clients, including a typically briefer duration of therapy; greater emphasis on immediate problem resolution, rather than determining the early-life origins of these problems; a more active and directive therapist role; and less emphasis on solely intrapsychic processes as the focus of change. Steuer (1982) outlines several themes commonly addressed in dynamic psychotherapy with the elderly: growing old; conflicts with children; conflicts with spouse; coping with physical limitations and disabilities; and death, dying, and grief. Literature documenting the effectiveness of these techniques with the elderly is typically found in case studies, rather than controlled, empirical therapy-outcome research.[19]

*Cognitive-Behavioral Therapy.* Two other promising therapy techniques that have been developed more recently are the cognitive and behavioral therapies for depression. These techniques can be provided separately, but are often combined into a cognitive-behavioral approach.

Cognitive therapy was initially developed by Aaron Beck in the late 1960s (Beck, 1973). Directive and time-limited in nature, its basic premise is that depression is caused by the individual's internal negative and distorted beliefs or *cognitions*. A nursing-home resident's belief that he is totally useless because he can no longer walk without supervision is an example of an exaggerated belief that can lead to depression. Other prominent types of distorted cognitions include themes of hopelessness and helplessness. (These concepts may be especially relevant for the elderly, at least partially dependent, nursing home resident, and the therapist needs to consider with his client to what extent they are, indeed, illogical.)

The therapist's initial task is to teach his client how to identify these illogical cognitions and their associations with his depressed moods. Then, he gradually helps the depressed client challenge and replace the beliefs with more logical and adaptive ones. Homework assignments are typically provided that stress rehearsal of the new, positive cognitions to enforce concepts presented in sessions and to generalize the techniques into the client's natural environment.[20]

Behavioral therapy, as defined by Lewinsohn (1974), proposes that depression is caused by the loss of positively reinforcing events that previously occurred in the individual's natural environment. This loss may be the result of new skill deficits within the individual, previously reinforcing stimuli losing their desirability in the eyes of the individual, or limited access to these former reinforcers. The theoretical basis of this therapy is particularly applicable to the elderly, especially institutionalized elders, with their greater physical limitations and restricted environmental experiences.[21]

Initially, the therapist teaches the client to monitor his daily activities and moods, in order to assess the correlation between his behaviors, their consequences, and his resultant emotional state. Next, clients are taught to develop self-change plans that include increasing activity levels and pleasurable experiences to optimize the likelihood of receiving positive reinforcement from the environment.

Another appropriate area of behavioral therapy is social-skills training, including assertiveness training.[22] The current cohort of elderly women may especially benefit from acquiring more-assertive and less-passive skills in interacting with staff and others. However, staff members also need training to respond in a prepared and reinforcing manner to newly assertive resident requests.

Another behavioral technique appropriate for residents is "environmental mastery tasks." Wetzel (1980) notes that these tasks should be selected by the elderly resident himself, to have personal meaning, and be broken down into attainable subgoals, to assure success. For example, the task can be as basic as reassserting choice over clothing worn each day, and if a withdrawn resident is truly hesitant or apathetic about picking an outfit to wear, starting with only two choices may be effective.

Goddard and Cartensen's (1986) case study exemplifies the use of behavioral techniques, as part of a multi-modal approach, for an eighty-six–year–old chronically depressed nursing home resident. The woman had recently suffered a broken wrist, and hence was unable to pursue some previously enjoyed activities. These losses of control and preferred, reinforcing activities appeared to be the cause of her subsequent further deterioration in mood. Treatment consisted of providing adaptive devices to allow the resident to read independently again (via the use of a special book stand), change her radio station (via an extension switch), and gain continual access to a preferred craft activity. A series of therapy sessions was also provided for two months, to provide the resident an outlet to discuss her emotions, reinforce her positive self-statements, and encourage her increased activity participation. Behavioral observations and self-reports of a significant improvement in mood followed implementation of the behavioral program.

By combining the two above approaches, cognitive-behavioral treatment can be an important intervention for late-life depression. Depressed elderly often demonstrate both negative, dysfunctional cognitions as well as the limited behavioral competencies that are the foci of change in cognitive-behavioral therapy.[23] A cognitive-behavioral intervention also has other advantages discussed earlier: the techniques are time-limited, problem-resolution-oriented, and address problems some theorists believe are shared by many depressed elderly—decreased environmental mastery, feelings of helplessness, and disengagement from previous activities.

Steuer (1982), however, suggests that cognitive-behavioral techniques should be modified for the elderly to include a slower learning pace, with more skill rehearsal. Fry (1984) also describes the success of a slightly modified version of this therapy. The basic components of this therapy were: (1) self-monitoring and self-recording of cognitions; (2) positive self-talk and cognitive restructuring to replace the negative and irrational beliefs with cognitions of independence, self-efficacy, self-respect, and outgoingness; (3) self-control procedures such as thought-stopping, relaxation training, and desensitization to specific anxieties; and (4) verbalizing self-reinforcing statements and rehearsing self-reinforcing roles.

There are several research studies that provide indications of the superiority of behavioral and cognitive therapies to other psychotherapies with elderly depressed clients.[24] Cognitive and behavioral interventions are superior to insight/relational therapy or no treatment according to Weinstein and Khanna (1986). However, they note that the cognitive approach may be more beneficial than the behavioral, at least with nursing home residents and exogenous depression. Additional research is needed to replicate and extend these findings to longer-term therapy before more definitive conclusions can be made. Further, because the cognitive and behavioral techniques are so often and easily combined, the relative efficacy of either used alone may not be an important consideration.

*Reminiscence.* Another individual therapy often used successfully with depressed elderly is life review or reminiscence, a process in which clients are actively encouraged to remember and discuss earlier life experiences and relate them to their current circumstances and behavior. The therapist's role is to assure, gently probe, and positively reinforce the resident during his life-review task, as well as to facilitate his insight into the usefulness of past coping strategies. Lazarus (as cited in Weinstein and Khanna, 1986) has suggested that reminiscence is especially helpful with depressed elders, because by promoting pride in past achievements, it offers hope for the future.

Limited therapy-outcome research is available for this intervention (e.g., Haight and Bahr, 1984), although many authors appear to recognize its benefits intuitively.[25]

***Group Psychotherapy.*** Group-therapy techniques for depression typically employ the same therapies outlined above for individual interventions, but have the added, interactive benefits noted previously in chapter 6. To the advantage of those working with the institutionalized elderly, most of the available literature on groups for depression addresses therapy groups within nursing homes. Unfortunately, this literature is comprised of case reports rather than more rigorous research studies, with a few exceptions.[26]

Gallagher (1979, as cited in Weinstein and Khanna, 1986), for example, compared behavioral group therapy with a nondirective group approach, most like supportive therapy in style. While the residents in the behavioral therapy exhibited a greater improvement in verbal interactions during therapy sessions, no significant differences were found between the two groups in self-reported depression or observations of interpersonal behaviors. Ingersoll and Silverman (1978, as reported in Weinstein and Khanna, 1986) compared the effectiveness of a reminiscence group to a behavioral group. They concluded that similar results were produced with both treatments, with one exception: at the conclusion of treatment, the reminiscence group reported significantly fewer somatic complaints. Thus, few useful empirical conclusions have been reached regarding the relative efficacies of various group interventions for late-life depression.

The advantage of the numerous case studies of therapy groups for depressed older adults is that they provide an indication of the diversity and creativity found in these psychotherapeutic techniques. One interesting example is psychodrama, a group intervention for depression that appears to be increasingly used with elderly clients. It is a technique of action-oriented role-playing of a variety of therapeutically relevant situations. Carman and Nordin (1984) believe that psychodrama is applicable for elderly clients because (1) it encourages them to interact with the environment, inhibiting social withdrawal and isolation, and (2) it serves to facilitate the resolution of old concerns identified within a therapeutic life review, allowing the resident to act upon and address old problems, make amends, and restore previous relationships. It is also particularly helpful in allowing those elderly who have lost verbal skills an opportunity for self-expression, according to Johnson (1985).

Another innovative group therapy approach is described by Kaye (1985), who led an eight-week Yoga course with depressed nursing home residents. She reports anecdotal findings of significant success in alleviating symptoms of depression in participants, as well as their apparent enjoyment of the program.

The new field of pet therapy provides a final example of such an innovative approach. Brickel (1984) describes a small study in which he compared "conventional therapy," which included discussion of significant issues, family involvement, and basic behavioral skills, to "pet-facilitated therapy." This second condition incorporated the same therapy process as the first group, with the one additional factor of bringing a pet dog into each therapy session. The dog was available for clients to hold or stroke as they desired. A no-treatment control condition was also included in the research design.

Brickel reports that while both the conventional and pet-facilitated groups evidenced significant reductions in depression, the pet-facilitated group's improvement rate was double that of the conventional therapy group. He theorizes that the pet served to facilitate conversations regarding past pets and other past life events by providing a frame of reference, as a catalyst for general disclosure, and as a safe means to interact with external reality.

***Psychotropic Medication.*** Another common treatment used with depressed elderly is antidepressant and other psychotropic medication.[27] Typical categories of medicines include the tricyclic and newer tetracyclic antidepressants. Less often, monoamine oxidase inhibitors (MAOIs), or lithium salts are prescribed. Antipsychotic medication or a medicine combining antidepressant and antipsychotic features is sometimes used if a psychotic process is theorized to underlie the depressive symptoms, or a psychotic process is observed. Antianxiety medications may be prescribed if anxiety or agitation are a prominent part of the clinical picture, and stimulants are infrequently given if the depression is manifest in severe apathy.[28]

Strauss and Solomon (1983) note that few sound empirical studies have addressed the efficacy of these various medication interventions. However, they are commonly used in the geriatric population, and particularly in nursing homes, so the consultant must be aware of their benefits and side effects, as noted in chapter 6.

***Electroconvulsive Therapy.*** One final treatment for geriatric depression, which is regaining popularity, is Electroconvulsive Therapy (ECT).[29] ECT consists of a series of administrations of electrical current to the skull, in order to induce a controlled seizure. While the specific mechanism of action is unknown, the intervention is often defended because it has been demonstrated to be more effective, with fewer risks of side effects, than even psychotropic medications, with a success rate of 80 percent to 90 percent according to Blazer (1982). Further, Gatz and Warren (1986) contend that it is effective in a very brief period, a potentially life-saving feature for suicidal or severely malnourished depressives.

Recent innovations in the technique, including the placement of the electrode onto the nondominant brain hemisphere, have served to decrease the likelihood of postseizure confusion and memory disturbance. However, at least transient memory loss of several hours is considered inevitable, and elderly clients treated with ECT do exhibit longer, though still generally temporary, periods of confusion following the procedure. This side effect is of considerable concern in elderly clients, who have a greater initial potential for memory problems or an otherwise-compromised cognitive status.

Additionally, ECT may produce profound disruptions in body systems, including hypertension, sinus tachycardia, extreme blood-pressure elevations, intracranial pressure, and cardiac arrhythmias. For these reasons, the use of ECT is generally considered to be a last resort, following attempted trials with psychotropic medications and psychotherapies.

## SUMMARY

The mental health consultant asked to recommend an effective and appropriate psychological intervention for nursing home residents with agitation, disorientation, or depression is faced with an incomplete and often empirically untested group of choices in each domain.

A review of the available (though sparse) literature on treatments for geriatric agitation indicates that the agitated behavior of elderly residents is typically addressed with medical interventions, if a physical cause is determined, or with psychopharmacological agents or behavioral therapies. As noted above, major disadvantages of psychotropic-medication intervention are the possibility of actually intensifying the agitation, as well as the frequent negative reactions elderly clients have to the medications. Furthermore, behavioral techniques appear to offer a more permanent resolution to the concern. However, as discussed in chapter 6, they have the disadvantages of initially being more labor-intensive for staff, as well as potentially delayed in effect.

The psychological consultant examining available treatments for disorientation within the nursing home is given few choices, and must therefore carefully consider which form of RO therapy, Validation therapy, or positive-reinforcement program, if any, is appropriate for the client. Important points in making such a decision include the resident's level of disorientation, whether the disorientation is serving an adaptive function as a defense mechanism of denial, and the resident's responsivity to more structured positive reinforcement techniques. A final consideration must be the staff members' level of comfort in correcting disorientation.

The treatment of choice in geriatric depression depends upon the individual resident's unique characteristics and presenting problem. In the area of individual psychotherapies, little research evidence is available for assessing the merits of three major types of individual therapy provided to depressed elders: supportive, insight-oriented/dynamic, or reminiscence therapies. The cognitive-behavioral approach to depression, however, appears particularly well suited for elderly clients, and there are some research indications that cognitive and behavioral therapies for depression are superior to insight-oriented, verbal psychotherapy.

Group psychotherapies for depressed elders typically employ the same techniques used in individual psychotherapy, but also include some innovative approaches, such as psychodrama, Yoga therapy, and pet therapy. Few empirical conclusions have been reached regarding the relative efficacies of various group interventions with depressed elders.

A variety of psychotropic medications are another type of intervention used for depression with elderly clients; again, little research has been completed that supports their effectiveness, although their use is common with this population. Electroconvulsive therapy is regaining popularity with depressed elders, and can be quite effective, though it has serious side effects that limit its use to a last-resort treatment. The possibility of combined psychological treatment techniques should be considered, and is often an effective intervention strategy, as exemplified below.

The case of Helen, this chapter's introduction, serves also as the chapter's conclusion, a true example of the significant, positive influence appropriate psychological intervention can have on the life of a nursing home resident.

---

Once Helen's depression was diagnosed, she and her treatment team developed a comprehensive program based upon her initial abilities, her needs, and the severity of her symptoms. She was initially placed on a course of antidepressant medication, and attended individual supportive-therapy sessions which incorporated gradually increasing expectations of client participation. After significant improvement had already been observed, she agreed to participate in the "therapeutic employment" program, and worked several hours daily in the nursing home's laundry, an example of an environmental-mastery intervention.

So much improvement in behavior and mood were observed that Helen and the treatment team agreed to discontinue her psychotropic medication after four months. Within the following six months, however, the antidepressant was reinstituted on a long-term, maintenance basis, due to an observable decline in mood, self-sufficiency, and activity level. Two years later, Helen married a fellow resident, and the couple moved out of the nursing home into a subsidized housing project for the elderly—a remarkable achievement for the "Alzheimer's" victim who would not initially respond to Sue's conversation.

---

## NOTES

1. While this symptomatic, descriptive approach is often beneficial, as argued in chapter 6, its cost may be a lack of attention in the research literature (see Cohen-Mansfield, 1986; Cohen-Mansfield and Billig, 1986).

2. Hussian and Davis (1985) list these common acute physical causes: hyperthyroidism, hyperglycemia, hypercalcemia, infection, myocardial infarction, congestive heart failure, arrhythmias, vascular insufficiency, trauma, fecal impaction, fractures, recent surgery or anesthesia, azotemia, cerebral tumors, Cushing's syndrome, hepatic failure, and reaction to medication. They identify common frustrating chronic physical conditions as immobilizing disorders or situations such as a cerebrovascular accident, and deteriorating conditions such as early Alzheimer's disease. Psychiatric disorders that include the symptom of hallucinations (such as schizophrenia and Alzheimer's disease) also often produce agitation, the resident's response to the panic the hallucinations may cause.

3. Williamson and Ascione (1983), in their review of contingency management programs with the elderly, describe a similar reinforcement program successfully used with an elderly "screamer."

4. The suggestions in this list are adapted from the work of Burnside (1980), Wattis and Church (1986), and Zarit, Zarit, and Rosenberg (1987).

5. Folsom's original description of RO was published in 1968. Other thorough overviews of classic individual and classroom Reality Orientation programs are provided by Taulbee (Burnside, 1978; Burnside, 1980) and a VA training guide (VA Hospital, Tuscaloosa, 1984). Hogstel's (1979) article provides a good, brief summary of the techniques.

6. Schwenk (1979) reported positive outcomes of the use of RO in research studies by Harris and Ivory (1976); Brook, Degun and Miller (1975); and Citrin and Dixon (1977). Studies in which RO was demonstrated to have little effect on disorientation were those of Zepelin, Wolfe, and Kleinplatz (1977); Zepelin and Wade (1975); and Barnes (1974). Powell-Proctor and Miller (1982) conclude that RO is more effective than nonspecific treatments.

7. See Brook, Degun, and Miller (1975) and Schwenk (1979).

8. See Hart and Fleming (1985), Hussian (1981), and Schwenk (1979).

9. Hogstel (1979), Schwenk (1979), and Zarit, Zarit, and Rosenberg (1987) comment on contra-indications to the use of RO. They explain how it can be harmful as well as ineffective.

10. Although the subjects in this research were not specifically designated as disoriented, those in a condition receiving secondary token reinforcers did dem-

onstrate more "cognitive improvement" on simple facts of orientation to self, space, and time than did control subjects.

11. A detailed description of this technique is provided in a manual written by Wetzler and Feil (1979).

12. This definition is provided by the Diagnostic and Statistical Manual, Third Edition (DSM-III) of the American Psychiatric Association (1980).

13. See Blazer (1982, chapter 2) for an extensive discussion of the symptoms of late-life depression, as well as discussions by Hussian and Davis (1985), Spar (1982), and Zemore and Eames (1979).

14. This endogenous-exogenous distinction is a theoretical issue and is not universally adopted as a useful concept. For example, it is not incorporated in the DSM-III diagnostic criterion for depression.

15. Institutionalization may still be a factor in waiting-list clients' depression; many are distressed regarding the impending admission and/or the conditions that necessitate it (Zarit, 1987).

16. See Weinstein and Khanna (1986) for an interesting and detailed summary of proposed psychosocial influences on depression in the elderly, as well as a reveiw of treatment alternatives.

17. See Steuer (1982) for a literature review outlining the historical development of individual-therapy techniques with the elderly.

18. Sundberg, Taplin, and Tyler (1983) discuss alternative individual interventions including insight-oriented/psychodynamic strategies.

19. See Weinstein and Khanna (1986, chapters 6–8) for a comprehensive summary of these case studies, and commentary on the modifications to traditional insight therapy noted here.

20. Gallagher and Thompson (1983) describe steps of behavioral interventions while Thompson and Gallagher (1984) outline cognitive interventions with depression.

21. See Goddard and Carstensen (1986).

22. Waller and Griffen (1984) describe such skills training for depressed elderly.

23. See Vezina and Bourque's (1984) article for a description of their research results on these negative cognitions and the behavioral coping strategies of depressed elderly.

24. See the article by Thompson and Gallagher (1984) for a comprehensive discussion of possible predictors of differential therapy success with elderly clients.

25. Haight and Bahr (1984) discuss life-review interventions and their usefulness. Other clinicians have suggested using psychodrama groups (Carman and Nordin, 1984), and interactions with young people (Weinstein and Khanna, 1986; Wetzel, 1980) to facilitate life review.

26. Weinstein and Khanna (1986, chapter 10) do an excellent job of reviewing the few such therapy-outcome studies, as well as several case reports.

27. See Lehmann (1982) and Strauss and Solomon (1983).

28. Blazer (1982, chapter 15), Strauss and Solomon (1983), and Lehmann (1982) provide good overviews of the types of antidepressant and other psychotropic medications used for depression, as well as related issues of administration.

29. See Gatz and Warren (1986) for current uses of ECT.

# 8

# Families in Long-Term-Care Settings

## *Margaret D. Cohn and Gina M. Jay*

Mrs. D.'s two daughters always come to visit her together and they spend the whole time arguing with each other. Their fights disrupt the entire wing and upset Mrs. D. so much that she can't sleep and doesn't feel like eating. I wish they'd do their arguing elsewhere.

*Carla, nurse's aide*

I wanted so much to help Mom with her physical therapy following her fall, but the nursing home wouldn't let me be directly involved in her rehabilitation. They said it had something to do with institutional rules and regulations. I know that Mom would recover more quickly with my help and encouragement, but there's nothing I can do. They're always complaining about being understaffed anyway, you'd think they'd appreciate some help.

*Sheila, resident's daughter*

Mrs. J.'s daughter Marie is helping organize this month's birthday lunch and has convinced Mr. G. [nursing home administrator] to allow alcoholic social hours once a month. She's done a great deal to boost morale among the staff and residents since her mother came to live here. I wish we had a few more like her.

*Margo, nursing home activities director*

My family is the most important thing in my life. I look forward to their visits. When things are going well with them, I'm happy, when they are having problems, I worry.

*John, nursing home resident*

I realize that Mrs. K. is concerned about her mother's health, but her constant phone calls are disrupting everyone's work. What can I do about her?

*Janice, nursing home administrator*

Mrs. H. is feeling so alone. She's been here for four months and her son still hasn't come to visit. I know he still feels guilty about not being able to care for her at home, but something must be done to bring him around. If Mrs. H. is going to be happy here, she needs to know her son cares for her.

*Barbara, nursing home social worker*

## INTRODUCTION

These quotes illustrate a few of the ways in which families can either positively or negatively affect resident, staff, and institutional functioning in the nursing home community. Think for a moment about how we deal with such situations at present. How can we encourage "helpful" family involvement in the long-term-care setting, and discourage disruptive or damaging involvement? What do we need to know in order to devise effective treatment plans and interventions to deal with family-related problems in the nursing home?

The answers to these questions lie in knowledge of two general areas: (1) the characteristics and experiences of the people involved either directly or indirectly in the problem (that is, staff, residents, and family) and (2) interventions and consultative approaches useful with these groups. Other chapters of this volume address staff and resident issues. The purpose of the present chapter is to aid the mental health community in understanding charcteristics of families in later life, and to sensitize them to the family process of placing an elderly member in a nursing home. This information serves as the foundation for designing intervention and treatment plans for family members in the long-term-care setting. Chapter 9 follows with a discussion of family interventions.

This chapter is divided into five major sections. The first section describes who our aging families are and the effects of demographic and social change on family life. Issues of family availability and contact with the elderly are also discussed. The second section focuses on the broad range of family functions and tasks. The third section centers on family support of the elderly and issues related to caregiving; here increasing care of the elder by family members is noted. The fourth section is concerned with the family's decision to place an elderly member in a nursing home. How do families come to place a member? What are the determining factors? The final section considers the characteristics and involvement of family members in the nursing home setting.

## WHO ARE OUR AGING FAMILIES?

Today's modern families differ from those of the past. Altered mortality and fertility patterns, changes in women's roles, and alternative family forms, have modified family life and family experience across the lifespan. For example, many grandmothers today are drawing paychecks rather than babysitting or homemaking.

---

Mary Lou, at fifty-two, is a very successful real-estate broker, wife, mother of four, and grandmother of three. She alternates visits to her grandchildren in upstate New York with visits to the nursing home where her eighty-year-old father now lives. Her mother-in-law and father-in-law live in Arizona and make annual trips East every Easter. Long-distance phone calls have become a special part of every weekend for the entire family.

Charlie and Carol became grandparents at forty, and custodial parents again at forty-one when their daughter Susan returned home after her divorce. Now their commuting careers and their daughter's work out of town have led them to hire live-in household help to provide twenty-four–hour help with their four-year-old granddaughter and Charlie's seventy-one–year–old Dad. They feel that they run their own home as paid day-care for both generations. They do get the assurance that Dad's emphysema and the baby's development are being well cared for.

---

Family patterns, like those characteristic of Mary Lou, Charlie, and Carol have resulted in part from broad demographic and societal change. These trends are discussed in greater detail below.

***Demographic Trends.*** There are at least three major demographic trends that have influenced the structure of the family: (1) increased average longevity; (2) smaller distances between generations coupled with declining fertility; and (3) the widening gender gap in mortality rates. Ample statistical evidence underscores the first demographic trend—increased average longevity.[1] As indicated in chapter 2, the segment of the population age sixty-five and over has grown twice as fast as the rest of the population in the last twenty years. Moreover, the oldest age group (those aged eighty-five and over) represents the fastest-growing segment. As one consequence, the membership profile of the family has become more heavily weighted at the older ages, or "top heavy."[2] Families in later life today have more older family members than in the past. In fact, it is not unusual for a middle-aged couple to have more surviving parents than children. Given this scenario, it is increasingly probable that families will be required to provide even more care to larger numbers of elderly members.

A decrease in the age distance between generations, coupled with declining fertility, also influences family life.[3] Four generations can now be conceived in the time it used to take for only three, a phenomenon that has been termed "generational acceleration." As a consequence, children of the aged are themselves old and may also be experiencing functional decline associated with age. As many as 10 percent of those age sixty-five or over have at least one child who is also at least sixty-five. This change in family structure raises new care questions: Will old children be able to provide care for their very old parents? Will young or middle-aged children be capable of caring for multiple older generations?

Generational acceleration also influences the individual's conception of age and generation. Simply knowing a person's age no longer automatically indicates the person's generation. People of the same chronological age may be members of different generations while persons of different ages may be members of the same generation. Consider yourself and others you know. At forty-five, are some of your friends grandparents and others still attending elementary school PTA meetings?

In addition, people are generally having fewer children. There is some concern that this decrease in family size will result in a smaller pool of children available to provide support to the elderly, and further decrease the proportion of young family members to those that are older. The implication is that fewer relatives will be available to care for increasing numbers of older family members.

A third demographic trend affects family life of older adults: the widened gap in mortality between men and women. This gap has resulted in a seven-year gender differential in general life expectancy, favoring women. As a result, the majority of the very old population are women, in and outside of the institutional setting: "The world of the very old is a world of women, both in society and within families" (Hagestad, 1986, p. 147). Thus, the majority of those requiring care are women. Later in the chapter we will see that women are also the most likely candidates for providing care to elderly relatives.

***Social Trends.*** In addition to these demographic trends, two broad societal trends influence the family: (1) the changing social roles of women in the world of work and (2) variations in family form. Women's labor-force participation is increasing at all age levels, with large numbers of women in the middle-age range—those most often responsible for care of elderly family members—working for pay outside the home. There is some concern that this employment picture will limit the family's ability to care for its elderly members. However, little evidence is available to support this argument. Rather, evidence suggests that women are organizing their work lives around elder-family-care responsibilities, much as they do in periods of child bearing and rearing (see Hagestad, 1986). It appears that labor-force participation may fluctuate while family care of the elderly continues.

The emergence of variant family forms resulting from divorce, remarriage, and alternative lifestyles represent a second societal trend. These changes give rise to a whole new series of family relations and support issues.

Consider the following dilemmas: Are divorced persons responsible for the care of their ex-in-laws when no one else is available? Are natural children more responsible for parent care than stepchildren? Is a child of divorce (who has not had contact with a parent for fifty years) responsible for that parent's late-life care? Should midlife-divorce alimony payments cover elder-care costs—elder-support payments? These questions would not have been posed thirty years ago, but are not uncommon today. The impact of divorce on family patterns of support and exchange can be severe and far reaching.[4] Economic and other forms of assistance may be halted entirely, resulting in an inability on the part of divorced children (particularly women) to care for their elderly parents. In addition, the complex kin networks resulting from divorce and family reconstitution may blur family relationships, and cause ambiguity surrounding who is responsible for older relatives. As a result, the structure of these families and of family relationships in late life may become quite confusing to nursing home personnel.

***Family Interaction.*** Just as family forms vary in later life, the interaction patterns and internal supports that families share vary from family to family. The national patterns or norms of family interaction provide a framework for working with more specific, individual situations. Our discussion of family-interaction patterns is organized around two critical areas for those working with older adults: (1) family availability and contact and (2) family functions and tasks. These provide a background for later discussion of family caregiving. Caregiving represents a very important function of the family in late life, one that endures both within the community and after an elder's move to a hospital or nursing home.

*Family Availability and Contact.* The degree to which family members are available to and have contact with their older members in the community has implications for their involvement and contribution in the long-term-care setting. If relatives are not available or do not have contact with their elderly members prior to institutionalization, they will probably not become closely involved after institutionalization. Conversely, if the family is actively involved in elder care prior to nursing home placement, it will most likely want to continue involvement following placement. Thus, background information on family availability and contact can be very useful to the mental health consultant in designing residents' care and treatment plans.

*Marital Status and Living Arrangements.* Marital status and living arrangements of the elderly vary by gender and age. Older men are much more likely to be married and living with a spouse than are older women. Women, particularly very old women, are most likely to be widowed and living alone. The 1980 census revealed that 30 percent of the community-dwelling elderly lived alone, 53 percent lived with a spouse, 15 percent with children or other relatives, and 2 percent with nonrelatives (see figure 8.1). When considering only those age seventy-five and above, a larger proportion live alone (39 percent).

Older adults prefer to live independently, but near their children—what is sometimes termed "intimacy at a distance."[5] In 1975, only 18 percent of the noninstitutionalized elderly lived with their children. However, 52 percent of the elderly lived either with or within ten minutes of a child. Among those who lived alone, half of those with children lived within ten minutes of them. Moreover, a full three-quarters of the elderly with children either lived with them, or within thirty minutes of them. Approximately 20 percent of the elderly had no children.

*Frequency of Interaction.* How often do older parents see their children? In 1975, more than half of those over sixty-five with children had seen at least one child the day they were interviewed or the day before, while over three-quarters had seen a child in the past week. In addition, the proportion who had not seen a child in the past month or more was only 10 percent. Thus, older adults generally see some of their adult children often.

*Siblings and Other Relatives.* Most older adults have and see their siblings. Approximately eighty percent of persons over the age of sixty-five have at least one living sibling, while 70 percent of those age seventy-five or over report at least one surviving brother or sister. In reference to the frequency with which they see one another, one-third of those with siblings report having seen them in the past week while more than one-half report having seen one in the past month. Widowed persons and those who have never married are more dependent on their siblings than married persons and are more likely to see them. Thirty percent of the elderly also report having seen some relative other than a child, grandchild, or sibling in the previous week. For childless elderly, this other relative is most often a niece or nephew.

***Summary.*** The dominant family form for older Americans is the modified extended family, which is made up of immediate family members, nephews, nieces, and other persons related either by blood or marriage. In general, older adults live close to other family members and have frequent contact with them. When working with the elderly and their families, it is important to know who makes up the family and where they live, as well as what it is that they do. The following section explores the role of the

**Fig. 8.1**

Living Arrangements
Community-Dwelling Elderly

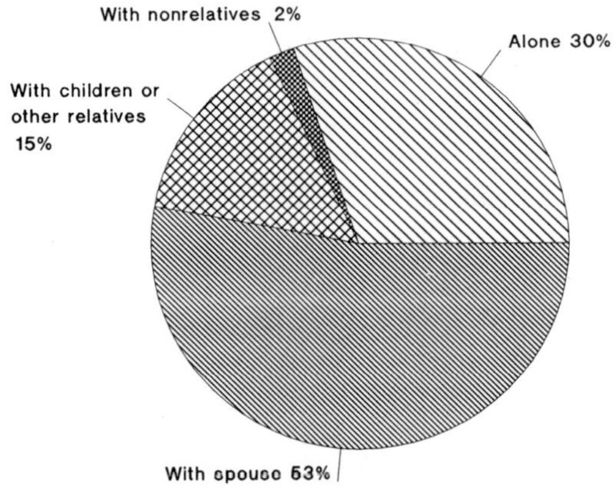


Source: U.S. Census Data (1980).

family in later life, emphasizing (1) select developmental tasks faced by the family in late life and (2) the functions of the family.

## FAMILY TASKS AND FUNCTIONS

The functions that families perform do not cease to exist after an elderly family member is institutionalized. However, the manner in which the functions are carried out may be altered in this new setting. Knowledge of family functions and tasks prior to institutionalization can aid in understanding their translation into the nursing home environment.

***Developmental Tasks of Later Life.*** One perspective on family functioning focuses on the developmental tasks of the family. These tasks represent major issues or processes that families must resolve in order to master the changes that life presents. In later life, these tasks are multiple, complex, and difficult to enumerate completely. They emerge as the family changes over time, and are constantly modified by the interplay of forces inside and outside the family.[6] However, there are what may be termed normal processes, or tasks, that many older families experience as elders become increasingly debilitated. These tasks are often confronted by families simultaneously and include the following:

1) Grieving for losses in the elder's independence and functioning, as well as the loss of the roles this elder once assumed and the functions he once performed.
2) Maintaining family integrity/identity in the face of vast change in the form and function of the family.
3) Coping with the physical and emotional demands of caring for a dependent elder, as well as caring for the needs of all other family members.
4) Managing resources that may be fixed or diminishing (as often occurs at retirement, or when demands on the resources increase); such resources may be in the form of assets, energy, time, or human labor.
5) Supporting individual growth and development of all family members (children, teens, adults, and the aged) in the face of multiple competing demands that erode self-esteem and thwart personal growth.
6) Providing increasing and continual emotional and physical support to elderly family members as well as to other family members.

These tasks represent ways in which the family fulfills its basic functions. Primary among these functions are socialization and fulfillment of the physical and emotional needs of family members. These functions differ somewhat in nature and focus in an older family (that is, one with a dependent elder) than in a younger family.

***Socialization.*** In the young family, socialization is geared toward guiding children and young adults to be responsible members of society—tasks for which there exist common knowledge and established norms for families to follow. Socialization in the context of the older family focuses on other life situations. Families become concerned with such issues as, What is the appropriate way to deal with the demands of an increasingly dependent elder? How do you cope with competing demands for resources from several generations? How do you provide long-term care for a dependent elder in the home? Who should assume primary responsibility for a dependent elder?

The need for education and guidance in these individual and family circumstances has a more recent history, and normative strategies and role models to aid in dealing with them are lacking. Circumstances like these have been termed cultural lags—aspects of life for which there are no clear culturally shared expectations.[7] Family members find themselves in a situation without historical precedent or cultural guidance on which to rely. As a result, older families struggle with their circumstances, often without sufficient knowledge or experience to guide their decisions.

***Emotional Support.*** Emotional needs are what hold families together. All family members have emotional needs that other family members can usually fulfill. However, older family members may have additional emotional needs. While most people have a basic need to feel loved, respected, and secure, older family members may find their needs colored by their increasing dependence and inability to reciprocate assistance as they have in the past. As such, elders may feel inadequate, unproductive, and burdensome. In these circumstances it is important for the family to assure the elders that they are loved and still vital family members.

***Physical Support.*** Physical care needs of the older family also differ from those of the younger family. The focus of care shifts from dependent children to increasingly dependent elderly members (although other family members may require physical assistance as well). Further, care in an older family is most often provided by middle-aged and older family members who may themselves be experiencing health problems, activity limitations, and difficulty dealing with competing demands from multiple generations. Often referred to as the "middle-generation squeeze," these individuals are faced with the challenge of simultaneously meeting the needs of both older and younger generations, while maintaining their own individual development and growth. Jean's experience illustrates this squeeze.

---

Jean sits feverishly knitting in the care givers–support group. "Boy, I can sure tell you, they're 'right on' when they call us the 'sandwich generation.' Between Tommy whining about no school today, what can he do, and Dad screaming about how the aides aren't doing his exercises, I feel as sticky and creamed over as peanut butter. I can't do anything but get chewed up or pulled apart."

---

Provision of support to the elderly is a central task of the older family that affects all members—those providing the support, those receiving the support, and the family as a whole. This process of care giving almost invariably precedes the elder's move to an institution and may have implications for the elder's care plan following placement. Before proceeding to a more detailed discussion of caregiving and family decision making, consider the true/false quiz below. Following this exercise we will address the implications of these issues for family care and involvement in the long-term-care setting.

*Family Support and Caregiving Quiz*

| | *True* | *False* |
|---|---|---|
| 1. Families provide 50 percent of the care to dependent elderly in the community. | — | — |
| 2. More than twice as many bedfast/homebound elderly are cared for at home than in institutional settings. | — | — |
| 3. Men are more likely to be caregivers than women. | — | — |
| 4. For married elderly, spouses are usually the primary caregiver. | — | — |
| 5. Financial strain is reported by caregivers more often than emotional or physical strain. | — | — |
| 6. Most caregivers experience some burden or psychological stress. | — | — |
| 7. Children caregivers are more likely than spouse caregivers to provide a variety of tasks ranging from transportation to bathing and clothing their dependent elder. | — | — |

8. Choice of caregiver generally follows a principle of substitution with spouses first, followed by children, relatives, and nonrelatives. ___ ___
9. Dependent childless elderly who are not married do not have anyone to serve as caregiver. ___ ___
10. Family history, family values, and past filial conflict patterns can influence choice of caregiver. ___ ___

## CAREGIVING FAMILIES

The family is the primary support resource for the elderly. It has been estimated that families provide between 80 and 90 percent of the care to dependent elderly in the community (see Shanas, 1979). More than twice as many bedfast/homebound elderly are cared for at home than in institutional settings. The following section provides a discussion of family caregiving in the community—who the caregivers are, what they do, and how they experience their roles. This information enables caregivers in the institution to understand the experiences of their community-dwelling counterparts better. Many of the relatives of institutionalized elderly have been caregivers for a substantial period prior to the nursing home placement.

***Who Are the Caregivers?*** Determination of the primary caregiver generally follows a principle of substitution with reference to closeness of family relationship.[8] For married elderly, spouses generally fill the primary caregiver role first, followed by adult children (who are most often daughters), other relatives, and finally nonrelatives (see figure 8.2). For childless elderly this pattern is altered somewhat. For childless marrieds, spouses are most often the primary caregivers; for unmarrieds, it is usually another relative (such as a sibling, niece, or nephew).

Family history, established family ties, geographic availability, past and present conflict patterns, and the value system of the family may also influence the choice of primary caregiver. For example, family history may dictate that a particular family member (for example, the eldest daughter) provides care for aged family members as such care becomes necessary. Deviation from this pattern would violate family norms and could cause family conflict and confusion. The quality of family relationships may affect caregiver choice as well. For example, if certain family members have had distant, cold, or conflict-ridden relationships with their elders in the past they may be less willing to provide direct or indirect care to them, particularly if conflict patterns become reactivated in old age. Local family members may be chosen by convenience. Finally, the value system of the

**Fig. 8.2**

Caregiver's Relationship to Elderly Recipient

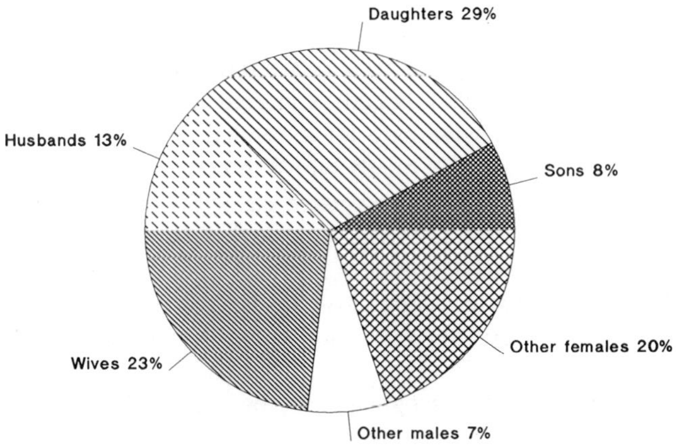


Source: Subcommittee on Human Services of The Select Committee on Aging, House of Representatives (1987).

family may influence the how, when and by whom care is provided to dependent elderly members. A family with strong familism feelings may be more likely to provide care than one that places less value on the family's ability to care for its own. In sum, several factors influence caregiving decisions in families, including the relationship of the caregiver to the care recipient, the availability of alternative social supports, and family history and value systems.

***Nature of the Care.*** What is it that care givers do? They provide both instrumental and emotional assistance to the care recipient.[9] Instrumental assistance can range from simple perfunctory care (such as assistance with shopping or transportation), to more personal physical care (such as grooming and feeding). As an individual becomes increasingly debilitated he or she requires more comprehensive care for extended periods of time. Caregivers who have the closest filial bonds with the care recipient are also most likely to provide the most comprehensive care. Spouses invest the greatest amount of time in the caregiving role and perform the widest variety of tasks, ranging from management of finances to bathing and clothing their spouse. Caregivers who are less close (other relatives and nonrelatives) generally perform perfunctory care, and spend far less time doing so.

***Impact of Caregiving.*** Caregiving can be stressful for all parties involved, no matter what their relationship to the elder. Emotional strain is most often reported by caregivers, followed by physical strain and to a lesser extent financial strain. The level of strain experienced is related to the closeness of the bond between the caregiver and care recipient, with spouses generally reporting the greatest strain, followed by children, other relatives, and friends/neighbors (see figure 8.3). Caregivers also report that caregiving has negatively affected their lives, by requiring them to give up leisure time and opportunities to socialize. Additional caregiving stresses on the family include (1) demands on time, spent in actually performing tasks and in managing responsibilities; (2) demands on space in the home; (3) demands on financial resources, both in providing quality care for the elder and in possibly giving up income from outside employment; (4) psychological stress; and (5) physical stress, particularly for caregivers who are old themselves.[10] The experience of burden in caregivers has been the focus of extensive study.[11] The findings from this research indicate that (1) most if not all caregivers experience burden; (2) burden can take many forms (subjective and objective); (3) burden is a complex construct requiring careful conceptualization and measurement; and (4) stress and burden may be decreased through supportive and educational interventions.

A new perspective on caregiving examines caregiver actions in terms of

**Fig. 8.3**

## Caregivers Reporting Caregiving as Emotionally Difficult

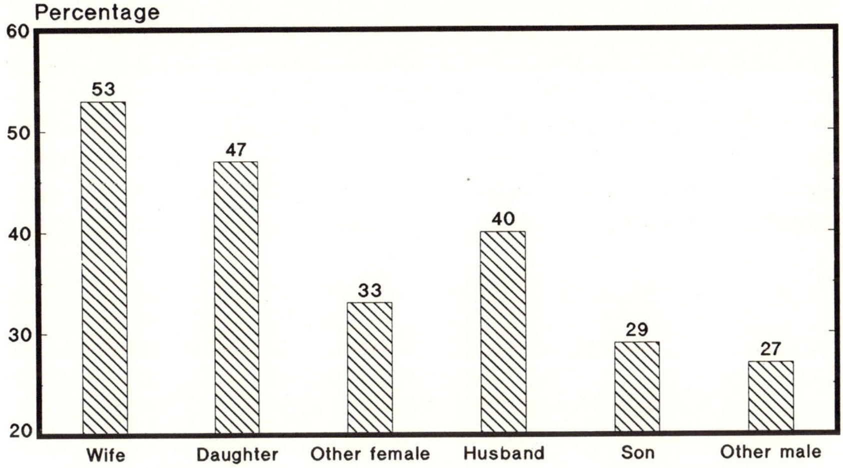


Source: Subcommittee on Human Services of The Select Committee on Aging, House of Representatives (1987).

their purpose rather than as tasks themselves. In a recent study, Bowers (1987) identified five categories of caregiving: anticipatory, preventative, supervisory, instrumental, and protective (see table 8.1 for definitions and examples of each type). In this study, instrumental care was reported by caregivers as the least important, while protective caregiving was deemed most important. Essentially invisible, protective caregiving requires that caregivers use idiosyncratic insights and tact in order to protect elders from the awareness that they are being cared for, and to maintain the older parent–younger child relationship. Unfortunately, as a function of their job requirements and relatively brief history with each resident, protective caregiving is rare among paid caregivers. Problems may result in the long-term-care setting from these differing family and staff care goals. It is important that both parties become aware of one another's goals and resources so that an effective and mutually satisfying care plan can be devised. Bowers (1987) describes this as a need for greater collaboration between family and staff, wherein the staff and family can benefit from each other's expertise and experience. The mental health consultant can aid in clarifying overlapping and distinct contributions.

TABLE 8.1: Caregiving Activities Defined by Purpose

| *Category of Caregiving* | *Definition/Example* |
| --- | --- |
| Anticipatory | decisions or behaviors based on the possible future needs of the care receiver (e.g. turning down a new job requiring relocation) |
| Preventative | activities aimed at preventing illness, injury or deterioration of the dependent elder (e.g. changing the physical environment to enhance safety) |
| Supervisory | active and direct involvement of the caregiver, which is recognized as caregiving activity (e.g. making sure that the elder is taking his medication properly) |
| Instrumental | hands-on caregiving of doing for, providing, giving, and assisting (e.g. preparing meals, shopping) |
| Protective | protect the parent from the consequences of that which could not be prevented, consequences which could damage the elder's self-image (e.g. eating a meal prepared by an elder with cognitive and sensory impairment in order to protect his/her self-image) |

Source: Bowers (1987).

***Summary.*** Family members serve several functions and support one another across the lifespan in a variety of ways. Long-term care of older adults has become a normative experience for individuals and families. However, as older family members become increasingly impaired and dependent, a shift occurs in the types of support required by the elder and in filial or informal patterns of assistance. Even the terminology used to describe family relationships alters; *care recipient* and *caregiver* replace the parent-child or other-elder dyad. Helping patterns are altered in four major ways:[12]

1) The required assistance time frame changes from acute and intermittent to long term and constant.
2) The degree to which the family is involved on a constant day-to-day basis increases.
3) Assistance flows more clearly from the family to the elder, rather than being balanced and reciprocal as it is throughout much of adult life.
4) The nature of the tasks that are performed change from being peripheral (e.g. occasional transportation) to more central (e.g., direct household intervention, personal care).

In general, more types of care are needed, for longer periods of time, and more often. In addition to these direct forms of assistance, an increasingly important function of the family is to serve as a mediator or liaison betweeen the aged and bureaucratic structures. Families directly meet the needs of their elderly members, and also identify needs for other institutions to address.

Whether viewed in terms of the physical tasks involved or the purpose of the activities carried out, caregiving represents an increasingly burdensome enterprise for the caregiver and the entire family. Given the demanding and stressful nature of this support, it is impressive that families continue to assume this responsibility. Nonetheless, families are often unable to maintain their dependent elders in the community indefinitely. At some point the demands on personal, family, and even community resources become too great to assure optimal care and well-being of the dependent elder and their caregivers outside of an institutional setting. At this time, families are faced with new tasks. They must recognize their limits to continue care of the elder in the home. They must cope with several issues at once: the distress of placing a loved one in an institution; the stigma associated with institutionalization; and the guilt and shame of being unable to care for their own flesh and blood. The time has come for the family to begin to move toward alternative help.

## THE FAMILY DECISION

The admission of an elder to a nursing home is a difficult task for most families. The people who make this decision are generally family members who have been actively engaged in the elder's care. Smith's research indicates that the typical decision maker is a married daughter who has a high-school education and is currently employed or retired (Smith, 1984). These individuals are the "consumers" of nursing home care and the "gatekeepers" between the community and the institution. They struggle to find appropriate care for their elders when they can no longer provide it themselves. In their distress, such families often fail to explore all care options or significantly involve the future nursing home resident in the decision.

Families' motivation to maintain responsibility for their elders is apparent; their ability to find sound solutions is less evident. Perhaps it would be helpful to look at how these families make their decisions, and the obstacles they encounter along the way.

***The Decision Process.*** Crises, such as a significant deterioration in the health of the elder (hospitalization, more than likely) or a loss in informal supports, are the events that most often push families to consider nursing home placement.[13] In fact, preliminary results from the 1985 National Nursing Home Survey (see Hing, 1987) found that 75 percent of residents transferred to the nursing home from another health facility. Families who have already restructured many aspects of their lives to meet the demands of daily support for a loved one, may not be physically or emotionally able to increase care as their elder's dependency escalates.

---

Sixty-year-old Sarah accumulated dental and medical expenses herself as her stress overwhelmed her. For six weeks after her sister Ellen was hospitalized with hip and pelvic fractures, she struggled to decide whether to retire to Florida with her husband or to insist on resuming the responsibility for daily meals and companionship for Ellen. Ellen was barely ambulatory before her hospital stay. Sarah's own back problems forced her to acknowledge she could not care for her sister, and that she had to take care of herself and her husband. She guiltily sought nursing home options and made plans for Florida.

---

When crisis forces a care decision, most families seek advice and do not examine a wide range of options. Research indicates that most families make decisions in a very short intense period of time, often less than one month.[14] Yet, families don't want more time since they are unable to determine feasible alternatives and have been counseled to accept nursing home placement by respected "authorities." Most frequently the decisive advice comes from a physician, or a social worker. Families frequently lack experience in systematic decision making and often fail to explore the formal support alternatives available. This omission may stem from three sources: a lack of knowledge of service availability; a lack of experience in making joint parent-child decisions; and the disabling emotional chaos produced by the personal conflict the decision itself represents.[15]

*Information Needs.* The first obstacle to sound decision making—lack of information—seems easily remedied, but most families today have had little or no prior experience with elder care. They have few family role models to demonstrate how to meet the needs of an increasingly dependent aging family. Families believe in managing as best they can. Sources of information and support are not "common knowledge." It is not always evident to caregivers that others may be available to help—even just for a few hours. Programs providing such assistance—Meals on wheels, "friendly visitors," and respite centers—do not advertise on television. And it is not unusual for people to fail to consider the Yellow Pages as a source of assistance. Community education is seldom directed toward showing families how to use the directories, guides, and handbooks to elder services, or how to apply this information to their specific situation. Since the choice of a nursing home is best made from a well-informed set of alternatives, it is important that mental-health professionals make certain that information is available.

*Problem-Solving Skills.* The second obstacle to sound decision making is families' lack of skill, experience, or confidence in family problem solving. When families have not prepared in advance for their health and resource changes, they feel pressed for fast action. Too often elders themselves are excluded from the search for care because of family members' reluctance to add problems to their loved ones' already distressed circumstances. Without guidance or prior experience with such long-term-care decisions families cannot weigh their options fully. Instead, they rely on the advice of their physician, social workers, or clergy who have provided counsel at other difficult times. While these professionals may be very helpful, each family must seek its own understanding of the situation and special set of values in order to make a sound decision. Often poor problem-solving skills are further eroded by the third obstacle, emotional turmoil.

*Emotional Chaos.* Faced with pressing change, families may struggle with loyalties, doubts, need for relief, and fear or guilt. These disabling conflicts force family members to seek remedies and absolution from familiar authority figures rather than seek their own answers from reflection and deliberation. Thus, making the decision is usually not a rational step-by-step process, but a series of emotionally charged reactions. Consider the example of Sis.

---

Sis, as she was known to all her friends, had taken her mother in to her home to die two years ago. Her mother's neurological deterioration had lingered on month after month. While Sis believed that she had a calling to care for her mother in this way (giving up most of her work and her social activities out of the home), the daily, hourly call upon her to feed, bathe, toilet, love, and distract her mother became overwhelming. Friends and local nursing agencies repeatedly suggested that additional assistance and relief in the home would make Sis's life more tolerable, but she took her caretaking role as a spiritual mission. Finally after twenty-seven months, the intractable pain that her mother was suffering around the clock became more than Sis herself could stand and she called the local nursing home inquiring about room availability, costs, and so on. When she described her mother's needs the intake worker acknowledged that she was more than eligible. The usual wait for a bed at this county facility was several weeks, but miraculously a place was to become available at the end of the week. The incredibly fast answer to her long-delayed request for help appeared to Sis as a definitive sign that she was destined to "give up her Mother." Within three days Sis's mom had moved and Sis began to wonder at her own inability to see and prepare for this change months before.

---

Most families fear involving the deteriorating elder in the discussion of nursing home options. They seek rapid resolution because they are unclear about the nature of available help. In this situation, a counselor can be most helpful by creating an environment for the family that is conducive to making a clear-headed decision. It has been found that satisfactory adjustment of both the elder and the family are greatly enhanced when the elder participates in the choice and all alternatives have been thoroughly examined. Inadequate information, lack of experience, and heightened anxiety and guilt can contribute to a precipitous, and less-than-adequate experience. Within the time constraints, and emotional pressures of this crisis, families need the information and support to explore choices together skillfully rather than merely make do with an offered solution.[16]

***Who Helps Plan for Nursing Home Care?*** Personnel most likely to participate with the family in the decision-making process include the family physician, hospital social-service personnel, and the admissions staff of the long-term-care facility. They all can contribute to encouraging early planning for elders who are becoming increasingly dependent. Clearly, it is better to plan ahead but the fact that nursing home placement is distasteful to most families leads to procrastination.

Physicians appear to have the greatest influence in the final decision to seek placement. As the person in charge of predicting the patient's medical future and prognosis, they are best able to determine the medical care required. Individual physicians have varying approaches to their patient responsibility. This personal/professional perspective will determine the counseling strategy used. Mental health collaboration with doctors often modifies physicians' advice giving from a prescriptive to an educative mode. Enabling physicians and social workers to recognize and support families working through their own decisions is one route to more effective and emotionally sound family transitions.

Within the nursing home, social-service personnel take the lead in communicating with families considering placement. However, all personnel, from nursing staff to dishwashers, contribute to the impressions families use in making caregiving decisions. In their roles as "surrogate family members," staff often have the most daily contact with elders. Families will carefully look at staff behavior in weighing the intangible qualities of a facility.

Ultimately, families make choices based upon a variety of nursing home features. Many guides are available to assist in the evaluation of nursing home adequacy.[17] Since families often make decisions immediately before admission, their contact with the staff begins with the decision phase. Thus, it is important that the staff be prepared to work as a team and collaborate with families in the decision and transition process. Additional skills in contributing to collaborative decision making may be helpful for both the staff and family. In addition, opportunities to increase mutual understanding of each other's experience are desirable.

During this time of transition, new issues face the older family. They must learn to accept their decision, deal with the guilt and grief that often surround the decision, reorganize their homes and lives without the elder immediately present, and plan for their continued involvement with the elder in the long-term-care setting.

## FAMILIES IN THE LONG-TERM-CARE SETTING

According to the *1976 Survey of Institutionalized Persons* (U.S. Department of Commerce, 1978),[18] most elderly living in institutions have family. In reference to next of kin, approximately 55 percent have a child, 8 percent a spouse, and 15 percent a sibling. Of those aged sixty-five to seventy-nine, nearly 28 percent report no family, while 38 percent of those over eighty report none. Preliminary data from the 1985 National Nursing Home Survey indicate an even higher proportion of nursing home residents having children (63 percent). This proportion increases with age and is greater for women (66 percent) than for men (56 percent).[19] Of all nursing home residents surveyed, approximately 62 percent received daily or weekly visitors, while only 13 percent received no visitors, and 25 percent received visitors with some other frequency. Not only do institutionalized persons receive visitors, but these visitors are often family members: 7 percent were visited by spouses, 50 percent by children, 51 percent by other relatives, and 36 percent by nonrelatives (see figures 8.4 and 8.5) (total exceeds 100 percent because multiple responses were possible). Several factors are associated with frequency of nursing home visitation, including (1) shorter distances that the visitors must travel (proximity), (2) close kinship relationships between the visitor and resident, and (3) a shorter length of residence in the facility.[20]

***Family Involvement.*** The literature suggests that families are very interested in being involved in the lives of their elderly institutionalized members. For example, one study found that 83 percent of the families wanted to participate in a program to help their elder. Sixty-five percent were interested in meeting the staff, 53 percent said they would attend classes on aging, and 47 percent reported that they would welcome advice on how to have productive and enjoyable visits. In another study, family members volunteered for an educational program that provided instruction on ways to participate with their institutionalized elder, and contracted for certain types of involvement with them. In general, families sought interactions with their relative that stressed family cohesion/connectedness, rather than involvement with the staff or the facility.[21]

Although families want to help, their involvement may be limited by the policies of the long-term-care facility. A recent study found that institutional family-care policies sensitive to the needs of the family had the greatest positive impact on family relations. Institutional policies that extended services to families, included families in facility activities, and made

Fig. 8.4

## Nursing Home Visitors
### Type of Visitor

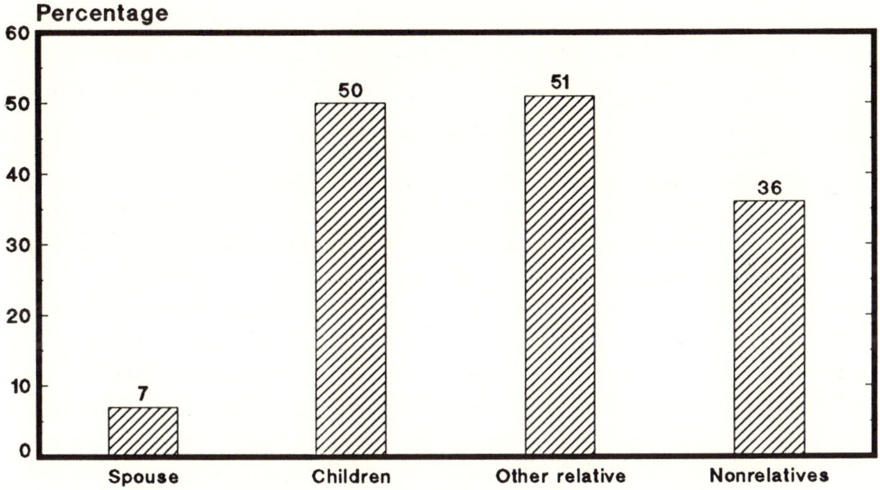


Source: National Center for Health Statistics (1979).

Fig. 8.5

## Nursing Home Visitors
### Frequency of Visits

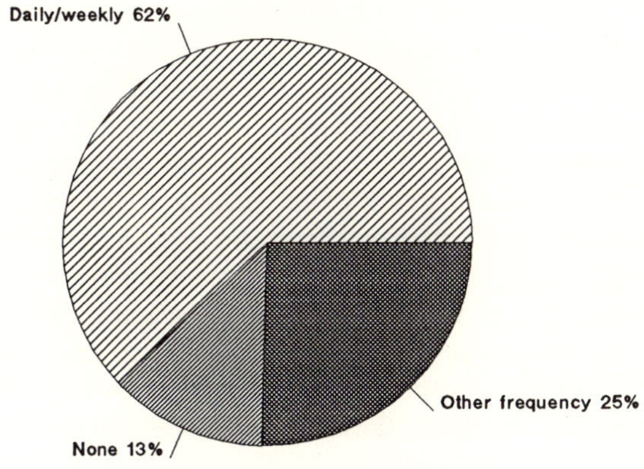


Source: National Center for Health Statistics (1979).

regulations with the family's well-being in mind, were associated with greater family integration (for example, the degree to which family members oriented their behaviors toward the interests of other family members). Conversely, institutional policies that did not actively consider the residents' families were associated with less family integration. In other words, families may only become involved to the degree that institutional policy allows them to.[22] This points to the need to include mechanisms in the institutional environment to recognize family contributions to care and reinforce effective involvement.

***The Family's Role in Long-Term Care or Role Ambiguity.*** As noted in chapter 1, ambiguity surrounds the roles the family should play in the long-term-care setting. Research on staff and family expectations concerning responsibility for tasks in the nursing home indicate discrepancies between the two groups.[23] Although both groups assign primary responsibility for technical tasks, such as housekeeping and cooking, to the nursing home staff, there is substantial variation in assigned responsibility for nontechnical tasks (for example, clothing selection). In general, where differences occur, both family and staff assign responsibility to themselves. In other words, families believe they should have the responsibility, and staff believe they should. The areas in which the most ambiguity was reported were (1) personalizing care, (2) clothing needs, (3) grooming, (4) assuring provision of care, and (5) providing reading materials. These discrepancies concerning care responsibilities in the nursing home may hinder effective cooperation of staff and family. This is one important area in which the mental health consultant can aid in defining problems and suggesting solutions.

***Positive Impacts of Institutionalization.*** Much of the literature concerning institutionalization concentrates on the negative aspects of this experience, and the dependency problems of the residents and their families. However, research indicates that institutionalization may have some positive effects on the elderly and their families. For example, one study found that residents who were visited more frequently had significantly lower psychosocial impairment, suggesting that visitation may enhance residents' well-being. Another study found that institutionalization was associated with enhancement or continuation of close family relationships. Reasons cited for these positive results were alleviation of preadmission strains on the family caused by the needs of the parent, and the improved health and well-being status of the parent resulting from the twenty-four–hour care and skill provided by the institution.[24]

The research findings noted in the previous paragraphs are consistent with Litwak's (1985) theory of shared functions and balanced coordination. As discussed in chapter 1, Litwak contends that the dependency needs of the elderly may be best met if there exists a proper balance between formal and informal systems of support. These two systems provide the support for which they are best suited. The formal system (nursing home) provides routine technical support, while the informal system (family) provides nonroutine, nontechnical, emotional supports, and highly personal biographical insights. In the case of the nursing home, the institution provides for and maintains the physical health of elderly residents, while the family emphasizes protective care and provides emotional support, which fulfills the unique needs of the elder (for example, bringing the resident items from home). Working as a team, the needs of all involved can be met satisfactorily.

In sum, a sizable proportion of nursing home residents have family who visit them, and who are willing and able to continue involvement in their lives. All nursing home community members—residents, family, staff—can benefit from family involvement. However, the linking of these community members requires guidance and education to work effectively. Planning and guidance in this identification and coordination effort is where the mental health consultant can be of great assistance.

## SUMMARY

Changes in the form of family life as well as in patterns of late-life family caregiving have been presented here. They illuminate the importance of providing responsive nursing homes as alternatives in long-term family care. Additional mental health attention is suggested to help families "care ahead" to meet the stresses surrounding admission and support of elder members in long-term-care facilities.

Most families provide life-long support through resources and relationships that have evolved into complicated networks of interdependence and assistance. The nature of this caring however is as idiosyncratic as the diverse personalities involved. We cannot make simple generalizations about the nature of families participating in long-term care or the roles they might play because the history of affection and assistance as well as the expectations of each individual interact to heighten variability in the nursing home setting. Family roles will be modified upon admission to long-term care, but affectionate exchanges and highly personal support can continue and even improve. Family concern and contributions can be strengthened with strategic mental health interventions.

There are several distinct points in the course of late-life family experience where mental health consultation can prove most helpful: (1) in confronting the role shifts and personal losses attached to increasing disability in a parent, sibling, or spouse; (2) in decision making around long-term-care alternatives; (3) in accomplishing the transition to long-term care; (4) in preparing for return to the larger community (that is, discharge planning); and (5) in coping with chronic or progressive problems. The consultant may directly consult with families, but more often the consultant will work with administrators and nursing-home personnel. Thus, the consultant is challenged to present a well-informed, and practical perspective on families, to encourage inclusion of families in care planning and institutional programming, and provide strategies for nursing home personnel to undertake to strengthen the family community. The importance of attending to families is generally appreciated, but variability of family needs and potential as well as the means for efficiently engaging with families is less-well understood. The process and outcomes of consultation around family issues are more fully discussed in the next chapter.

## NOTES

1. Our discussion of the demographic and social trends influencing the family in late life derive primarily from Aizenberg and Treas (1985), Horowitz (1985), and Seelbach (1984). Refer to these sources for a more detailed discussion of these trends and their implications for filial responsibility toward older family members.

2. See Hagestad (1986) for a thorough discussion of the roles and experiences of older female family members.

3. Hagestad (1981) provides a comprehensive discussion of the concept of "generational acceleration" and its impact on the family. Other issues of concern in intergenerational relations are also presented. Troll, Miller, and Atchley (1979) also discuss the "aging" of children in current society.

4. In a paper presented at the National Symposium of Alimony and Child Support, Smyer and Cooney (1987) discuss the implications of family relations across the lifespan for alimony and support decisions in later life. Cicirelli (1983) examines specific caregiving differences of divorced and nondivorced children.

5. The data reported in the following paragraphs on family relations and frequency of interaction derive from a study by Shanas (1979). These data were collected in 1975 on a national sample of noninstitutionalized elderly age sixty-five and over. More recent supportive data are reported by Blieszner and Mancini (1987) on smaller convenience samples in the southern United States.

6. Many textbooks on family development provide a discussion of developmental tasks and functions of the family across the lifespan. The present discussion of these concepts is based on the writing of Duvall (1971).

7. See Hagestad (1986) for a discussion of cultural lags and their impact on family experience.

8. Johnson (1983), Johnson and Catalano (1981), and Soldo and Myllyluoma (1983) report studies on family support of the elderly, including consideration of who fills the caregiver role.

9. See Johnson and Catalano (1983) for a report on the nature of family supports to the impaired elderly.

10. Cantor (1983) provides an interesting report of the dimensions of strain experienced by caregivers in the United States. Kingson, Hirshorn, and Cornman (1986) outline additional caregiving stresses placed on the family.

11. See Brody (1985); Hooyman, Gonyea, and Montgomery (1985); Kahan et al. (1985); Montgomery, Gonyea, and Hooyman (1985); Poulschock and Deimling (1984); Rakowski and Clark (1985); Zarit and Zarit (1982); Zarit, Orr, and Zarit (1985); and Zarit (in press) for a discussion of various aspects of caregiver burden and intervention research.

12. See Cantor and Little (1985) and Sussman (1985) for a more detailed discussion of social and family care of the elderly.

13. See Arling and McAuley (1983) for information concerning issues surrounding family vs. institutional caregiving.

14. See Smith (1984), Furse (1983), Johnson and Van Meter (1985a, 1985b) and Johnson and Werner (1982) for additional discussion of the selection of long-term-care facilities, and those who make that decision.

15. See Janis and Mann (1977) for elaboration of decision making in crises.

16. Johnson and Van Meter (1985a, 1985b) discuss points of support for family decision making.

17. Silverstone and Hyman (1983) and Cohen and Gans (1978) are two such useful guides written to aid families in making long-term-care decisions.

18. These data are reported in Tobin and Kulys (1981). More recent data from the 1985 National Nursing Home Survey (see Hing, 1987) are available for only a limited number of family variables. When possible, data from the 1985 source is cited.

19. These data derive from a preliminary report of the 1985 National Nursing Home Survey (NNHS) provided by Hing (1987). Complete reports of the 1985 NNHS are currently not available. Most data reported here refer to the 1977 National Nursing Home Survey (National Center for Health Statistics, 1979).

20. For further discussion of the influence of these factors on frequency of nursing-home visitation see Hook, Sobal, and Oak (1982).

21. See York and Caslyn (1977) and Miller, Linsk, and Pflaum (1986) for reports of their studies assessing family involvement in institutional settings.

22. See Montgomery (1982) for a more detailed discussion of the role long-term-care policy plays in family involvement.

23. Rubin and Shuttlesworth (1983) and Shuttlesworth, Rubin, and Duffy (1982) report on their studies examining family and staff role expectations in the nursing home setting.

24. See Greene and Monahan (1982) and Smith and Bengtson (1979) for more detailed descriptions of these studies and their findings.

# 9

# Consultation Strategies with Families

*Margaret D. Cohn*

> I've helped my four children getting started in nursery school, elementary school and summer camps. I've gone through their farewells before going off to college and trips overseas. None of these difficult parenting experiences was as emotionally trying as the recent experience I have had in helping my elderly father adjust to living in a residential facility for older persons.
>
> *Bernard Reisman, director of the Hornstein Program in Jewish Communal Service*[1]

## INTRODUCTION

Good nursing home care is a continuation of family life, not the end of it. Whether a resident has children or siblings nearby, or only long-distance special visits, the meaningful participation of helpful, healthy families is an important mental health goal for long-term care communities. The goal of this chapter is to describe strategies for improving family functioning in nursing homes.

Caring for families who care for residents is a relatively new and important element in nursing home services. As reviewed in chapter 8, changes in family functioning over the lifespan clearly affect the interpersonal, emotional, and economic resources available to older adults, both at home and "in a home." Family problems and family-staff conflicts are well recognized in the institutional setting, but specific preventative or therapeutic interventions for families of residents are rarely reported.[2] In contrast, community-based family caregivers have received considerable attention. Similarly, as noted in chapters 5, 6, and 7, individual assessment and treatment have been emphasized by researchers and clinicians.

This chapter builds upon the overview of elder-caring families, described in chapter 8, and considers the specific problems of families of institutionalized older adults. After discussing the limited attention given to nursing homes' families, we focus on their most common concerns. We then highlight the preparation and perspectives of personnel who work with families and existing family services in nursing homes. Next we point out two different consultative strategies, case centered and administrative, which are appropriate for approaching family problems. Finally, we focus on specific assessment and intervention strategies for family-centered care. This includes individual casework approaches, group programs, and institutional changes. Our suggestions emerge from familiar community-based interventions or well-accepted therapeutic efforts with individual residents, as well as the work that has been documented with families in the nursing home setting.

## FORGOTTEN FAMILIES

Specific problems faced by residents' families in nursing homes are receiving increasing attention: the disruptiveness of role changes; the conflicts generated in relinquishing caregiving responsibility; the unfamiliarity and bewilderment of approaching a new bureaucracy; the continuity of unresolved family issues; and the painful feelings of fear, guilt, powerlessness, and distrust that often accompany a relative's entry into a nursing home.[3] Despite greater attention, however, ways to work with families in this setting have only begun to be addressed.

---

Bob spent two hours every evening after work with his dad, cleaning up after the TV dinner, watching the news together, talking over the sports events of the day, and helping the ninety-two–year–old get ready for bed. Once a week he checked with the visiting nurse about his dad's condition and care and a couple of mornings a week he checked in with the aides to see if there were things his dad needed or he should know about. Bob ran his own distributing business, had a wife and three adult kids to worry over, and ran a staff of five people caring for his dad as well. He enjoyed the hours he spent with his dad, and worked well with all the community services available. But when Bob had a heart attack himself at sixty-one, Dad had to enter Fairway. Bob no longer had direct information from all the people working with his father. He missed seeing him on a daily basis. Bob and his wife argued repeatedly about the quality of the care given since many of the nurse's aides "weren't Americans." Talking to the social worker only made him more upset, because she repeatedly dismissed him with reassurances that everything now was fine. Things did not seem fine to him at all. If "the nursing-home family" could now do everything he had done before, what good was he? Bob found fault with most of the nursing staff, and didn't hesitate to tell them.

---

As this example illustrates, the family is a pivotal element in community-based long-term care, but is often neglected once older adults are institutionalized. Numeroff (1983) describes this family exclusion as the "identified patient syndrome." She notes the tendency of staff to view families as merely tangential to resident care. Although nursing home families are "the real consumers," they are "forgotten clients."[4] Family issues are often defined as irrelevant to resident concerns, and therefore, inappropriate targets for staff attention. However, not only the mental health of families, but also the residents' own longing for absent family may be unrecognized.[5] Thus some of the best collaborative outcomes for residents and their families are overlooked.

Systematic exploration of family needs and of effective ways to collaborate with families needs to be incorporated into practice in long-term care. In doing so, important concepts from community experience (such as peer support and family-group problem solving) can be initiated institutionally. Innovation in family care will draw on current information regarding older families and strategies for family counseling and group or system interventions.

## WHAT ARE FAMILY PROBLEMS?

Problems faced by families in nursing home settings include problems in maintaining hope, family connections, and resident dignity and control over the environment.[6] These problems are experienced by both families and residents and emerge most frequently at times of transition, that is admission, when significant deterioration in the resident's health occurs, or with impending death. Families are puzzled, in pain, inexperienced, and poorly informed about the roles, routines, relationships, and routes within the bureaucracy.[7] They need and may not know how to find information that can guide their "acculturation" to the nursing home. They are emotionally and often economically strained by the increasing dependence of their older relatives. They are often unskilled and lacking in confidence about how to retain their family integrity.

---

When Martha, (eighty-three), was admitted to the local nursing home following her spontaneous hip fracture, her two sisters anxiously conferred with each other but did not know how to reach anyone at the home or in Martha's home town to help others help her. Martha was widowed and childless and lived one-thousand miles from her sisters, but they had always used the phone and frequent visits to feel close to each other. Now the distance was impenetrable. Neither sister was strong enough to travel much anymore and yet they felt responsible and lonely for Martha. They had never even visited one of "those homes" and became increasingly agitated about their own helplessness. Finally they each called their own local minister to see if he knew what might happen to their sister and how they could find out and help. Indeed, the ministers not only guided the sisters to the nursing-home case worker and local nursing services and aging programs, but provided sensitive support for their continued caring and concern.

---

Thus, family problems found in nursing homes reflect the full range of family life issues: from strained finances to conflicted relationships, to inability to act in helpful ways.

Family difficulties appear to create trouble within the institution in a variety of ways. For example, recurrent financial delinquencies may indicate that a particular family is financially unprepared, or they may be troubled and resistant. The underlying family issue needs to be explored. Disruptive behavior by family members, such as drunken episodes, argumentativeness, misuse of other residents' property, and other emotional outbursts are easily labeled as family problems. They create difficulties for staff, residents, and other families. But the underlying issues of guilt over placing a parent or concern with how to communicate with a confused sibling are less often appreciated. Staff-family conflicts are extremely common, such as disagreements over lost items, or treatment schedules, or visitation. These may be seen as staff problems by the family and family problems by the staff. They are problems that deserve attention for both family and staff well-being. In addition, when staff performance and/or resident functioning appears affected by such differences, further attention to preventing as well as resolving these conflicts can be provided by an outside consultant.

## WHO IS THERE TO HELP FAMILIES?

The preparation and perspective of staff working with families are as important to problem resolution as the nature of problems themselves. Whether families demonstrate intolerable life-long patterns of overt conflict or predictable confusion and/or resistance to admitting a parent, the perspective and skills of staff are constantly tested. The diversity of personnel available to support families is important to understand.

It is worth noting that there is a far greater potential for family help than there is a reality. Community psychologists and psychiatrists are well prepared to work with families but are rarely called into nursing-home settings to provide service to residents, much less their families. Professionally prepared social workers and nurses have considerable training in family intervention. But staff performing these roles in nursing homes are rarely professionally trained. In many nursing homes, nurse's aides have the most day-to-day family contact while an administrative person, generally called a family service worker or family caseworker, is assigned the responsibility for admission procedures and family contacts.

***Family Caseworkers.*** The family caseworker bears the major responsibility for orienting and facilitating family interaction within the nursing home. Often these practitioners function like social workers but have little formal preparation for working with families and insufficient administrative or policy support for this role.[8]

A social casework approach to resident problems has historically focused on both individuals and their social-economic (family and/or institutional) environment. The social worker generally manipulates environmental conditions to support the needs of the "client" better. This social perspective contrasts strongly with both medical and psychological perspectives that examine intrapersonal dynamics to alter physical, cognitive, or emotional patterns for the "patient." Thus the untrained caseworker may have little skill in understanding or enacting many strategies when surrounded by medically oriented personnel.

The National Nursing Home Survey of 1977 (National Center for Health Statistics, 1979) found that social workers or social-work assistants were on staff in only a little over half of all nursing homes (see table 9.1). In the other 45 percent of homes we have to assume family casework is managed by nonprofessional, alternative, or untrained personnel. Even when professional social workers are on the staff their role as family advocates may be questionable.

TABLE 9.1: Percentage of Nursing Homes Employing Social Workers and/or Social-Work Assistants

| | *Full Time* | *Part Time* |
|---|---|---|
| Social workers | 16.4 | 30.1 |
| Social-work assistants | 4.8 | 3.7 |

n = 18,900 homes. Percentages do not add to one-hundred since multiple categories can apply and only homes employing such personnel are shown.

Source: National Center for Health Statistics (1979, p. 16).

Often social workers have been hired to assure regulatory compliance and thus reimbursement by Medicare and Medicaid programs. It is evident from table 9.2 that the availability of these personnel for counseling varies significantly according to the care level of the institution and, more importantly, its certification status; that is, Medicare–certified skilled-care facilities will be *required* to have social workers on staff or as consultants to complete routine social-evaluation procedures, rather than programmatic services. These patterns of staffing suggest that the employment of social-work consultants is undertaken to effect Medicare compliance, not necessarily to assure high-quality services.[9] Thus, families may be seriously underserved.

***Nursing Personnel.*** Nursing practice has emerged from patient-centered medical models of care, but has historically involved collaboration with family caregivers. Present staffing patterns in nursing homes, however, are weighted toward nursing assistants and aides with little training in family or environmental interventions. Registered nurses and nurses with advanced education and broader perspectives are found only in supervisory and administrative positions. These supervisors are sought out by families, but the day-to-day interactions occur among families and patient-centered aides. Thus the care perspective and job orientation most common to nursing personnel can be best described as individually oriented with a medical emphasis. This results in families' being considered as adjuncts to care, not as central.

***Summary.*** Most disciplines represented in nursing homes now prepare their practitioners to consider both the internal and the external environment in planning client care, and to address families and special groups as clients themselves. Social work has developed more complex models of

TABLE 9.2: Nursing Homes with Counseling Available by Social Worker or Other Mental-Health Personnel According to Skill Level of Facilities

| | *Skilled* | *Intermediate and Skilled* | *Intermediate* | *Not Certified* |
|---|---|---|---|---|
| Social Worker | 78% | 78% | 67% | 28% |
| Other mental health pers. | 36% | 41% | 28% | 17% |
| n | 3600 | 4600 | 6000 | 4700 |

Note: Percentages do not total one hundred since only homes with these services are shown.
Source: National Center for Health Statistics (1979, p. 11).

human behavior and intervention.[10] Psychologists have expanded their theories and practice to embrace a number of family-therapy models and nursing also practices holistic forms of individual care attending to environmental and family issues.[11] However, today's young professionals who have the greatest potential for assisting families are least likely to be found on the nursing home staff. They may be providing consultation. The staff, instead, are likely to be less formally educated caseworkers or caregivers who learn their roles and responsibilities for families "on the job" from older systems of practice.

Nursing homes, thus, embrace a mix of both social and medical perspectives, employing representatives of differing disciplines.[12] In this setting the apparent goal of both social and medical models is to support the resident, not the family. Therefore, introduction of a family-systems and/or psychological perspective will require explanation and reconciliation with different personnel views, as noted in chapter 3. The appropriate consultant can approach identified family issues at both the case-centered and administrative levels as discussed below.

## LEVELS OF FAMILY CONSULTATION

Minimal staffing, untrained staff, and client-centered philosophies are strong deterrents to the development of family interventions within nursing homes. Roberta Greene describes intergenerational forms of family treatment as being "in their infancy."[13] Certainly, application of these treatments within nursing homes is even younger, perhaps embryonic. A true "systems" perspective, which views resident problems as issues for the whole family, may appear novel to both nursing home staff and families themselves. Indeed, effective management of family concerns may require both case-centered and administrative changes. Both levels of consultation were discussed at length in chapter 3. In this section we address opportunities for consultative change at each level separately.

***Case-Centered Consultation.*** When a family's behavior interferes with resident care or when family needs and anxieties have not responded to previous attention, professional family intervention is needed. Here the consultant can work directly with the family or indirectly guide the staff in exploring and resolving family problems. Such a family situation is illustrated by the Rappaports described below.

---

Jerome Rappaport, (seventy-nine), was admitted to Fairway with minimal responsiveness to people or events in his environment. His forgetfulness had become hazardous at home where his daughter had cared for him and his two school-age grandsons. Ever since his wife died in 1981, Mr. Rappaport's daughter had very closely ordered his daily life and provided the same routine and activities he had known in his retirement with his wife. But his tendency to turn on all the lights and occasionally leave the wood stove open and lit became frightening. Although Jerome had visited Fairway before admission and had been included in discussions about moving, he became very quiet and "removed." On visits from his family he was more silent and "downcast" than ever and they, in turn, spent much time coaxing and cajoling him to tell them what was bothering him and attempting to get him to interact. They were worried that the decision to move had driven him crazy, they feared that he would not recover, and repeatedly expressed their concerns to the nursing and administrative staff. Reassurances that he was cooperating and progressively more active were rebuffed. Mr. Rappaport's daughter visited more frequently and could be seen pacing worriedly when she wasn't imploring some response from her dad. The family caseworker was unable to alter the daughter's self-criticism and anxiety.

---

New behaviors among family members will occur when expressed belief systems and well-rehearsed patterns of interaction are altered. In this example the goal of family consultation would be to identify these elements and plan for ways for staff members and family members to adapt to change. Clarification of how "the problem" is viewed by all participants as well as a good family process assessment is required to illuminate the target beliefs and interactive responses. A concrete, behavioral perspective helps define the problem and structure the family assessment in detail. We will return to this assessment process after introducing another consultative strategy for family support: administrative consultation.

***Administrative Consultation.*** Systems-level or administrative consultation has three potential products of benefit to families: (1) programs or protocols directly supportive of families; (2) strengthened practitioners who develop both family-centered and behaviorally sound programs; and (3) clarified policies that can alter the interaction patterns of groups within the institution, enabling the caregiving staff to collaborate more effectively with disrupted families. These changes involve the management of the institution as well as the community of families within the facility.

Administrative change is called for in two general cases: (1) when it appears that management or staff practices and family concerns are irreconcilable and escalating tensions appear between personnel and family members; or (2) when basic family support mechanisms appear inadequate.

Administrative support for changes in protocol or subcommunity practices is essential. Changes are very welcome if they proceed quietly, inexpensively, and without "making waves." This is not always possible. Therefore, documentation is needed of specific changes: what their benefits are, and what "costs" are involved in time, personnel, and other resources. An institutional assessment is a good place to start. Both individual-family data collection and institutional assessments may need to be designed by the consultant.

## FAMILY ASSESSMENT

Nursing home records are extremely useful when it comes to family data. Family caseworkers gather this information to meet legal requirements and to direct decision making to the appropriate, responsible family member, rather than to provide direction for counseling. Nursing-care records contain little family information, except occasionally noting visitors, family requests, outings or suggestions on the care plan from family.

Most family data are found in narrative form on the discharge planning reports, or on the face sheet of the resident records. Records may not provide complete biographical or interaction data, but they are a good place to start to avoid redundant inquiry. Typical family data are summarized below.

*Family Data Found in Nursing Home Records*

| | |
|---|---|
| Family composition: | Members, genealogical (not personal) relationship, address for spouse, children, parents, and sometimes siblings |
| Next of kin: | Family member who is responsible for family decision making (e.g., bills, medical issues, emergencies) |
| Family resources: | Often incomplete (including only data on family informant, and other nearby family members):<br>Savings, income, and investments of spouse/self<br>Time available for caregiving if resident discharged (caregiver specified)<br>Living arrangement of potential caregivers<br>Burial arrangements |

Family history: Marital history
Living arrangements prior to resident admission
Dates and cause of death of near relatives (parent, spouse, children)

Family visitation patterns: Who, when, general response of resident

Caseworkers may keep additional counseling records, but such records are usually anecdotal and individualistic. The regulatory demands upon social workers in nursing homes require descriptive quarterly discharge summaries, which define the limits of data obtained. The time demanded by these reports often precludes other record keeping. Therefore, the introduction of additional documentation may be met with understandable resistance.

Some caseworkers believe they have little opportunity to safeguard resident/family confidentiality—often at risk in the intimate interactive community of the home—if they document family interactions and observations. However, one of the most important contributions the caseworker can make toward facilitating family-staff communication is to complete and share good preadmissions and follow-up interview data. Staff respect for family confidences is most likely when staff roles in family support and collaboration are clear, and the rationale for open communication is explicit.[14] This communication can be improved first by clearly defining identified problems.

***Problem Definition.*** As noted earlier, nursing home personnel describe many issues as family problems while families often describe the same issues as management problems, staff problems, or resident problems. It is important to determine the following initially: What are the specific behaviors that are seen as difficult? Who is defining this as a "problem"? Who are the actors involved? What is the duration and extent of the situation?

The resident or the family rarely experience a problem as belonging to the whole family.[15] Thus, the consultant and consulter must explore very specifically what the problematic circumstances are, who is involved, and how a pattern of interaction among family members, resident, and staff can be further observed and approached. A family meeting together, "to share input," creates the opportunity to have the family involved in communication and problem solving and defining their own goals.[16] A family group interview may be planned with specific guidelines, objectives, and supervision. Such an interview constitutes both the family process assessment and the beginnings of family intervention.

***Family Process Assessment.*** Procedures for assessing family functioning and dynamics can be found in the literature on health practice with children and young families and in texts for family therapy practice.[17] In contrast, protocols for family assessment are very rare in the literature on aging or intergenerational therapy.[18] This contrasts sharply with the extensive development of individual gerontological assessment procedures reviewed in chapter 5.

Questions framing family interviews are provided below.[19] These are not totally structured. They afford an opportunity to organize data collection in a concrete, narrative form consistent with the social-work tradition, but efficiently concise in an effort not to overwhelm the recorder or reader.

*Family Assessment Questions*

1) What is functionally wrong with the resident (not just diagnoses, but functional restrictions)?
2) What is the family composition—geographical and genealogical positions?
3) How did the family decide to come and work on the problem? (Who initiated the discussion? What was the decision-making process? Who speaks for the group?)
4) What is "the problem"—according to each member of the family, including the resident?
5) What kind of change does each member expect? (How hopeful are they? What would "improvement" look like?)
6) What are the developmental needs of individuals and family groupings? (For example, are there issues of "middle-generation squeeze," or problems with the "children" planning their own retirement?)
7) Who is involved now in the resident's life?
8) How do family members see *each other* in relation to the resident? (What kind of relationship have they had; for instance, are they highly protective, critical and blaming, superreasonable, or removed?)
9) What events and circumstances led up to the admission?
10) How did the family try to solve similar problems before? (What did they try? Who was involved? Why did it fail—according to them?)
11) What kind of help was exchanged prior to admission?
12) How often are visits made? By whom?
13) What occurs on visits? (What is difficult? What is pleasant or gives pleasure?)

14) Who in the family makes plans for future needs? How and when?
15) Who in the family monitors staff performance or other care adequacy? How and when?
16) Who in the family helps with day-to-day personal care? How and when?
17) Who in the family can provide staff guidance, offering highly individual "biographical" information and personal items? How and when?
18) What kind of help do family members expect from the caseworker or other staff? (Do they want information, different routines, changed attitudes?)
19) How can expectations of help and change (i.e., the goal) be met? (Do family members expect to change themselves or only ask for others to act differently? What intermediate steps can be determined? What will be the measure of "success"?)

Since these data ideally are obtained in group family meetings, including the resident when cognitive impairment does not preclude meaningful participation, the *process* of managing family meetings deserves comment. It requires planning and skill. Family-therapy techniques provide the basis for approaching families in a straightforward problem-solving way.

Coworkers or a consultant and consulter jointly undertake such family meetings in order to assure attention to meeting process as well as content and to provide guidance for the consulter. Under most circumstances, when meetings involve more than four family members such collaborative leadership is important. The family interview will most often occur at the facility except when preadmission planning allows for a home visit to explore the placement issues fully. A meeting room where family and staff members can sit together in a comfortable circle will put people at ease and encourage dialogue. Herr and Weakland (1979) and Zarit and his colleagues (1985) suggest the following pointers for conducting family interviews:

1) Model open communication skills (e.g., good listening).
2) Be genuine and open, but not overinvolved.
3) Recognize that messages sent are not messages received—check and recheck differing understandings.
4) Observe family leadership and participation patterns.
5) Agree to disagree, and acknowledge family members right to see things differently.
6) Explore family history straightforwardly.
7) Make concrete, realistic, behaviorally described small suggestions as goals.

8) Mutually identify the events that trigger "the problem" and seek means to circumvent these.
9) Mutually find rewards for changed behaviors.

The skills involved in gathering data about complex family interactions can be directly applied to exploring institutional patterns. The assessor not only obtains diagnostic and baseline evaluative data in this process, but also initiates collaborative relationships essential to undertake change.

***System or Community Assessment.*** Determination of the nature and extent of family concerns within a specific nursing home will require the review of policy and program materials as well as talking with staff and families. Programs "on the books" are not necessarily as good as (or as bad as) they might appear. Interviews with differing participants particularly the administrator, the program leaders and family participants will provide concrete answers to the questions posed below.[20]

*Nursing Home Community Assessment Questions*

1) What is the specific community-wide issue? (Give several concrete examples.)
2) Which community or subcommunities are involved (i.e., families, or families and staff)?
3) What family-centered programs and resources are presently in place in this facility (e.g., preadmission groups, tours, new family groups, orientation programs, family-staff-introduction procedures and/or events, aging seminars, family information centers, buddy systems, joint-care planning conferences, "worry reports" to communicate family or staff concerns, family-shared events, staff in service on family needs, family-visiting rooms, a library of resources on aging and retiring families, family-photo boards)?
4) What are the institutional constraints or "red tape" that currently prevent change?
5) How flexible and open are the community or the subcommunities of the home to innovative programs?
6) What external or family-community pressures for or against change exist?
7) How can new practices be described and integrated with existing concepts of community behavior?
8) How can each community be involved in planning and implementing change?

9) What are the alternative ways the present community-wide need can be met or prevented?
10) What are the predictable costs of a systems change?
11) How will the community of interest know when change has been useful? What will be your measure of success?

In the process of exploring these issues a vast amount of data on the functioning of the facility are accumulated. The information makes it easier to discuss the importance of moving beyond individual-case-management issues to more systemic approaches. But we will start the next section dealing with case-specific interventions and move then to more systems-wide alternatives.

## INTERVENTIONS WITH FAMILIES

Present family interventions range from the most common (that is, counseling surrounding admissions) to the most rare (family-staff therapeutic collaboration).[21] Family counseling is often the *only* form of family intervention. It usually focuses upon orientation concerns, family expectations, and resident adjustment and health issues. Economic and other family-health issues are common problems as well. Caseworkers provide information about the facility, and about the predicted course of a resident's stay. They serve as problem solvers and community liaison in this counseling, but they are rarely prepared to offer structured family therapy. The consultant can either offer additional direct family-counseling assistance or provide guidance and supervision for on-site staff to upgrade their family-counseling skills.

In providing guidance and support for more extensive family counseling the consultant will assist the identified counselor in initiating the family assessment. As noted, this assessment is best begun in a family meeting, which also begins the process of family change.

During the first family meeting the documentation of past actions and their consequences (good and bad) can direct family attention to how family members have learned to be together. The description and verification of caring, caretaking, and problem solving can affirm individual worth and perhaps interrupt scapegoating. The illumination of problem characteristics, individual alienations, problem-solving efforts, and present goals provide the structure for the design of alternative new steps.

Following the family-assessment meeting a decision must be made whether to refer a family for additional family therapy or to carry out a specific support program surrounding a single problem. An on-site family-care plan involves articulating stepwise family goals and contracts for contingency management of target behaviors, events, or conditions. Only one problem at a time should be singled out for attention within the case plan, illustrating how to organize and simplify the problem-solving process for the family.

The *principles* of family problem solving and behavioral management should be highlighted for future applications with other family issues. The further involvement of family members, individually or together, is emphasized in this plan. For example, the problem faced immediately may be family adjustment to admission, but the way to deal with significant cognitive losses by the resident in the next few months or emerging financial disagreements among the siblings may be independently handled if the process is emphasized, rather than specific solutions offered. The following case illustrates the case consultation method, emphasizing a family interactive problem-solving approach.

---

Sarah Upton had been a resident in Fairway for four and a half years. She was ambulatory and managed some self-care but was very limited cognitively and had only minimal recognition of her children when they visited. Until seven months ago her husband was responsible for decision making and bill paying. He visited quite regularly but died rather suddenly and their daughter Jenifer Ryan assumed responsibility for her mother's affairs.

Jenifer lived thirty minutes from the home and had been visiting regularly on a weekly basis for the first six months after her dad died. However she stopped visiting and many of Mrs. Upton's bills remained unpaid. Frances Gorley, the social worker, called to remind Mrs. Ryan on three occasions with no success reaching her after the first call, and no resulting payments. Information in the files indicated that Mrs. Ryan had access to adequate money for support of her mother, but had a disabled child and other family demands upon her time. Mrs. Upton's only other child, Arthur, lived two-thousand miles away. When Mrs. Ryan stopped returning phone calls the social worker turned the matter over to the administrator for direction to a collection agency. The administrator however thought that perhaps there were some unresolved family issues here and that the social worker could use some support in approaching Jenifer differently. He suggested a mental health consultation.

The first meeting between the consultant and the social worker involved a review of information on the family and on the social-work interventions to date. Ms. Gorley described her perceptions of the family and her role as facilitator of family-home business exchanges and planning for Mrs. Upton's present and future care. The mental health consultant supported this role and suggested that another approach involved supporting the *family* in handling troublesome issues in order to assure that the requirements of both the family and the nursing home could be met. All family members were contacted suggesting a joint meeting to discuss mutual concerns.

The consultant met again with Ms. Gorley before the family interview to explore the goals for change and the process of the interview. At this time, the position of the consultant as counselor and resource was further reinforced and the skills of the caseworker in managing family-centered problem solving were reviewed.

The family meeting took place about two weeks later when Arthur was scheduled to be in the area on business. Mrs. Upton was present for the first few minutes but became restless and rambled incoherently, interrupting meaningful exchanges between the others. She was taken back to her room for the rest of the meeting.

Arthur and Jenifer were initially angry with each other and with the caseworker for insisting that things be faced together. A history of rivalry between the now-adult children emerged as did long-standing conflict between Jenifer and her mother. The responsibilities of managing the resolution of Mr. Upton's estate as well as ongoing details of Mrs. Upton's care were overwhelming.

Jenifer didn't see any urgent need on the part of her mother. She not only found visits unpleasant and disheartening, but she preferred to forget about that part of her life entirely. She also refused help from her brother rather defiantly. (He always could do *more* and *better*.) She wanted to prove she could manage herself, and if that meant ignoring Mother, so what! She didn't believe her mother noticed. Besides, the friends who had been around right after Mr. Upton's death were not so concerned any longer and so neither encouragement nor child-care assistance for her visits were readily available now.

Arthur himself found his sister and his mother so distraught and discouraging that he felt useless, and so he withdrew, only making an occasional call. What else could he do? His mother didn't seem to recognize him; and his sister was unwilling even to talk to him. Even his offers to handle specific details or visit were rebuffed, so he offered less often.

The social worker helped both Arthur and Jenifer to see that they were continuing to interact as they had for years. The patterns of action, reaction, and resistance were not easy to accept, but the result in isolating Jenifer, isolating Arthur, and then isolating Mrs. Upton was acknowledged. Now the three could more calmly discuss what each wanted in the future and how a different pattern of interaction might look. Both

Arthur and Jenifer wanted to visit only occasionally and to find ways to make those visits seem useful: to know better why they were there, even if their mother didn't know who they were. They wanted concrete tasks that were personal. Paying bills was hardly personal. The social worker indicated she wanted the family contact to be meaningful. She suggested that the business affairs could be taken care of regularly perhaps automatically through direct bank-payment services.

Further planning with this family involved the identification of ways each individual could benefit from new interactions with each other and the nursing staff. Both nursing home functioning and family interaction benefited.

---

Repeated referrals for case consultation may reveal concerns that can be best accomplished through programs addressed more comprehensively across the institution. This institutional or administrative approach is discussed next.

## SYSTEMS OR PROGRAM INTERVENTIONS

Educational and support groups for family members are becoming more common today, especially for new families adjusting to residential life. Various members of nursing and social-service staff convene these groups, which can relieve admissions personnel from total family responsibility and provide an efficient way of interacting with multiple families. These forms of peer support have several benefits, such as diminishing family isolation and generating new ways for members to communicate with staff and residents within the home.[22]

A selection of group programs, focusing on a variety of family needs, from personal growth to collaborative support skills are presented in table 9.3. The literature describing such interventions is limited, however.

The initiation or revitalization of family-specific programs is another important strategy for directly addressing family issues. Orientation groups, support groups, newsletters, family events, and routine family involvement in care planning can be initiated or reorganized. The form of such family interventions appears limited only by resources and commitment.

Buckwalter and Hall (1987) describe a series of collaborative therapeutic roles for family members. They suggest a nursing liaison to work with families in a variety of common resident interventions, such as reality therapy or music and movement exercises. However, the existing nursing staff, like the existing social-work staff, may find it hard to add family-care responsibilities without additional resources, preparation, and administrative support. Facilities require specific resources and policy to direct these efforts.

***Family-Staff Interventions.*** When family-staff patterns have become dysfunctional alternative programs or policy changes need to be considered. Using specific case examples, clinical conferences or programs can be proposed, involving both families and staff. The goals of these meetings are (1) to illuminate persistent "problematic" behaviors, their interconnectedness, and their consequences; (2) to introduce observational protocols that are simple and clear for use by the staff and/or family to record the sequences of disruptive situations; (3) to brainstorm alternative responses to "classic" problems; (4) to formalize or agree upon new, more helpful desirable behaviors; and (5) to identify the time and means for evaluating the usefulness of new practices. Breslin (1978) describes other staff- and family-focused seminars designed to increase dialogue between groups within the facility and to solve problems together.

When staff morale and performance issues appear to contribute significantly to ongoing problems with families, additional staff development should be considered.[23] Chapters Ten and Eleven of this volume discuss approaches to staff oriented mental health interventions.

TABLE 9.3: A Sample of Intervention Groups with Families in Nursing Homes

| *Author* | *Program Form* | *Program Focus* |
|---|---|---|
| Horsman & Echtenacher (1981) | Family council & Family Involvement Team (FIT) | Communication of family concerns and political activism in behalf of families in long-term care |
| Hausman (1979) | Eight weekly community-based sessions; families all preadmission or undecided about placement | Individual and family self-understanding of decision making, interaction patterns, and needs with aging |
| Manaster (1967) | Ongoing support group for resident's families and those on waiting list | Increasing self-awareness, understanding of aging and aged family members, peer support |
| Safford (1980) | Six two-hour group sessions; families of both community-based and admitted elders | Specific knowledge and skills for supporting elders during admission adjustment and life in a long-term facility. |

Source: Adapted from Smyer and Frysinger (1985).

When lack of skill in responding to dysfunctional elders is identified as an issue for families and/or staff during consultation a proposed intervention may ultimately involve the development of training-program protocols. For example, when family members or evening staff provide forbidden cigarettes in Mr. Rollin's room because he begs pitifully, the day staff feel sabotaged. Staff efforts to encourage sociability and safety need to be shared with everyone who helps the resident. Training in behavioral technology may then be appropriate to assist nursing staff who need both guidance in recognizing family-staff interaction patterns and information and preparation in altering their own responses. It can also be most useful for families who require more effective ways to respond to their elders and each other.

***Training-Focused Programs.*** Another form of family intervention involves the identification of family informational and behavioral "gaps," which can best be bridged through planned instructional interventions. General informational needs, interpersonal skills, and behavioral-management skills are potential topics for training. The administration of the nursing home may need help in recognizing the belief systems, thought processes, and interaction patterns that guide family behavior in relation to institutionalized relatives. Interpersonal communication skills and behavioral-management programs can enable the residents and all their caregivers (family and staff) to be more confident, comfortable, and effective in their caregiving.

No published programs that provide such training to family caregivers of adults have been found. When behavioral-management strategies are being carried out with residents, the importance of behavioral training for family members is evident. Hussian and Davis (1985) point out that problems of noncontingent reinforcement introduced by uninformed visitors create frequent errors in behavioral programs. It is here that new and innovative efforts can be most helpful.

Evaluation of existing family participation and skills precedes the design of curricular strategies that will reinforce mutually rewarding collaborative relationships among residents, staff, and families. Family awareness of social-learning principles, their effectiveness in communicating with staff and each other, and their readiness to participate actively in nursing home programs determine the appropriateness of including family members in training sessions.

The majority of behavioral family training has been carried out with parents of disabled or difficult children where predictors of family success in mastering behavioral strategies have included income, education, attendance, and involvement.[24] Families of institutionalized elders should be similarly evaluated. Short programs that introduce concepts and provide practice in role-playing situations may allow consulters and/or trainers to evaluate participants best for further programs.

The content of training must extend beyond the principles of behavior management to include insight into cognitive changes and emotional issues of aging. Introductory sessions on basic communication skills and interpersonal helping strategies can well be adapted from Guerney's (1987) work with relationship enhancement and family-communication training. The information below helps family members understand the practices that shape more acceptable/comfortable behavior.

*Steps to Understanding Problem Behaviors as a Learned Process*

1) Question the need to intervene in behavior.
   Is it harmful to self, others, the care giver?

2) Recognize that behavior occurs in a context and in a sequence.
   The sequence = A B C.

   A = antecedents or things that precede a behavior.
   1. Physical sensations
   2. Psychological experiences
   3. Other people's actions
   4. Physical environment

   B = the behavior or actions themselves
   1. Motor
   2. Verbal
   3. Psychological/emotional

   C = consequences
   1. Personal: reinforcing
      extinguishing/punishing
   2. Social: acceptable
      problematic: disrupts others, interferes with care, harms self

3) Recognize ways to change behavior.
   Alter contingencies (antecedents or consequences)
   Change conditions that provoke behavior
   (e.g. simplify environment, limit stimulation, redefine meaning, avoid troublesome events and experiences).

   Change rewards
   (e.g. ignore behavior, timeout, substitution, etc.).

4) Recognize the family members' role in and reactions to supporting (changing) behavior—teaching vs. manipulating people.

## SUMMARY

Attending to family needs in nursing homes requires the coordination of practitioners with varied preparation and job descriptions. Interventions may range from individual-family-problem resolution to thorough program design. Therefore, understanding of both family and nursing home functioning is critical. Consultants can be most useful in helping practitioners assess family issues, in directing nursing home personnel and families to appropriate resource materials, and designing supportive programs and instructional opportunities.

In conclusion, the area of education and skills training for families of nursing home residents is a new and promising field for development. A consultant who is prepared to address individual family issues with a variety of intervention strategies, or one who has experience with the development of other training programs will have much to contribute to institutions ready to support families in new ways. The readiness of families and nursing homes for further support and consultation is not in question. The availability of funds and personnel to provide such consultation will continue to be a challenge.

## NOTES

1. Bernard Reisman (1986) not only gives a touching description of his own experience in this article, but he provides four strong and helpful suggestions for use with other families.

2. Staff-family problems are discussed by Buckwalter and Hall (1987), Kramer and Kramer (1976), Pratt et al. (1987), Silverstone and Hyman (1976), Tobin and Kulys (1981), and Wentzel (1979).

3. Issues of involvement, burden, and satisfaction are the most frequent subjects for study of families in nursing homes. See Hatch and Franken (1984); Linn and Gurel (1969); Hook, Sobal, and Oak (1982); and Braun and Rose (1987) on the subject of family satisfaction; Rubin and Shuttlesworth (1983); Shuttlesworth, Rubin, and Duffy (1982); Smith and Bengtson (1979); and Bowers (1986) on the issues of family roles and attachment; and Pratt et al. (1987) on continuing family burden.

4. See Furse (1983), Buckholdt (1983), and Pratt et al. (1987).

5. Blieszner and Mancini (1987) redirect our thinking to the enduring ties older adults want or expect from their families. This community-based study reminds us to consider the wishes for connectedness from the perspective of the older adults as well as from their families.

6. Bowers (1986) contends that family protective caregiving within the nursing home involves carrying out these tasks, which are often in direct conflict with institutional norms.

7. Taken, with liberties, from Reisman's (1986) suggestions for family participation in the adjustment to a nursing home. See also Solomon (1983).

8. See Garner and Mercer (1980) and Mercer and Garner (1981).

9. Goldmeier and Mannino (1986) provide a brief but thorough overview of the evolution of social-work consultation in the face of changing professional standards and settings for social work. Their questions about the roles and impact of social-work consultants have relevance for mental health consultants from any discipline.

10. Several casework models have emerged in the past decade that direct social-work practice to more systems-centered, developmental, and problem-solving procedures. Further exploration of these newer models can be found in Germaine and Gitterman (1980), Reid and Epstein (1977), Roberts and Northern (1976), and Silverstone and Burack-Weiss (1983).

11. For additional reviews of family-therapy approaches with the aged see Eyde and Rich (1983), Herr and Weakland (1979), and Qualls (1987). Nursing models for gerontology have been discussed most recently in the September 1987 *Journal of Gerontological Nursing.* These papers do not expand upon family components. See Riehl and Roy (1974) or Kreiger (1981) for more extensive attention to advanced-nursing practice.

12. See Buckwalter and Hall (1987, p. 181) for a simplified comparison of social and medical models of nursing-home organization.

13. See Greene (1986, p. 337) in her discussion of a functional age model of intergenerational therapy. Intergenerational in this context refers to relationships between at least two adult generations.

14. Buckwalter and Hall (1987, p. 185). Table 11.3a in their book contains a concise rationale.

15. See Greene (1986).

16. See Stamm (1972).

17. Examples of family assessment can be found in Moos family environment scales (Moos, Insel, and Humphrey, 1974), in the McCubbins's work with families of chronically ill children (McCubbins, McCubbins, and Cauble, 1979), and in Smoyak (1975). Satir (1967) and Bandler, Grinder, and Satir (1976) provide additional ways to understand family interaction patterns and dysfunctional communication systems.

18. See the preadmission format introduced by Buckwalter and Hall (1987).

19. Herr and Weakland (1979), Silverstone and Burack-Weis (1983), and Qualls (1987) provide significant structure for exploring family interaction patterns. The questioning stance suggested by Herr and Weakland has inspired the expanded questionnaire format provided here.

20. Vernberg and Reppucci (1986) outline ten major problems encountered in behavioral systems innovation, from which the succeeding list of questions were drawn. For further discussion of systems change in human-service organizations they direct the reader to Brager and Holloway (1978), Goodstein (1978) and Reppucci and Saunders (1983).

21. Buckwalter and Hall (1987) describe suggested joint caretaking.

22. These kinds of family services are described further by Lewis (1980).

23. Eleven staff-specific interventions are reviewed by Smyer and Frysinger (1985) with attention to the approaches used as well as desired outcomes and evaluation strategies employed.

24. See Clark, Baker, and Heifetz (1982) as well as Dattilo and Murphy (1987).

# 10

# The Primary Caregivers: Aides and LPNs

*Diane Brannon and Joy Bodnar*

> You want to know what makes this place work? It's the aides. . . . They are the backbone of the nursing home.
>
> *An RN nursing home supervisor*

## INTRODUCTION

In this chapter we consider the nursing home community as a place of work for employee caregivers. This scenario is somewhat analogous to that of "townies" who provide the service foundation for resort communities. These service providers do not live in the community (by virtue of limited financial resources); they tend to have no role in civic affairs; yet their contribution, the quality of their labor, makes them essential. Just as a resort community cannot function without service personnel, the nursing home community's major source of cohesion is its cadre of caregivers. The centrality of these paid caregivers in the nursing home derives from the constancy and intimacy of the care they provide. Their potential role in improving mental health outcomes in nursing homes is the focus of this chapter.

Many nursing home residents could live in the community with intensive services provided by relatives or others. Thus, the staffs of nursing homes are, indeed, substitute caregivers and substitute primary groups for some residents (Litwak, 1985). The motivation, skill level, quality, and stability of these personnel dramatically affect the quality of life in nursing homes. The effective management of human resources, consequently, looms very large as an issue for mental health consultation.

While not all administrators are aware of the importance of caregiving staff in the mental health treatment process, they are well aware of the importance of the caregiving staff per se. Attracting and retaining both LPNs and nurse's aides (or nursing assistants), are probably the most persistent management problems faced by the nursing homes industry. Indeed, it is the unusual administrator who does *not* present staffing as an issue for consultation. Even when individual cases are the reason mental health consultation has been sought, the consultant will not have to probe very far to discover the impact of staffing problems in nursing homes.

Annual turnover rates vary greatly among facilities, but run in excess of 100 percent of staff positions in some areas. This means that there are more "quits" during a year's time than there are staff on an average day. The wage scale is clearly part of the problem, with aides' wages at or just above minimum wage. The economic structure of long-term-care reimbursement renders this a seemingly intractable problem. Consequently, other solutions are desperately sought.

Certainly, any efforts to increase the role of caregivers in mental health treatment must be sensitive to the issues of caregiving as a job, and one in a labor market that also has a variety of competitive jobs available.

Thus, we raise several questions in this chapter for considering these members of the nursing home community, the caregivers for hire:

1) Who are the caregivers?
2) What is their role?
3) What is the nature of their work?
4) Are caregivers motivated by their work?

These four questions structure our discussion of the primary caregivers' contribution to the nursing home community. At the conclusion of this chapter we suggest the viability of a mental health paraprofessional role for nursing home caregivers.

## THE CAREGIVERS: WHO ARE THEY?

---

Susan H. is the typical nursing home caregiver. She has been employed in her current job as a nurse's aide for less than two years and has less than five years' total experience as a paid caregiver. She is white, under thirty-five years old with twelve or fewer years education and little or no training in nursing skills.

---

According to preliminary data from the National Nursing Home Survey of 1985, LPNs and nurse's aides held 88 percent of full-time–equivalent nursing positions in nursing homes. Within this caregiver work force there were approximately 4 aides for every LPN and 1.5 LPNs for each RN in 1985. More detailed data from the 1977 survey showed that almost all (94 percent) of this work force was female. Seventy-six percent of the caregivers were white in the 1977 survey, though nonwhites predominated in some areas. People younger than thirty-five years of age made up 53 percent of the work force, 18 percent were ages thirty-five to forty-four, 14 percent were ages forty-five to fifty-four, and 15 percent were age fifty-five or older. Sixty-eight percent of the caregivers had a high-school education or less (primarily aides), and another twenty-six percent had thirteen to fourteen years of education (primarily LPNs).

More than half of the caregivers at the time of the 1977 survey had been employed in their current position for less than two years, and only 8 percent had job tenure of ten or more years. In terms of total experience in the caregiving "field," 60 percent of the work force had less than five years of total experience, and only 19 percent had been in the field for ten or more years.

As of 1985, only seventeen states had minimum requirements for nurse's-aide training (Institute of Medicine, 1986). Of these seventeen, only two states, Maine and New Hampshire, required preemployment training. Maine required thirty classroom hours of training prior to employment, and New Hampshire required a combination of thirty classroom and seventy clinical hours of training. The New Hampshire requirement could be waived, however, if a facility had a certified training program. Therefore, it is unlikely that an aide has any training at all prior to entering her or his first position and most never have to meet any minimum training requirement to maintain employment.

SNF and ICF standards (as described in chapter 2) do require that nursing homes have ongoing staff-development programs. However, the topics that are required to be included in the programs are infection control, fire prevention and safety, accident prevention, confidentiality of patient information, and patient dignity. It would be rather surprising, therefore, if large numbers of nurse's aides had received any formal training in how to deal with mental disorders that are commonly identified in nursing homes. In a survey of nurse's aides and nursing home administrators conducted in Pennsylvania (Smyer et al., 1985), nurse's aides were asked whether they had received training in how to deal with eleven mental-health problems. For only one problem area—disorientation—did more than one-third of the aides perceive themselves as having received training. Over twice as many administrators consistently reported that that training had indeed been provided in these areas. This large discrepancy suggests it unlikely that the need for mental health skills training in nursing homes is being met. Consequently, the potential treatment role that caregivers might serve, by virtue of their proximity to residents, is not well developed.

## WHAT IS THEIR ROLE?

The Institute of Medicine's recent report (1986) on nursing home quality suggests the salience of the caregiver role:

> Nursing homes are "total institutions" in which care-givers, particularly nurse's aides, represent a large part of the social world of . . . residents and control their daily schedules and activities. This is the total environment for many . . . for the duration of their stay, which may be several years (p. 74).

For the majority of nursing home residents, the caregivers are their major social network, their primary group (Litwak, 1985). Since they comprise the largest group in the nursing home community, their influence on the social environment is profound. For the approximately 12 percent of residents who receive no visitors during their stay, the staff and other residents are their *total* social environment. The frequency of interaction between caregivers, most notably aides, and residents is suggested by the staffing ratios in table 10.1.

The quality of life for nursing home residents, then, is profoundly affected by the quality of care provided by the nurse's aides. In addition to the frequency of interaction between caregivers and residents, another major factor contributes to the overall role of the aides and LPNs: the qualitative nature of the interaction between staff and residents, which may be viewed as a sign of the institution's culture. The caregiving staff, then, are principle bearers of the values and behavioral norms of the facility. Variations in nursing home cultures across facilities have not been systematically studied. It is likely, however, that the way residents are managed and/or cared for reflects an institutional belief system which is demonstrated in the behavior of aides and LPNs. Not surprisingly, the quality of staff and staff/resident interaction was deemed the most important factor in a recent study of nursing home resident consumer satisfaction (Spaulding, 1985).

TABLE 10.1: Number of Personnel per 100 Beds: 1977 and 1985

| | *1977* | *1985* |
|---|---|---|
| Aides | 30.3 | 30.8 |
| LPNs | 6.1 | 7.4 |
| RNs | 4.8 | 5.1 |
| Physicians | 1.0 | Data not available |

Sources: National Center for Health Statistics (1981) and Strahan (1987).

Further confirmation of the important role played by caregivers is the relationship between staff behavior and resident behavior posited by Lawton and Nahemow (1973) more than a decade ago. Since that time, researchers and clinicians have found substantial evidence of the direct impact of staff behavior, both negative and positive, on residents' functioning.[1] The role of the caregiving staff, in promoting quality care is, therefore, pivotal.

## CAREGIVING AS WORK

> Taking care of helpless adults, their personal needs, is not a job for everyone.
>
> *A nursing home supervisor*

Nursing home caregiving is stressful in many of the same ways that family caregiving is. Aides, especially, have not been professionally trained to distance themselves emotionally from disturbing resident-related incidents. While intrafamilial roles are not an issue, other social roles, especially those involving personal privacy, are stretched, if not violated, in the provision of care. Without benefit of nursing education, "off-the-street" caregivers are often ill prepared for the emotional demands of their work.

The most likely support system for paid caregivers is their employer and coworkers. Thus, many administrators are vitally concerned with the effects of the job on the morale and satisfaction of caregivers. We will examine caregiving, therefore, in terms of the characteristics of the job itself—its context in the organization, its structure, and the technology it employs. Finally, we will examine what caregivers think of their jobs in addressing the question of motivation.

In the rest of this chapter, the caregiving job is examined as a collection of vital, if socially awkward, tasks linked in a service technology. It is helpful to separate the work from the characteristics of workers in order to identify a range of possible interventions. Thus, work is distinguished from working. Work, itself, is "energy directed at organizational goals, identifiable separately from the person who does it and (it is) analyzable" (Charns and Schaefer, 1983, p. 210). Working, in contrast, is an individual's response to the structure, context, and technology of work, influenced both by these characteristics and by the individual attributes of workers.

## THE ORGANIZATIONAL CONTEXT OF CAREGIVING

Litwak's (1985) analysis of nursing homes as formal organizations that attempt to substitute for disabled primary groups provides insights relevant to the societal context of caregiving as work. The nursing-home industry has emerged apologetically as a "necessary evil"—an embarrassment to the mobile nuclear family. Institutionalizing frail elderly relatives is perceived as another painful, if inevitable, step away from the family as the preeminent social unit. In this book we attempt to dispel the view of the family as "disabled" and treat the nursing home as a supplement to rather than as a substitute for primary groups. Yet we recognize that the weight of the "dumping" stigma remains a factor in the morale of the nursing home.

Another major factor in the organizational context is that nursing homes, as formal organizations, are characterized by specialization of functions, written rules, hierarchical authority, and economic incentives (Litwak, 1985). If you were to work in a nursing home as an aide, you would punch a time clock and refer to a posted schedule in determining which residents to bathe each day. Your schedule would be set by a supervisor and you would be paid by the hour for the care that you gave.

Primary groups, in contrast, are holistic, manage themselves by interpersonal commitment and face-to-face peer relationships, and are motivated by affective ties. Accordingly, if you were to serve as the primary caregiver for a family member, your work would proceed on a more *ad hoc* basis, as you would negotiate the scheduling and sequencing of personal-care tasks. Your rewards would be interpersonal and your duties would not end after an eight-hour shift. Because of these differences, Litwak points out, primary groups most effectively provide nonroutine (that is, personalized) services, whereas formal organizations best provide routine services that are not highly variable from client to client.

When formal organizations are required to provide nonroutine services that are normally offered by primary groups (for example, the preparation of meals), Litwak observes several responses that may occur: (1) service delivery is routinized; (2) primary groups continue to provide some services; (3) some services are eliminated; or (4) organizational structure is moderated to be more like a primary group (Litwak, 1985).

If the fourth response, organizational innovation, does not occur in a significant way, then some combination of the other three must occur. Even when a relative is in a nursing home, primary-group members are needed to provide the "extras" that affect quality of life. Table 10.2 provides examples of caregiving tasks that may be best performed by the family and nursing home staff, respectively, and those that may be performed by either.

Thus, according to Litwak's analysis, nursing homes are forced to routinize personal-care services to some extent or to eliminate some services entirely. Those services that are lost are those that cannot be routinized (and thus are not likely to be provided by staff), nor can they be provided by family members. Examples might include responding to special dietary preferences or planning for future events such as holidays. These are services that "require continual face-to-face contact and resources" (Litwak, 1985, p. 61). Clearly, mental health treatment in the nursing home setting requires continual responsiveness and fits Litwak's criteria for lost services. The scarcity of mental health services available in the nursing home setting has been documented elsewhere (Smyer and Frysinger, 1985).

What Litwak's analysis tells us about nursing home caregiving is that its context is one of perceived inadequacy. The staff are too few to provide personalized care to residents. The perception of not being able to do enough creates a highly stressful work environment. One issue that a consultant will want to pursue is the relative effectiveness of coping mechanisms employed by staff to deal with this stress. Examples of coping mechanisms that may be observed include depersonalizing resident relationships, the use of morbid humor, and infantilizing residents.

## THE STRUCTURE OF CAREGIVING WORK

While systematic job analysis that focuses specifically on the mental health aspects of nursing home care has not been done, it is clear from table 10.1 that nurse's aides have the most frequent opportunity to influence resident mental health status. The range of tasks they perform has been delineated in a scale-development process for a Behaviorally Anchored Rating Scale (BARS) of aide job performance in nursing homes (Sheridan, Fairchild, and Kaas, 1983). The behavioral anchors were selected and scaled based on the opinions of LPNs and aides regarding the centrality of the activities to

TABLE 10.2: Caregiving Tasks of Resident Family and Facility Staff

| *Family Tasks* | *Staff Tasks* | *Shared Tasks* |
|---|---|---|
| Lifespan continuity<br>Shared memory<br>Contact with future generations | Nursing | Socialization<br>Current events<br>Literature |
| | Personal hygiene | |
| Financial management | Assistance with activities of daily living | Transfer to other services |
| Funeral arrangements | Assistance with adjustment | Maintenance of personal identity<br>Gifts<br>Room decor |
| | Managing death | |
| | | Preparation for death |

five key performance dimensions. The following profiles are based on the BARS and job descriptions from nursing homes.

---

*Profile of Nurse's-Aide Activities*

The aide is expected to do passive range of motion exercises for stroke or paralysis patients. In the event of hemorrhaging, she would be expected to elevate the affected part of the body immediately and apply pressure before calling the nurse. She is required to seek help and/or use correct body mechanics in moving patients. The aide is expected to reconcile food-service deliveries with patients' dietary restrictions. Observation of changes in patient status is a responsibility of the aide. She is expected to observe whether a patient's toenails need to be cut and whether decubiti are present. She monitors food and water intake, emotional states, and patient ambulation. A capable aide would notice probable circulatory problems, changes in body temperature, and paralysis. Personal care of patients is another major category of job activities. Aides provide clean, wrinkle-free changes of bed linens. Aides receive and return linens to the laundry and, sometimes, food trays to the kitchen or cart. Aides are expected to initiate and facilitate interaction with and among residents and to assist in and encourage ambulation.

*Profile of LPN Activities*

The LPN gives and receives reports. She answers telephone inquiries and assists visitors. The orientation, instruction, and supervision of other nursing personnel are included in her duties. The LPN evaluates patient needs, condition, and care. She is expected to admit and orient new residents and relatives. She reviews physicians' orders, transfer and preadmission information, and the resident's medical and social history. In response to this process, she requisitions diagnostic and therapeutic services as ordered by physicians. She is responsible for maintaining patient and unit records and for scheduling services for residents. She may make rounds with and assist physicians. The LPN passes medications and gives injections. She assumes charge of the unit in the absence of her supervisor when so assigned. Where time allows, the LPN provides personal care to residents (that is, bathing, dressing, making beds, feeding, and so on). She may assist or perform such nursing duties as recording vital signs, measuring and recording fluid intake and output, doing clini-tests on specimens, giving enemas, changing dressings and drainage bags, and caring for the dying and dead.

---

An analysis of the structure of work requires specification and categorization of the activities included in the job. Are these activities primarily those of direct work, managerial work, or support work? Direct work in the nursing home setting is care residents receive from staff. Hands-on assistance with activities of daily living is a good example. Managerial work involves providing the resources and environment for the provision of personal and health services. Staff recruitment and selection are managerial work. Support work is that which maintains and sustains the direct provision of care and the management of facilities. Laundry service and accounting are both examples of support work in this setting.

While health-care providers focus most of their activities toward direct care, they are increasingly unable to avoid management and support functions. The most often cited reason for this intrusion is the documentation of clinical processes required by third-party reimbursement agents. Because RNs function primarily as shift supervisors or charge nurses, they have lost much of their direct-care role in nursing homes. LPNs typically are the primary health care providers in that they are generally allowed by state law to perform some professional nursing duties. They also are managers, however, and are expected, in some cases, to supervise the direct care provided by nurse's aides or assistants.

Nurse's aides provide the large majority of the direct care, the personal-care services, and are the staff in most frequent contact with the residents. While aides must contribute to record keeping and maintenance of physical facilities, they engage in a set of activities largely in response to the immediate needs of residents in their care. Consequently, a consultant may observe that the greatest potential for behavioral treatment of resident mental health problems lies with the nurse's aides. To the extent that chronicity requires tenacious, frequent, and consistent treatment, aides may well be the only therapeutic resource available. As family caregivers are being trained to respond therapeutically to Alzheimer's victims, so aides might be trained to respond therapeutically in the administering of personal-care tasks.

## CAREGIVING TECHNOLOGY

In the preceding sections of this chapter, we have identified the *who* and *what* of nursing home caregiving. Now, we turn to the question of *how* this work is done—that is, its technology. *Technology* refers to the manner in which inputs are transformed into outputs. It is not an easy phenomenon to observe in a service setting. A conceptual framework may be helpful. Organizational theorists have generally analyzed technology along two dimensions: uncertainty or predictability[2] and task interdependency.[3] Both of these analytic dimensions can be applied to caregiving as work.

Uncertainty may be characteristic of inputs, transformation processes, or outputs. A high degree of uncertainty in the work technology has been observed to impede the administrative goal of making work more routine. Nursing homes, like other human-service organizations, deal with highly variable inputs in the form of resident-care needs. As Litwak (1985) indicates, however, in the translation of personal care to bureaucratic work, the caregiving process becomes routinized and standardized to a considerable extent. Nursing homes have been unusually effective at routinizing their core technological processes (that is, providing personal care) despite highly unpredictable inputs (that is, residents; see an example of a shift schedule for nurse's aides in the appendix to this chapter). They have been able to accomplish this because they have nearly exclusive control over the skills and, therefore, the processes employed by their primary workers. Nurse's aides, especially, are bound by the knowledge they have gained on the job and not likely to challenge routine procedures.

Furthermore, nursing homes have not had to be greatly concerned about the effectiveness of their work outputs, which might be operationalized as therapeutic relationships. That their technology may be ill suited to their clientele's needs has not been a significant market factor for nursing homes. The demand for nursing home beds has been and continues to be high relative to the supply, with occupancy rates running in excess of 90 percent in most areas. Generally only flagrant neglect in the resident care is noticed by regulators. Lesser effects of routinizing personal care are tolerated as an unfortunate side effect of institutionalization. Thus, the lack of fit between uncertain or unpredictable inputs (residents) and routinized processes of care has become a "given" in the nursing home industry.

The issue of work flow or task interdependency can best be understood with an example. In facility A, a sequential technology defines the way care is given. A consulting physical therapist examines a resident and leaves orders with the RN charge nurse for an exercise regimen. The charge nurse attaches the order to the resident's chart or perhaps directly to a caregiver's task schedule. Thus, a stepwise progression of orders precedes the initiation of the exercises by the caregiver. In facility B, a batched technology prevails. Periodic case planning conferences include, at a minimum, caregivers, a professional nurse, and attending therapists. A care plan emerges from discussion of the resident's condition and life situation. The caregivers in homes A and B may end up with similar sets of orders, but the processes used to give them are very distinct.

A sequential technology works well when a positive outcome can be routinely produced without give and take among employees. A one-way linear flow of tasks and orders across different work stations and workers is appropriate for simple, routine tasks. Many nursing home administrators have recognized the liabilities of this approach to resident care and are using variations on the "patient-care team" model initiated some time ago by hospitals.

To conclude, nursing homes are in the enviable position of defining caregiving technology in ways that are organizationally rational. Litwak's (1985) bureaucratic analysis suggests that this rationality requires that care procedures be supportive of the organization's economic incentives and its need to control nonprofessional workers. Are these bureaucratic goals in conflict with that of strengthening the therapeutic role of caregivers vis-à-vis resident mental health? Not necessarily. Efficiency and effectiveness are mutually achievable goals in this instance under certain circumstances: (1) when the administration is able to take a long-term view of institutional wealth over short-term profit, and (2) when improved staff motivation and performance result in more independent (less care-intensive) residents. Performance is jointly determined by the workers (the caregivers) and the work (its context, structure, and technology), as shown in Figure 10.1.

## ARE CAREGIVERS MOTIVATED BY THEIR WORK?

Continuing with our primary focus on caregiving as work rather than on individual workers, Hackman and Oldham's (1980) model of work design is most relevant. This conceptualization details the processes by which the structure of the work itself affects the motivation and performance of workers and, in turn, the work outcomes.

Five job characteristics contribute to what Hackman and Oldham refer to as the motivating potential of the job itself. In other words, regardless of the personal characteristics of the job incumbents, how does the job design itself rate? Hackman and Oldham (1980) identify these five key characteristics of work as follows: skill variety, task identity, task significance, autonomy, and feedback. Each of these characteristics will be discussed below.

The Hackman and Oldham (1980) model suggests that these structural characteristics promote the corresponding affective responses of experienced meaningfulness, experienced responsibility, and knowledge of results. The worker then values and feels responsible for the work and understands how effective his or her actions are. These affective responses are theorized to affect performance and work outcomes, both qualitatively and quantitatively defined.

Fig. 10.1

**A Model of Caregiving Work Performance in Nursing Homes**

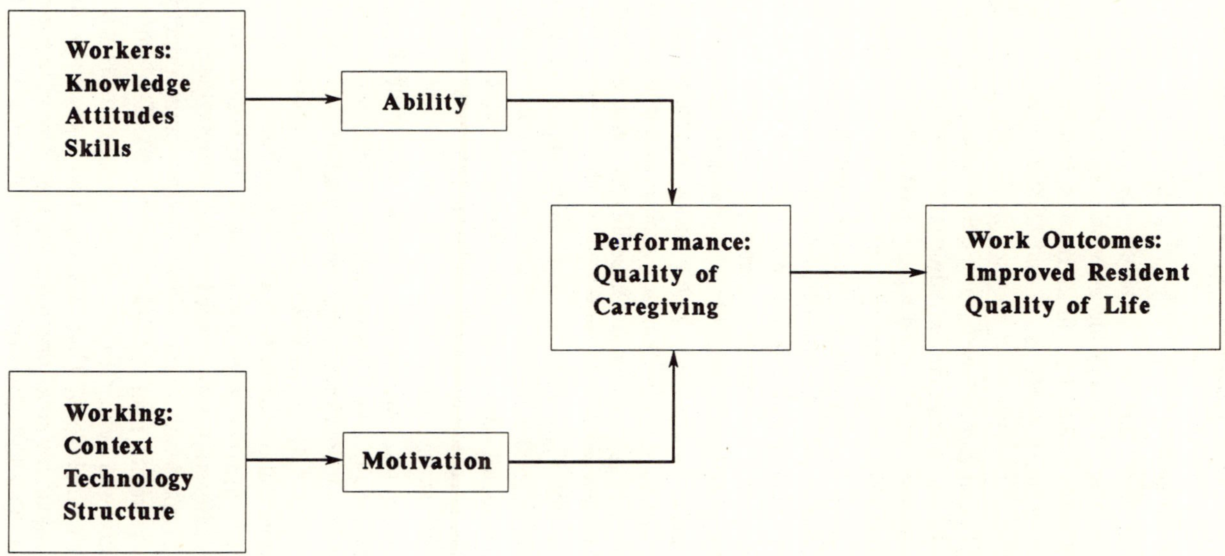

## THE PENNSYLVANIA CAREGIVERS' SURVEY

A recent analysis of nursing home aides' and LPNs' work (Brannon et al., 1986), using the job characteristics model, revealed the strengths and weaknesses of caregiving as work. This analysis was based on a survey of 498 aides and LPNs in 21 nursing homes in Pennsylvania. The Job Diagnostic Survey (Hackman and Oldham, 1980) and its companion instrument for supervisors were used in this study. The Job Diagnostic Survey (JDS) is an eighty-seven–item questionnaire designed for use in diagnostic activities to determine whether (and how) existing jobs can be improved. Having been widely used for the past decade, the JDS is useful in making comparisons with other job categories and published norms (Oldham, Hackman, and Stepina, 1979). The instrument is designed to measure each of the five job characteristics listed above. While the five scales do not always appear as expected upon factor analysis of sample data (only three factors were evident in the caregiver sample), the observed overlap is to be expected conceptually since the job characteristics are interrelated. Comparisons are made with available norms (Oldham, Hackman, and Stepina, 1979) for jobs that are similar to nursing-home care giving, from a labor-market standpoint. These include: women workers; blue-collar workers; hourly employees; employees of small organizations; for nurses' aides, those with high-school or less educational level; and for LPNs, technical-school-trained workers. For purposes of comparative analysis, we treat the job characteristics as discrete, though in practice they clearly overlap, as should be evident from the following discussion.

*Skill variety* refers to the range of activities requiring different abilities or behaviors. Assembly-line work, which employs the principle of work simplification and a sequential technology to increase standardization, is notoriously deficient in this job characteristic. The practice of medicine, at the other extreme, involves information processing, decision making, and communication, all in complex applications.

Nursing home aides and LPNs in the Pennsylvania sample viewed their jobs differently with regard to skill variety (see figure 10.2): LPNs (n = 101) experienced a considerably wider range of activities and related skill requirements than did aides (n = 389). The aides' mean score on skill variety was similar to that of other women, as well as to blue-collar and hourly employees. Their average was lower than that of other employees of comparably small organizations that tend to use employees in many functions. The LPNs' scores, in contrast, were higher than the averages for women, hourly employees, and blue-collar workers, and were similar to those of other employees of small organizations. This substantial variety

**Fig. 10.2**

Skill Variety
Aides and LPNs with Comparison Groups

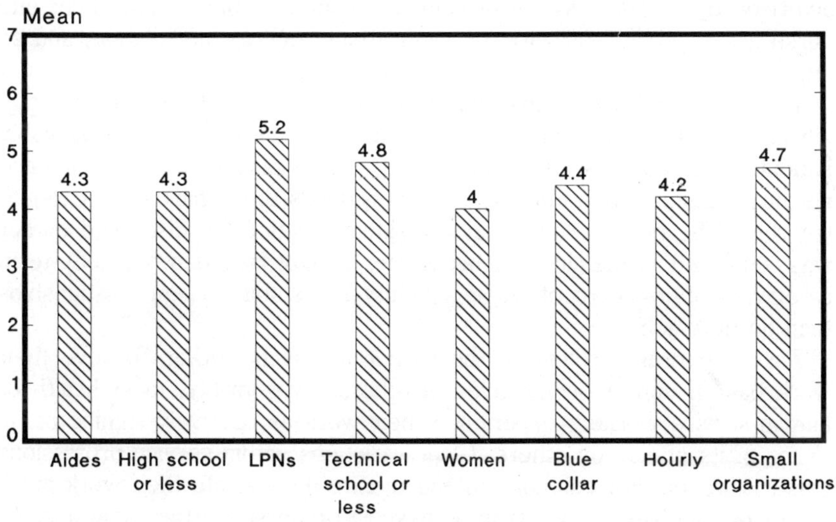


**Sources: Brannon et al. (1986) and Oldham, Hackman, and Stepina (1979).**

of LPN duties can be inferred from the profile presented above. LPNs do some of the same work as aides and some of the same work as RNs.

*Task identity* represents the extent to which a job includes an identifiable (if not actually whole) piece of work. Accordingly, a small-batched technology using work groups, each of which produces an identifiable output, is likely to be high in task identity. A long-linked, sequential technology, characteristic of mass production via conveyor-belt organization, offers its workers little task closure or identity and much alienation.

In the provision of health services, the most logical unit of work is the patient or resident. Such organization has not always been the norm, however, as evidenced by the popularity of functional nursing, which is characterized by a clear division of labor and limited scope of activities: one nurse assumes responsibility for medications, one for ambulation, and so on.

The caregiver survey revealed that aides have slightly, though not significantly, more positive identification with whole units of work, presumably patients, than do LPNs (see figure 10.3). LPNs dispense medications and perform administrative functions, which reduces their "hands on" caregiving role. The primacy of the aide-resident relationship discussed earlier was confirmed by the aides' higher perceptions of task identity: Long-term caregiving offers more of an opportunity to establish client relationships than do most jobs.

*Task significance* refers to the extent to which workers believe their work has an impact on the lives of others. Presumably, most health or human-service workers experience their work as relatively significant, in terms of its effects on others. Clear variations within service professions exist, however. For example, intensive-care nurses rate their work much higher on task significance than do psychiatric nurses in the same hospital (Joiner et al., 1982).

Perhaps the clearest message delivered by the 1986 Pennsylvania nursing home staff survey was that the caregivers were well aware of the importance of what they did (see figure 10.4). Given the primacy of the staff-resident relationship in nursing homes, it is not surprising that caregivers scored higher than any of the published norms for other job categories. LPNs felt the significance of their work more strongly than did aides, but both were very high. This finding may reflect a normative response or social-desirability bias rather than a definitive response to the operational reality of the work. Generally negative societal attitudes toward aging and nursing homes would suggest a likely counter bias, however. Furthermore, if this strong sense of task significance is a socially constructed perception, it may also be a socially constructed reality, thereby affecting behavior.

*Autonomy* is the most clearly understood, and in the health-care sector,

**Fig. 10.3**

Task Identity

Aides and LPNs with Comparison Groups

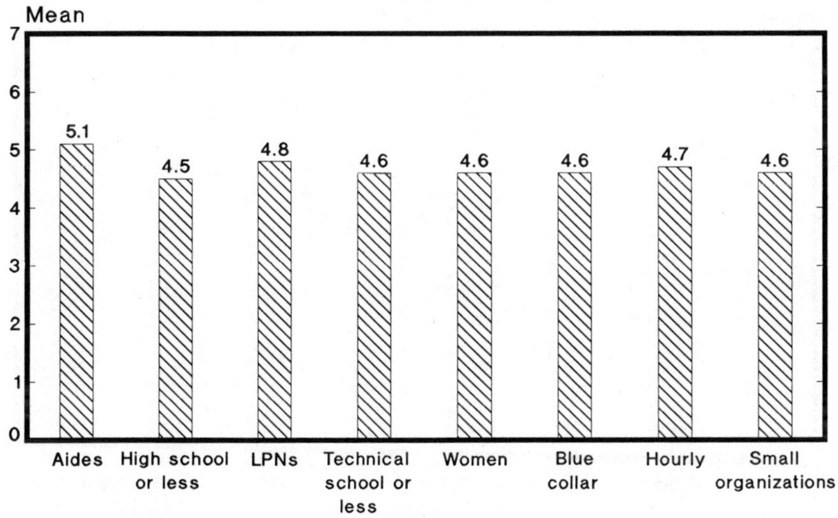


**Sources: Brannon et al. (1986) and Oldham, Hackman, and Stepina (1979).**

**Fig. 10.4**

Task Significance
Aides and LPNs with Comparison Groups

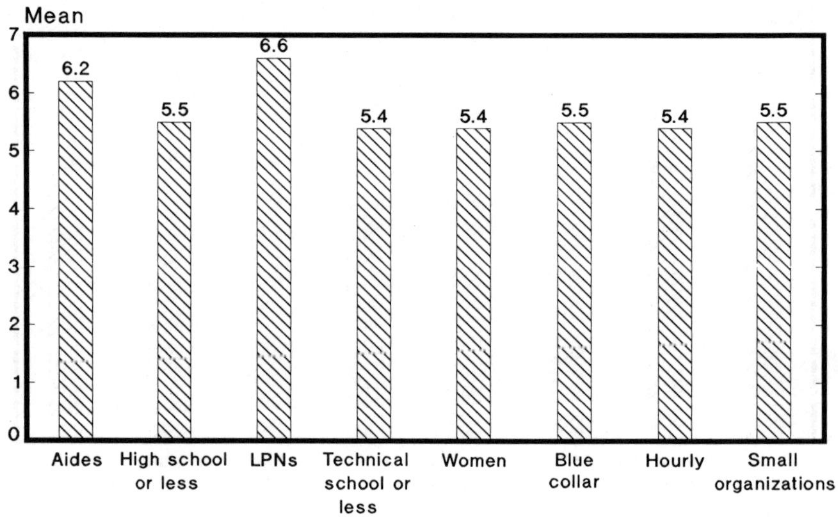


**Sources: Brannon et al. (1986) and Oldham, Hackman, and Stepina (1979).**

perhaps the most troublesome, job characteristic. Autonomy is discretion in the scheduling of work activities and in determining procedures to be used. Professionals have more autonomy than nonprofessionals because it is assumed that credentials limit behavior within a range of acceptable treatment approaches. Although behavioral responses to clinical, especially mental-health, symptoms are rarely prescribed with precision, this lack of precision has not resulted in widespread autonomy among nursing home care providers. Legal constraints, both legislative and litigated, result in a centralization of discretion at the top of the hierarchy of jobs. Physicians and professional nurses have the most apparent autonomy, though we will explore later the more subtle forms of discretion exercised by lower-level staff.

An analysis of the amount of flexibility or discretion associated with caregiving work reflects the bureaucratic structure that is typical of most nursing homes. Accordingly, lower-level employees experience less autonomy in the scheduling and implementing of their tasks than do their superiors. While aides' autonomy is similar to comparably low level jobs (see figure 10.5), the autonomy experienced by LPNs in nursing homes is exceptional. None of the other comparable job-category norms approached the level of autonomy experienced by LPNs in the caregiver sample.

Although aides perform a notable variety of tasks, nearly all of which are related to patient care, their performance of those tasks is largely organizationally determined. The scheduling of tasks and choice of procedures are fairly well prescribed by administrative staff. Aides are trained and supervised to operate within a limited scope of options. This limited discretion is typical of jobs filled by unskilled workers. Again, a discrepancy occurs, however, in that it is not typical of jobs designed to provide health and human services.

*Feedback* on task performance provides workers with knowledge of the results of their actions. Feedback is motivating in that it provides reinforcement, promotes self-correction and provides evidence of consequences of performance. Feedback from the work itself, derived from the flow of tasks, is generally valued more highly by workers than is feedback from supervisors. Likewise, objective, task-specific feedback is more significant than periodic performance ratings based on judgments. Feedback from the work itself is rarely perceived by workers in any job as adequate. It may be the case that more creative workers devise their own indicators for successful task performance.

The JDS measures both feedback from the job itself and feedback from supervisors or others. The Pennsylvania survey findings for both types of feedback are shown in figure 10.6.

With regard to feedback from others—supervisors, coworkers, resi-

**Fig. 10.5**

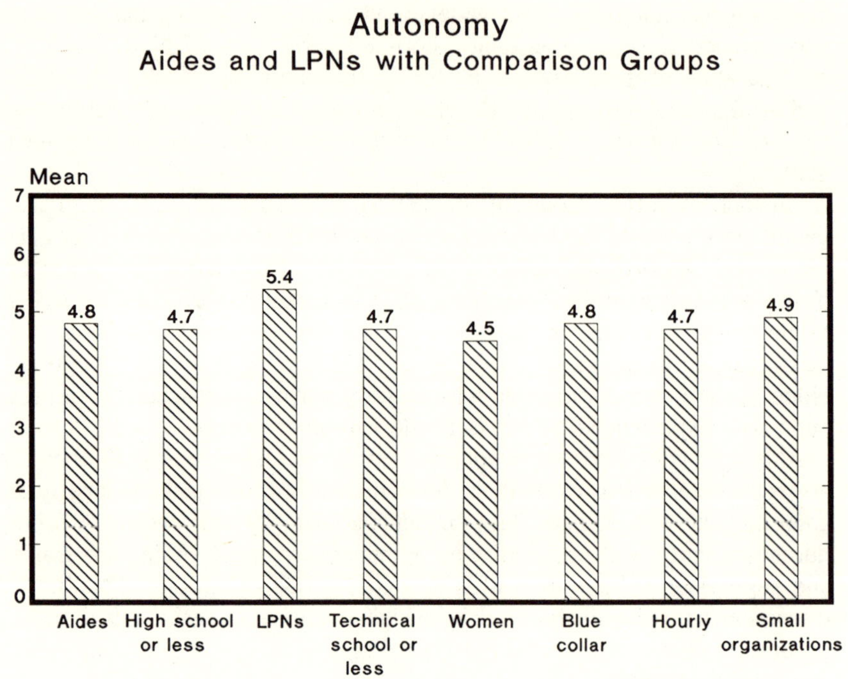


**Sources: Brannon et al. (1986) and Oldham, Hackman, and Stepina (1979).**

**Fig. 10.6**

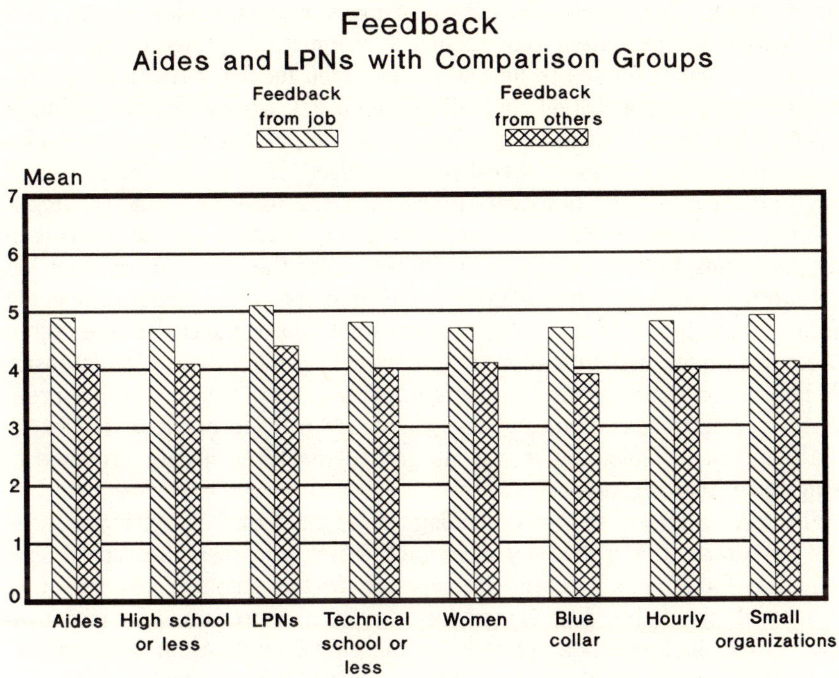


**Sources: Brannon et al. (1986) and Oldham, Hackman, and Stepina (1979).**

dents, and their families—both aides and LPNs were similar to women workers and employees of small organizations. LPNs were somewhat higher in their perceptions of feedback from others than were workers with equivalent education and hourly employees. While the long-term care provided in nursing homes might lend itself to extensive feedback from residents and their families, this job aspect is not perceived as a strength of caregiving work. The mental disabilities of many residents may impair communication to the extent that feedback is impaired. Joiner et al. (1982) found psychiatric nurses to be low in perceived feedback relative to other hospital nursing specialties. In addition, feedback from residents and their families has been difficult to separate from the practice of "tipping" to induce preferential treatment. Creative alternatives, such as the "Merit Gram" system, are emerging however (Reingold, Grossman, and Burros, 1987).

Feedback from the nursing home caregiving job itself was not perceived by the Pennsylvania caregivers as different from the norms from other job categories. LPNs reported slightly higher perceptions of feedback than did aides. In the Joiner et al. (1982) hospital study, coronary-care nurses rated their work quite high in feedback. The authors related this to the intensity of interaction not only with the patient and physician, but also to the presence of electronic monitoring devices, which provide constant feedback. To date, such equipment is not integral to the level of care provided in long-term-care settings.

To summarize these survey findings, it appears that caregiving work is not as bad as it is frequently described. When you read the typical shift schedule for nurse's aides in the appendix to this chapter, you may well react with sympathy, disgust, and/or a profound appreciation for your own job status. Such reactions have led professionals and researchers to perpetuate a negative image of caregiving as work. Yet the Pennsylvania survey data (Brannon et al., 1986) suggest that for these workers, caregiving in the nursing-home setting is at least as motivating as other types of work available to them. LPNs, in fact, find their work in nursing homes as intrinsically motivating as several types of professional hospital nursing. Aides' job perceptions are normative, albeit mediocre, on most job characteristics and are very high in task significance.

Since aides have the most contact with nursing home residents, their role in the nursing home community and thus, the nature of their work, deserves special attention. The challenge to nursing home administrators and mental health consultants is as follows: How do we make the most of our major human resource—the nurse's aides? The Pennsylvania survey results point to aides' perceptions of their work as more akin to professional-service delivery than one might think. Yet their work is viewed by outsiders and some administrators as menial. Surely facilities and residents stand to benefit from any approach that builds upon the positive aspects of caregiving work. One such approach is using aides as paraprofessionals in mental health treatment.

## NURSE'S AIDES AS MENTAL HEALTH PARAPROFESSIONALS

Alley et al. (1979) define the paraprofessional as a "regularly employed and fully salaried staff member whose formal degree does not exceed the baccalaureate" (p. 13). Although nonprofessionals have always been the core staff of mental hospitals, the term *paraprofessional* was coined in the 1960s in conjunction with war on poverty and community mental health programs. The belief was that the targeted underprivileged population could best be served by people with similar economic, social, and ethnic backgrounds. As such, indigenous paraprofessionals were hired based on personal traits and knowledge of a culture, not because of education or other credentials. These paraprofessionals were expected to act as mediators between lower-income clients and human-service agencies. With the deinstitutionalization of the mentally ill, which began in the late 1960s, a revitalization of community mental health services was needed. Paraprofessionals were to provide part of the answer to this need.[4]

The emphasis for paraprofessional involvement in mental health care has apparently shifted over time. Educated paraprofessionals are now less likely to assume the desired bridging function between clients and service agencies (Levine et al., 1979). There are clear differences between the paraprofessionals and the patients in terms of age, health, and social status. Increasingly, the role of the paraprofessional in the community and in institutions appears to be as part of a treatment team.

Although paraprofessionals were initially criticized as having limited capabilities for providing services to clients,[5] the various treatment roles they can effectively serve have been documented.[6] While research on paraprofessionals has focused primarily on mental health settings, many of the principles can be applied to nursing home environments as well. What about the nursing home staff? How should they be classified? The information provided by James (1979) categorizes LPNs at the paraprofessional level and RNs at the professional level. We agree with the aforementioned definition of *paraprofessionals* (Alley et al., 1979), and with the divisions identified by James (1979), but additionally propose that there is a hierarchy of paraprofessional roles in nursing-home settings. LPNs clearly have more training than nurse's aides, and, as was discussed earlier, often operate autonomously. In some nursing homes, LPNs may, in fact, be viewed as professionals. Table 10.3 outlines eleven such roles for paraprofessionals working in long-term-care institutions, with parallels drawn between com-

TABLE 10.3: Roles and Functions of Paraprofessionals

| *Function* | *Community Example* | *Specific Examples for Nursing Homes* |
|---|---|---|
| Represent client and community | Teach staff, administration, and policy makers about needs of local community while also educating residents about the available services of the center | Teach families and new professionals about the nursing home |
| Generalists and advocates in outreach work | Act as advocates in relation to variety of community centers (hospital, welfare, schools, etc.) | Promote patient activity; buffer effects of institutionalization; individualize service delivery |
| Community organization workers | Organize neighborhood projects and activities in response to mental health needs and problems; train community leaders involved in developing programs | Organize activities for nursing home residents |
| Advocates for citizens dealing with public agencies | Assist clients with various service bureaucracies; set up mutual-referral relationship between center and other service agencies | Help patient make contact with social worker, with doctor; channel information between client and administrator |
| Workers in primary prevention programs | Organize self-help groups in client population | Monitor nutrition; encourage participation in exercise program |
| Mental health education workers | Organize community mental health programs | Organize reality-orientation programs; participate in behavioral-management regimes |
| Workers in secondary prevention and case identification | Identify individuals and families in the community who need help in the early stages of the mental health program | Recognize early symptoms of mental health problems in patient and provide initial assessment and/or referral for assessment (see chapter 5) |
| Agents for reducing the social stigma of the illness | Help individuals and their families overcome the social stigma connected with mental illness | Help individuals and families deal with stigma associated with nursing home placement |

*Continued on next page*

TABLE 10.3—*Continued*

| *Function* | *Community Example* | *Specific Examples for Nursing Homes* |
|---|---|---|
| Workers for patient reentry | Assist client with reentry into community life, family life, work life | Aid in assessing the least restrictive environment for patient and move him to that level; follow up with phone calls if patient moved home or to a new location; help families' reentry into community without patient |
| Liaisons between professionals and the community | Contact prospective clients in the community | Recruit volunteers from church; help family with transition if death of patient occurs |
| Deliverers of clinical-intervention services | Provide therapeutic intervention and mental health counseling for individuals and families, under the supervision of professionals | Perform behavioral interventions in the processes of caregiving |

Note: The first two columns of information are based on the ideas of Tarail (1979).

munity mental health programs and nursing homes. We believe that these roles and functions can be handled effectively by nurse's aides.

The most commonly cited reasons for paraprofessionals' effectiveness are that they are warm, emphatic, and sensitive (see, for example, Kahn, 1981). Paraprofessionals have been observed to have the ability to establish peerlike relationships with clients, the ability to take an active part in the clients' life situation, to empathize more fully with the clients' style of life, to teach the client successfully using the client's own frame of reference, and to help with transition (Gartner, 1979).

The innovative roles often assumed by paraprofessionals (see table 10.3), their flexibility and spontaneity (Sobey, 1970), as well as their cost effectiveness, may be seen as primary assets to a nursing home setting. In general, Sobey (1970) reports that paraprofessionals tend to be ready and willing to learn and undertake more than is expected of them. She studied 10,000 paraprofessionals in 185 mental health programs, and concluded that they contributed in two ways: "filling new roles based on patient needs which were previously unfilled by any staff, and performing parts of tasks previously performed by professionals, but tailoring the task to the nonprofessionals' unique and special abilities" (p. 174).

What is suggested here is a new role to address the needs of chronically mentally impaired nursing home residents. The proximity of nurse's aides to problematic resident behaviors makes them key to the constant and consistent treatment required. Two alternative strategies for implementing such a role are (1) training all aides in observational and behavioral-management skills or (2) creating a new job category—a mental health technician position—for which aides could apply.

Clearly, there is institutional work to be done in establishing a mental-health paraprofessional role. New job responsibilities in the area of mental health without the commensurate skills, training, and job redesign could prove to be demoralizing to aides and thus, counterproductive to the nursing care institution. With appropriate training, nurse's aides could provide valuable mental health–related services. The following criteria, adapted from Alley et al. (1979), are guidelines for successful use of these appropriately trained paraprofessionals:

*Criteria for Successful Utilization of Paraprofessionals*

1) Paraprofessionals are regular paid employees with bachelor of arts degrees or less education.
2) At least two full-time paraprofessionals comprise the service team.
3) Paraprofessionals work with staff members from a variety of disciplines.
4) Paraprofessionals carry out a significant proportion of the service delivery for the program.
5) The responsibilities of the paraprofessional staff are meaningful.
6) There is an awareness of the unique experience and skills that paraprofessionals contribute to a program; cost efficiency is not the only concern. Paraprofessional tasks extend beyond supplementing professionals and broaden the types of services available.
7) Staff members are recruited with consideration to the community being served.
8) Skills and experience, rather than academic qualifications are emphasized in the selection process.
9) Training is an ongoing process, with academic credit available from local colleges and universities.
10) Regular, formal supervision exists.
11) Opportunities for career development or advancement exist.
12) Evaluation is an ongoing process.
13) There are mutual learning and interaction between professional and paraprofessional staff members.

14) When appropriate, paraprofessionals are assisted and encouraged to continue formal educational development.

In considering the use of nurse's aides as paraprofessionals, it is also important to learn from others' experiences regarding their misuse:

> Telling him (her) that his sustained relationship with the patients is extremely important, we sit by while the aide is transferred to another ward. Attempting to give him our additional recognition by calling him an important member of our team, we practically insult him by ignoring, or showing disinterest in, what he says. We tell him how interested we are in him and his development, and then fail to learn his name, his background, or what interests him in his work. Encouraging him to take initiative, we fail to defend or support him when something goes wrong. Without considering the fact that aides help patients get better, we publicly attribute patient improvement to drugs or psychotherapy. We tell the aide that the hospital (nursing home) could not run without him, and then pay him so little that he has to take an outside job to support his family (Ellsworth, 1968, p. 46).

There has been a common resistance among professionals towards the employment of paraprofessionals, which Austin (1978) has attributed to feelings of threat to the professionals' expertise, anxiety about role blurring and loss of identity,[7] and the presumption that a lowering of standards would result due to the limited competence of the paraprofessional. The consultant should therefore be aware of possible resistance to an increased role for nurse's aides by staff RNs and LPNs. This may be less of a problem, however, if the focus is on a mental health treatment role, since there is not likely to be existing in-house mental health expertise to be threatened. A new service is being suggested, not a role transfer.

If the paraprofessional program sets out to "change the roles, interaction patterns, and power of the professional, then the outlook for success is dim." Similarly, "the greater the ambiguity of purpose for paraprofessionals, or the greater number of functions desired of a paraprofessional program, the less likely it is to succeed" (Wagenfeld and Robin, 1981, p. 352). It has been repeatedly suggested that new paraprofessionals be supervised closely for the first several months since this is the stage when role conflicts often arise (McPheeters, 1979; Sobey, 1970). This supervision also allows for the teaching and/or refinement of skills related to the paraprofessional role (McPheeters, 1979).

Conflict with professionals in conjunction with general disregard by management may result in paraprofessional job dissatisfaction, which could potentially lead to serious problems in job performance and attendance. As was previously mentioned, absenteeism and turnover have significant consequences for the nursing home community, resulting in disruption of care for residents.

As summarized by Moffic et al. (1984), the success of paraprofessionals depends on their basic human potential, appropriate training, and active participation in a team of professionals and nonprofessionals alike. Paraprofessional development occurs through exposure to and monitoring by professionals. Interviews with administrators in the statewide nursing home survey provided clear statements that better integration of aides into the case-planning process would improve patient care.

## SUMMARY

In this chapter, we viewed the quality of resident life in nursing homes as being significantly influenced by the job performance of paid caregivers. That performance is jointly determined by the ability of the caregivers and the motivational quality of the job itself. We progressed in this chapter from an apologetic view of what staff can and cannot do in institutional settings to a more hopeful statement of what may well be feasible. In chapter 11 we invite the reader to explore ways of operationalizing a mental-health-paraprofessional role for primary caregivers.

## NOTES

1. Baltes and Reisenzein (1986), through a series of observational studies, have documented the role staff play in maintaining and changing dependency behaviors among nursing home residents. Patterson et al. (1982) have demonstrated that staff behavioral interventions can be effective in improving the functioning of regressed elderly mental patients in a wide range of areas. These include self-care skills, social interaction, basic tasks, and self-esteem.

2. For a fuller discussion, see March and Simon (1958), Hage and Aiken (1969), or Perrow (1967).

3. The work of Joan Woodward (1965) is considered the classic treatment of how task interdependency affects technology.

4. For more comprehensive histories of the paraprofessional movement, see Levine et al., (1979) and Nash, Lifton, and Smith (1978).

5. Austin (1978) presents a thorough discussion of the perceived limitations of the paraprofessional.

6. In an early review by Karlsruher (1974), twenty-seven studies of paraprofessional programs were examined, and it was concluded that paraprofessionals were effective in creating positive psychotherapeutic change, and that no particular group of nonprofessionals appeared to be the most effective. Additional evidence for effectiveness comes from a frequently cited review article by Durlak (1979), in which forty-two studies, representing a wide range of client populations and outcome

measures, were examined. Comparisons between relatively untrained paraprofessionals and highly skilled, doctoral-level professionals across the studies led to the conclusion that paraprofessionals achieve clinical outcomes that are equal to or significantly better than those obtained by professionals. Durlak's research has been criticized on several grounds (see Nietzel and Fisher, 1981), yet his review does support the viability of a clinical role for paraprofessionals.

7. As Kahn (1981) points out, both professionals and paraprofessionals need to recognize the differences in their values, taking into account the things that are important in each other's value system as well as those things each considers to be most important in caring for the patient. Paraprofessionals who come from a lower socioeconomic class may have difficulties in dealing with middle-class professionals. Professionals may see themselves as representatives of the system, superior due to their training and status. Their perceived authority and decision-making power can lead to feelings of worthlessness, powerlessness, and resentment among the paraprofessional workers.

## APPENDIX

### NURSE'S AIDES

7:00–3:00 Routine

7:00 Report from 11–7 nurses—listen attentively
Receive assignments for the day from the nurse-in-charge
Check nursing care plans.
Prepare patients for breakfast:
- A. Wash hands and face
- B. Elevate head of bed
- C. Put on bibs

7:00–8:00 Serve trays and feed those who require it, assisting others as needed.

8:00–11:00 Routine morning care for all patients assigned:
- A. The nurse's aides are assigned to lists, each being responsible for her list.
- B. Daily baths are given to all bed patients who need them. Ambulatory patients are assisted with tub baths, two or three times a week, according to their individual needs. All other days they are to be given partial baths.

C. Special attention is given to eyes, reporting any abnormality or discharge to charge nurse.
D. Dentures are cleaned and oral hygiene given.
E. Wash genitals thoroughly and dry well to prevent chaffing and decubitus ulcers. Any areas that may be irritated or any breaking down of skin must be reported to charge nurse or supervisor.
F. Linen should be changed as needed each day.
G. Beds should be made with mitered corners and linens well tucked in to insure comfort of the patient. Be careful not to bind toes. Complete instructions for bed making is found in the Procedure section of nursing manual.
H. Fresh water and ice in pitchers to all patients who can handle them.
I. Patients to physical therapy or activities as scheduled.

11:15 Cleaning duties as assigned to each list:
A. Laundry Cart #1
B. Laundry Cart #2
C. Clean utility room
D. Dirty utility room
E. Tub room

Cleaning and sanitizing equipment is done on a different day for each list.
A. Bedpans
B. Wash basins
C. Emesis basins
D. Water pitchers and glasses

Bedside stands, dresser drawers, and clothes cupboards are cleaned and tidied as the need arises.

11:30 Early dinner for those assigned.

12:00 Take patients to dining room in preparation for dinner. Put on bibs.

12:00–12:30 Dinner for all other personnel.

12:35 Serve trays and feed or assist patients as needed.

1:15–3:00 A. Wheelchair patients taken to bathroom and put to bed for naps.

B. Back rubs given to each bed patient.
C. Ambulatory patients are walked for exercise.
D. Incontinent patients should be checked at least every two hours and cleaned as needed.
E. Bed patients should be checked every two hours and position changed, or oftener, as the situation requires.
F. You are responsible for your assigned patients during your tour of duty.
G. Take patients to scheduled activities.
H. Attend in-service programs as scheduled.

3:00 Report by charge nurse to 3–11 shift.
All nurse's aides remain on the unit until report is over.

### GENERAL INSTRUCTIONS

1. Remember to leave your area in good condition, neat and clean.

2. Each shift is responsible for the cleaning and returning of all equipment to its proper place. Always replenish supplies.

3. Remember—the information you hear is confidential and should not leave the facility.

# 11

# Job-Design Interventions for Improving Caregiving

*Larry Borchardt and Diane Brannon*

> Ninety percent of direct patient care in nursing homes is delivered by aides, a category that by law and usage implies no formal training or education. Just under half of all nursing home employees are aides. It is aides who rouse the patients in the mornings, escort them to the bathroom and to meals, assist them in dressing, clean up after them, and as a general rule administer—illegally—at least some of their medication. When residents are incontinent, aides clean up after them. When residents cannot bathe themselves, aides assist them. When residents cannot speak or make themselves understood, aides must divine their meaning.
>
> Few jobs in this society are worse than those of aides in nursing homes.
>
> *Bruce Vladeck*

## INTRODUCTION

In chapter 10 we identified caregivers within the nursing home community and described the nature of their work. The mental health-paraprofessional role was suggested as a way to meet treatment deficits within the nursing home community. However, low morale and an exacerbated turnover problem can be expected if caregivers are given increased responsibilities without careful preparation, participation, and the commitment of the entire organization.

In this chapter, we suggest a strategy that will maximize the likelihood of successfully implementing such an expanded role: a combination of a job-enrichment intervention and skills training. To prepare the consultant or other change agent to implement such a strategy, this chapter will (1) introduce job enrichment as a behavioral intervention appropriate for use in the nursing home setting; (2) explore the elements that enhance the probability of a successful job-enrichment project; (3) explain why caregivers are an appropriate target population for job enrichment; (4) suggest a job-enrichment strategy specifically for the jobs of caregivers in nursing homes; and (5) consider the importance of skills training as a parallel intervention.

## BASIC CONCEPTS IN JOB DESIGN

Job design is the deliberate, purposeful planning of a job, including all of its structural and social aspects. Over the past twenty-five years the basic philosophy of job-design theory has evolved into one that implies that more satisfaction can be derived from work where the structure of tasks is designed to increase the individual's motivation, facilitate his use of a greater variety of skills and increase participation in relevant areas of decision making. This evolution has resulted in the development of a behavioral-science-based approach to job design that is commonly labeled "job enrichment."[1]

Job enrichment has its roots in the work of Herzberg and his colleagues and is intended as a means of increasing the motivation and satisfaction of people in their work place and consequently improving productivity. A strategy of job enrichment is consistent with the other interventions recommended in this book since it is based on a behavioral model. Generally, people do the tasks they are given. How well they do them depends on many factors, however, including how the tasks themselves are designed. On the other hand, people do not always behave in a manner consistent with their attitudes, their levels of satisfaction, or what they have been told they "should" do. Indeed, it is now well established that an individual's attitudes often are determined by the pattern of behavior engaged in, rather than vice versa. Job enrichment, then, may have a twofold benefit. First behavior itself is changed. Second, there is usually an increase in levels of autonomy and personal discretion at work, thus increasing the likelihood that workers will develop attitudes that are supportive of their new on-the-job behavior.[2] Job enrichment does not rely on changing attitudes and hoping that the attitude change will generalize to work behavior. Instead, the strategy is to change the behavior itself in a way that gradually leads to a more positive set of attitudes about work, the organization, and the worker's self-image.

Although job enrichment has become the dominant job-design approach, it is not the only approach that is espoused. There exists also the mechanistic approach based on "classic" industrial engineering, the biological approach based on biomechanics and work physiology, and the perceptual-motor approach based on experimental psychology. There have been nearly seven hundred "rules" for job design identified in the literature relating to these four different approaches.[3] These different approaches do contain some overlap but there is considerable divergence in focus and direct conflict in some of the advice offered. For example, the recommendations that derive from a job-enrichment approach and from a mechanistic approach are almost opposite concerning the complexity of a job and the mental demands contained in a job.[4]

Therefore, not everybody agrees what job design is, or should be, so care must be taken to define terms when discussing the concept. Two elements have contributed significantly to job enrichment's popularity over the past two decades. First, it contains a more socially attractive value orientation than other job-redesign approaches. It views people as working toward personal fulfillment and self-esteem through their intrinsic motivation rather than solely in response to external rewards, such as money. In this way, it is consistent with the popular sociopsychological theories of Maslow, Herzberg, and McGregor. Second, it holds out to organizations the possibility of increasing productivity without raising salaries, increasing benefits, or making costly investments in new plants and equipment.

## RESULTS OF JOB-ENRICHMENT INTERVENTIONS

Hackman and Oldham's (1976; 1980) job-characteristic model, introduced in chapter 10, holds that four beneficial effects will be derived from a job-enrichment strategy: (1) internal work motivation, (2) reduced turnover and absenteeism, (3) work satisfaction, and (4) enhanced quality of performance. Hackman and Oldham identified five key job characteristics: task identity, task significance, skill variety, autonomy, and feedback. These characteristics are dimensions of job design and subject to intervention. Strategies for intervention, or job redesign include the following, according to the Hackman and Oldham model: vertical loading with authority and responsibility, combining tasks, establishing client relationships, forming natural work units, and opening feedback channels.

Kopelman (1985) has reviewed the results of thirty field experiments involving behaviorally based job-redesign interventions in settings ranging from assembly-line workers to Internal Revenue Service tax examiners. The interventions studied employed at least one and up to all five of the implementing concepts prescribed by Hackman and Oldham. Studies were reviewed only if they gave a clear indication that either productivity or quality of production in the work place had been affected.

For the thirty interventions that clearly demonstrated the impact on productivity, the median result was an increase in productivity of 6.4 percent. Eleven cases, however, produced results that were either zero or negative which supports Hackman's assertion that job redesign will not consistently improve productivity. In the nine studies that provided a clear indication of effect on absenteeism, the median result was a 14.5 percent decrease in absenteeism. In twenty-one cases the impact of job enrichment on work quality was measured. The median result was a 28 percent improvement. The indicator of improved quality was generally reduction in errors. In twenty of twenty-four experiments that measured job satisfaction an increase was reported. Feedback was found to be a particularly important implementing concept. In summary, the results indicate that job enrichment can have a positive impact upon job satisfaction, absenteeism, and quality of job performance in varied settings, but the results are not consistent. Later in the chapter, we will examine methods of enhancing the probability of a successful job-enrichment effort in organizations in general and nursing homes in particular.

Although the field studies above include interventions in a wide range of organizational settings, none of the job-enrichment projects involved jobs that required the worker-client interaction that is present in the jobs of caregivers. Kopelman (1986), however, reviews the results of job-design interventions that focused on one of the implementing concepts described by Hackman and Oldham (1976), opening feedback channels. Job enrichment can be unidimensional, such as simply improving feedback.[5] Several of the interventions involved workers responsible for the direct provision of services in mental health care settings. These cases are described in some detail below.

---

*Case I* (Shook, Johnson, and Uhlman, 1978).
*Sample and Setting.* Six therapists employed at one health-service center.
*Intervention.* (1) Job simplification; (2) individual feedback on completion of tasks and verbal reinforcement in the form of one or two sentences.
*Results.* Reducing the amount of response effort needed increased performance levels slightly. Individual and group feedback along with instructions were clearly more effective in controlling behavior although there was a high degree of variability. The researchers demonstrated effective techniques for increasing the rate of low-rate, everyday behaviors.

*Case 2* (Prue et al., 1980).
*Sample and Setting.* Approximately 750 staff delivering services to approximately 950 clients in a state mental hospital.
*Intervention.* (1) Weekly summary of each unit's treatment activity was sent to the unit's treatment coordinator; (2) same as (1) with the information that results would be posted at some future time; (3) public display of the number of staff hours spent on treatment, number of hours of client participation, number of programs meeting description and correspondence criteria.
*Results.* All three methods of feedback were followed by large increases in treatment activity. Performance feedback increased the frequency of

staff conversation regarding treatment and interlevel staff interaction. Treatment information served an instructional function. The inducement to avoid "punishment" of posting a poor performance level was created. Interunit competition may have been brought on by public posting. The study demonstrated that systematic use of feedback can produce increased performance levels even in large complex organizations.

*Case 3* (Kreitner, Reif, and Morris, 1977).
*Sample and Setting.* Eight mental health technicians in a mental health facility.
*Intervention.* Public posting of an interoffice memo of each technician's frequency of target behaviors for the week. Each week's performance was added in another column. No other reinforcement outside of the public posting was used.
*Results.* Improvement in performance levels occurred for all eight technicians across all three target behaviors. Group-therapy sessions doubled, individual-therapy sessions tripled, and daily-routine performance doubled. A marked decrease in staff conflict and a decrease in patient complaints were also noted.

*Case 4* (Quilitch, 1975).
*Sample and Setting.* Seventeen mental health technicians in four residential child-treatment units.
*Intervention.* (1) Administrative memos directing staff to lead daily recreational activities; (2) workshops designed to show staff how to lead recreational activities effectively; (3) public feedback on staff performance of leading activities.
*Results.* Neither the memos nor in-service training had an effect on level of performance, although staff evaluations of the workshops were overwhelmingly favorable. Public feedback, however, increased the average number of residents involved in recreational activities from 7 to 32 in the 4 units (out of 95 total).

*Case 5* (Pommer and Streedbeck, 1974).
*Sample and Setting.* Nine staff employees in a residential child-treatment facility.
*Intervention.* Feedback on performance by publicly posting notices of staff efficiency in completing assigned duties. One-dollar tokens were also given for meeting specified performance criteria.
*Results.* Performance levels increased during the time that they were posted and performance quickly dropped to baseline levels once the postings were discontinued. The combination of posting and tokens produced the highest levels of performance.

## WHY JOB ENRICHMENT IN NURSING HOMES?

> I do not find that job satisfaction, improved job attitude, happiness or for that matter, mental health are saleable quantities in and of themselves. As a consultant, I have found it difficult, if not impossible, except in rare instances, to sell job satisfaction or mental health; so I sell human resource utilization in the form of job enrichment (Whitsett, 1971, p. 31).

Nursing homes are fundamentally not unlike other organizations, and we would expect that Whitsett's comments are applicable to them. While the perspective presented in chapter 10 makes clear that job redesign may be useful in improving caregiving, there must be other incentives for nursing home operators and administrators to undertake a job-enrichment project. Similarly, improving the job satisfaction or the mental health of the work force may be less than compelling reasons. One primary incentive involves the substantial turnover within the care-giving staff in the nursing home industry. The high attrition rate in nursing homes has economic consequences for owners and administrators, work load and social consequences for the coworkers of staff that leave, and medical, social, and financial consequences for nursing home residents and their families.

The cost of recruiting, hiring, and training replacement staff can be as high as four times the salary of the caregiver who has departed. These costs are, of course, for the most part passed on to consumers, but are a problem over which owners and administrators would like to have better control. In addition, much of supervisors' time must be devoted to continually training new personnel. This affects the supervisors' job satisfaction and reduces the amount of time that they are able to devote to patient care.

The importance of the social aspects of the jobs of caregivers was pointed out in an earlier chapter. Loss of friendships and uncertainty of what to expect from replacement staff compounds the problems that are caused for coworkers due to added work loads when a colleague leaves. These conditions may interfere with the staff's ability to render care that would be possible with a more stable work force.

The costs to residents and family go far beyond the financial ones incurred when charges are raised to reflect the cost of high turnover to the owners of the nursing home. Patient care suffers when those with valuable knowledge about the medical condition and likes and dislikes of residents leave on a regular basis. Disruption of daily routines due to the constant introduction of new staff can only add to the distress felt by many nursing home residents. Finally, the importance of the caregiver–patient relationship has been pointed out earlier. The close, personal emotional contact and support that caregivers are in a position to provide is lost when caregivers leave for long enough or must be constantly moved around the institution in order to plug gaps caused by the departure of others.[6] Also, there is a growing competition among facilities on quality of care issues, which expands the importance of these issues for nursing homes.[7]

Although job-enrichment projects have produced inconsistent results in terms of improving productivity, their track record in improving organizational commitment, as manifested by low turnover and absenteeism has been more impressive.[8] In nursing, high turnover reduces productivity by at least 50 percent.[9] Therefore, by making a commitment to a job-enrichment project, the administration of a nursing home makes a commitment to attack a problem that is costly in terms of dollars, quality of care, and strain on remaining staff with a strategy that has proven effective in other settings in reducing turnover, requires little capital expenditure, and may also increase the satisfaction and mental health of the workers. Job enrichment and nursing homes seem a natural combination.

## OBSTACLES TO JOB-ENRICHMENT IMPLEMENTATION

> Aides are often ill at ease with and intimidated by the verbal fluency that comes much more easily to professionals, not only because of their limited education and opportunities for verbal discussion, but also because so many of the skills needed and nurtured in their work are nonverbal. Words are instruments of power, instruments that aides, as a rule, wield badly (Dawes, 1981, p. 273).

From the results reported in the preceding section, it is clear that the effects of job-enrichment interventions are inconsistent. Job redesign, when done correctly, is not easy. It is hard work that requires the total commitment of the organization.[10] What causes job-enrichment project to be successful in one setting and to fail in others? Sirota and Wolfson (1972) present a summary of confounding categories of variables that may be obstacles to implementation:

***1) Educational.*** Managers often lack the knowledge and skill required to implement job enrichment successfully, and this, along with some false starts, can quickly discourage them from persevering.

***2) Ideological.*** Belief in the principles of scientific management still prevails in most organizations. Job enrichment is viewed by many managers as an employee benefit that returns nothing to the organization. Introduction of job enrichment is likely to encounter resistance from at least some managers on these grounds.

***3) Organizational.*** Job enrichment represents a current cost for which there will be a future return. Most organizations are under pressure to produce results today so there is limited interest in the future. There is also a problem with managers' leaving an organization while a job-redesign project is in progress. The interruption this causes can be detrimental. Finally, the jobs of more people in the organization are affected than just those whose jobs are redesigned. Therefore, the cooperation and support of the entire organization, with no personal gain, is sometimes necessary.

***4) Managerial.*** There are at least two reasons why a manager may resist a job-redesign effort. The manager may feel threatened by any sort of change, feeling safer with the status quo, and/or the manager may feel a loss of control as workers assume more responsibility for their own actions.

***5) Technological.*** Sometimes (although not in the case of nursing homes) a considerable investment in new equipment must be made in order to implement a job-redesign project. Since there can be no guarantee of success, this cost will always be an obstacle when such action is necessary. Nursing licensure laws will constrain the job activities of unlicensed caregivers, however.

***6) The Employee.*** Employees may be incapable or unwilling to perform the jobs as redesigned. Obviously the job redesign needs to be tailored to individual capabilities. Generally, however, workers have been described as eager to participate in job-redesign endeavors. Union endorsement, however, is critical.

***7) The Consultant.*** When job redesign involves an outside consultant, he or she is likely to blame the organization in which the project is taking place or its employees for any failures rather than examine the strategy or the methods being used to implement it.

***8) Diagnosis.*** Job enrichment is not right for every organization and changing work content does not automatically solve problems in the workplace. There are instruments, such as the Hackman and Oldham (1976) Job Diagnostic Survey (JDS) and, alternatively, the Sims, Szilagyi, and Keller (1976) Job Characteristics Inventory (JCI), which can assess the appropriateness of job enrichment, and they should be used before any intervention is attempted.

***9) The "Prove It Here"*** and

***10) The "Nothing New Here" Attitudes.*** These attitudes, which stress the uniqueness of an organization and the good management techniques that an organization has always used, can result in managers' only going through the motions without any real commitment to the job-enrichment project.

***11) Time.*** Job enrichment, when done correctly, will require weeks of planning, implementation, and evaluation. Even managers who begin a project enthusiastically will be drained as time goes on if they are ill prepared for this degree of commitment. Time presents an obstacle to keeping the process of job enrichment going once it has begun.

## HOW TO IMPLEMENT JOB ENRICHMENT SUCCESSFULLY

In order to overcome or avoid these and other obstacles, Frank and Hackman (1975) developed four prescriptive guides for the successful implementation of a job enrichment strategy. Table 11.1 summarizes the prescriptions and suggests how they might be applied in a nursing home setting.

Every organization that initiates a job-enrichment project will be unique in some manner. Thus, some of the obstacles that will be encountered will also be unique to that organization. However, careful diagnosis intended to expose those differences combined with a flexible, theory-based strategy that undergoes frequent evaluation and necessary changes is a more important determinant of success or failure of a project than the organizational setting in which it is implemented.

## ARE CAREGIVERS READY TO BE ENRICHED?

> Aides were frequently referred to as "kids" (even though many of them were middle-aged) by the nursing staff. They were openly called "dumb," "stupid," or "lazy" before their peers. Although they were responsible for most patient care and performed the more difficult tasks, they were generally not perceived as being part of the staff. The majority of the nursing staff were often perceived by the aides as "cold," and "insensitive," or "selfish" (Sbordone and Sterman, 1983, p. 245).

The introduction to this chapter quotes Bruce Vladeck, "Few jobs in this society are worse than those of aides in nursing homes" (Vladeck, 1980, p. 20). If this is true, what are the implications for affecting the jobs of caregivers through job enrichment? Job enrichment is largely built upon

TABLE 11.1: Applications of the Frank and Hackman (1975) Guideline in Nursing Homes

| *General Guidelines* | *Nursing-Home Applications* |
|---|---|
| 1) There should be a theoretical base to job-redesign efforts.[a] | The job-characteristics theory is an appropriate model for nursing home caregivers. It states that the more an individual experiences meaningfulness, responsibility, and knowledge of results, the greater will be his personal work motivation, quality of performance, and job satisfaction. The theory also has the advantage of providing a diagnostic model for measuring both job characteristics and employees' attitudes and needs prior to the redesign of work. |
| 2) Before any intervention is initiated, a diagnostic evaluation of the jobs that are to be redesigned and the social and technical environment must be made. | Consistent with the recommendation of using the job characteristic approach as a theoretical base, the Job Diagnostic Survey should be used to determine if the jobs of caregivers are suitable for job enrichment. The degree of support of management and other nursing personnel must be determined. The impact upon the jobs of supervisors and other nursing personnel must also be determined and these personnel made aware of what to expect. The potential impact upon clients and their families must also be developed. |
| 3) Given the results of the diagnostic task, contingency plans should be developed in advance to deal with anticipated and unanticipated problems that will inevitably occur. | The entire nursing home staff must be made to realize that job enrichment is not a panacea and problems will occur. A project-coordinating committee including members from all affected work groups within the nursing home should be established to which problems can be taken and which has the authority to initiate action to overcome these problems. |
| 4) The consultant or other change agent must be prepared for setbacks and set up mechanisms for continuous evaluation and be flexible enough to change implementing plans as the project unfolds. | Short-term operationalized goals must be set, such as incremental reductions in absenteeism or increased input from caregivers in patient-care planning that is measured in some way. These items can be tracked by an in-house coordinating committee but the consultant must be prepared to meet with this group on a regular ongoing basis in order to maintain momentum in the implementation process. |

[a]There are four theoretical approaches to the redesign of work activation theory (see Schwab and Cummings, 1976), motivation-hygiene theory (see Herzberg, 1968), job-characteristics theory (see Hackman et al., 1975), and socio-technical systems theory (see Trist et al., 1963).

Herzberg's motivation-hygiene theory. According to the theory, hygiene factors must be satisfied before motivation factors could have any effect (Herzberg, 1966). The implication is that workers must be reasonably satisfied with their work context (that is pay, job security, and coworkers) in order for job enrichment to have a significant impact. Oldham, Hackman, and Pearce (1976) found that if a worker is too dissatisfied with his work context, job enrichment may in fact produce negative results. If caregivers concur with the feelings of Bruce Vladeck, that their job is one of the worst in our society, it is unlikely that they would be good candidates for job enrichment. Chapter 10 describes a survey of caregivers in nursing homes in Pennsylvania using the Job Diagnostic Survey (JDS). We will now highlight these findings in relation to the Hackman et al. (1975) four-step approach to using the JDS to determine if a job-enrichment strategy is appropriate. We apply this approach to the Pennsylvania survey results:

*Step 1. Are motivation and satisfaction central to the problem?* The results in the Pennsylvania survey clearly demonstrate room for improvement, but these areas are not so bad that they are beyond help.

*Step 2. Is the job low in motivating potential?* The results show again that the motivating potential score is low for caregivers, but not very different from workers in other job categories in which job enrichment has been used effectively.

*Step 3. What specific aspects of the job are causing difficulty?* Subscores on the JDS can then be used to identify the specific strengths and weaknesses of the target job. For the caregiver sample, "feedback" was a weakness while "task significance" was clearly a strength.

*Step 4. How "ready" are the employees for change?* Once it has been documented that there is need for improvement in the job and the particular problem areas have been identified, the specific action steps that will be taken to enrich the job can be considered. An important consideration is the level of growth needs of the employees, since workers high in growth needs should respond more readily to job enrichment than those with little need for growth. The JDS has a direct measure of growth-need strength (GNS). In the caregiver sample, the GNS score was relatively low. The implication is that job enrichment should be introduced more cautiously for caregivers than the average worker. However, there is evidence that the GNS increases once a job-enrichment project is introduced as well as evidence that brings into question whether it is a moderator at all.[11]

Therefore, based on a survey of over four hundred caregivers in Pennsylvania, one can conclude that the jobs of caregivers have need for improvement in satisfaction and motivation, show a particular problem in feedback, and that a job-enrichment project should be implemented cautiously, due to the low GNS scores.

## NURSING HOME ADMINISTRATORS AND JOB ENRICHMENT

> The aides perceived the administrator as a "nice person but blind to what was really going on," the nursing staff perceived the administrator as "generally on top of things." The administrator perceived the poor morale of the aides as being due to their poor salaries (Sbordone and Sterman, 1983, p. 245).

It was stated earlier that job enrichment must have the total support of management in order to be effective (Sirota and Wolfson, 1972). There is no reason to think that the situation in a nursing home would be any different. Does a consultant have any reason to believe that the operator or administrator of a nursing home would be receptive to the suggestion of a job-enrichment project in his or her nursing home?

As part of the effort that involved administering the JDS to caregivers in the state of Pennsylvania, seventeen nursing home administrators or their assistants were interviewed. The principle purpose of the interviews was to determine if administrators felt that there was room to improve the job design of the work of caregivers according to the five elements of the job characteristics model of Hackman and Oldham (1976) within the context of that nursing home. The administrators were also asked for specific suggestions as to what could be done within their facilities to accomplish this.

All of the administrators identified at least one job characteristic that could be improved for nursing home caregivers and some identified all five. The most frequently identified were feedback and task identity. Most administrators felt that caregivers already viewed their jobs as significant and felt that legal and licensing questions constrained what could be done in terms of skill variety and autonomy. When asked for specific ways improvements could be implemented an overwhelming number of responses fell within the implementing concept described by Hackman and Oldham (1976) as opening feedback channels. The responses included giving more feedback to caregivers, encouraging more opportunities for formal feedback *from* caregivers, giving caregivers more opportunity to receive feedback from residents, and also providing opportunities for feedback through interaction with the families of residents. The idea of increasing feedback from residents and their families overlaps with the implementing concept of establishing client relationships.

Therefore, without any introduction to the concepts of job enrichment or their potential benefits these nursing home administrators were able to identify areas where they felt the jobs of caregivers could be improved and how these suggestions could be implemented within the nursing home setting. It is reasonable to believe that a carefully prepared presentation of the concepts of job enrichment as well as their applicability and potential for nursing homes would be met with considerable interest. In addition, the industry journals reflect what appears to be a growing interest in making optimum use of its largest component of "human capital," the nurse's aide.[12]

## THE PROCESS OF A JOB-ENRICHMENT PROJECT IN A NURSING HOME

> Language difficulties made direct communication between many aides and supervisors difficult. Even when language was not a problem, messages to aides by the nursing staff were often confusing or later contradicted. A strong "grapevine" or informal communication system within the facility also tended to alienate aides and nursing staff. Aides were rarely included in decisions regarding patient care, nor were they permitted to verbalize their opinions about patient care. In general, the strong need to create a strict, hierarchical structure discouraged or at times punished constructive feedback from lower level to higher level employees (Sbordone and Sterman, 1983, p. 245).

On the surface, the situation in the nursing homes described above appears appropriate for job enrichment using at least the implementing concept of opening feedback channels. If a consultant felt this were the case, how would he proceed from here?

The specific nature of a job-enrichment project for any organization, including a nursing home, can be designed only after a thorough diagnostic effort has taken place. However, experiences from other organizations in which job enrichment has been implemented can give some direction about the process that should be followed, if not specific job-design changes.

The consultant or other change agent must be certain that there is commitment at the top of the organization to a job-enrichment program, if a diagnostic evaluation indicates such a project would be useful.[13] For this commitment to have meaning, key managers within the nursing home must have an understanding of what job enrichment is, what results can and cannot be expected, and the amount of work that it will require. Therefore, these people must receive training in job enrichment. This could be accomplished by the consultant's assigning relevant readings to this group and leading several discussion sessions on the topic. If the type of commitment necessary for a successful job-enrichment project is present, this activity should not meet resistance.

After this training is complete, these managers will be in a position to decide if job enrichment is something to which they wish to commit the energy and resources of the organization. Given the types of job changes that may need to take place, they should start to consider now if they think the technology of the work within that particular nursing home is amenable to change, even though recommendations for specific changes will not be made until later.

If the key managers still feel that they are interested in job enrichment, a careful diagnostic evaluation of the nature of the work in that nursing home should take place. The Job Diagnostic Survey (JDS) (Hackman and Oldham, 1980) is a useful tool in this regard. Supervisors can be administered the companion Job Rating Form (JRF) in order to validate the responses of caregivers. As much as possible must be done in order to satisfy employees that all of their responses will be kept confidential and that there is no sinister motivation behind the testing. At the same time, announcing that job changes will or will not be made contingent upon the results of the survey will certainly bias the results. How much one needs to disclose is probably contingent on the amount of harmony between administration and staff and could be an indicator of problems in and of itself.

If the results of the JDS indicate that the jobs are low in motivating-potential score, and reasonably high in contextual satisfaction and growth-need strength, there is reason to believe that a job-enrichment project would be of some use.[14] The JDS should also illustrate which job characteristics need improvement. There is some disagreement about the process of deciding what job changes should be made in order to bring about the desired improvements. Some feel that employees should not participate since they do not know enough about the total organization or would be too inhibited to make suggestions for real change. Others feel that the employees whose jobs will be changed should participate because of their ability to make reality-based substantive contributions.[15] Seeborg (1978) performed a direct test of these two methods and concluded that the participation method was preferable, especially where coworker interaction was valued.

It is important to remember, however, that not only the jobs of the target workers are affected by a job-enrichment project. The immediate supervisors of the caregivers will probably also find their jobs altered in some significant way.[16] It is essential, therefore, to make them feel a part of the redesign process as well. One method for accomplishing the active participation of caregivers and supervisors is to have caregivers brainstorm ways to implement the desired improvements and prioritize the changes that they would like to see take place, and then allow supervisors to review these results, ranking them according to difficulty of implementation. All of these results would then be reviewed by a job-enrichment committee of key managers and a consultant if one is used. This could be an iterative process if necessary. The committee could select a number of suggestions it deemed most appropriate from those suggested and send them back through the process. The committee, of course, would hold final responsibility for what changes would be made and when.

The final step in the process, evaluation, and modification, would be an ongoing one. Job enrichment is not an end in itself. If the desired outcomes are improved resident care, reduced turnover, and improved worker satisfaction, and they are not met, the project needs to be redesigned or at worst abandoned.

## SKILLS TRAINING FOR CAREGIVERS: A PARALLEL INTERVENTION

> Knowledgeable assistants who know more about disease and symptoms assume more responsibility. They feel good about their job and they develop high levels of self esteem. No longer are they "just" nursing assistants (Lindeman, 1984, p. 65).

Organizational policies and practices in such areas as training and career development can essentially neutralize the effect of job-enrichment changes if they are not congruent with and, supportive of, the kinds of behavior that employees are expected to exhibit on their enriched jobs.

Training programs can increase the persistence of changes caused by job enrichment, sometimes substantially. Two types of training may be especially useful in association with a job-enrichment project. The first is technical training, to ensure that employees have the knowledge and skills necessary to perform the new tasks competently. If job enrichment has been successful, then employees will care more about performing well than they have previously. They should experience enhanced self-esteem when they have done well and feel displeased with themselves when they fail. A good technical-training program for employees with enriched jobs can increase the likelihood that their work experiences will be characterized more often by self-reward than displeasure.

Another type of training that often is needed when jobs are enriched has to do with the management of interpersonal relationships and decision-making processes. When work is designed in accord with the recommendations of the mechanistic approach discussed earlier in the chapter, employees have little need to coordinate and negotiate with others to get the work done or to make decisions about work processes or scheduling. All such matters are decided by management and specified in clear detail for those who will actually perform the work. On enriched jobs, however, a higher level of decision making and coordination may be required, and the prior work experience of the employees may have provided them with few chances to use or develop their skills in carrying out such activities. Thus, even when employees are competent to execute the technical aspects of their enriched work, problems may develop because of insufficient knowledge and skills in carrying out such activities. Training in this regard should be welcomed by affected employees since it should increase the degree to which enriched work is accepted and becomes permanent within the work unit.

Current literature on paraprofessionals in the mental health field emphasizes training. In contrast to the nursing home environment, the contribution and effectiveness of paraprofessionals is recognized in the mental health area. Thus, the focus has turned toward training issues, that is, on how to make these paraprofessionals *more* effective.

Training programs are considered to be responsible for the optimal functioning of paraprofessionals. Moffic et al. (1984) note that excellent training programs consider the apprehension of the paraprofessional concerning formal education, avoid overly academic or merely vocational training, involve educational leaders who respect paraprofessionals, and use a longitudinal method for training, rather than a "stop-gap" method. Gartner (1981) cautions against allowing the other extreme to occur in an attempt to move away from an overly academic model that results in paraprofessionals who are only trained to perform simple, specific functions without being educated with any kind of professional knowledge.

Santos et al. (1983) designed a series of successful training programs to improve mental health outreach to the elderly over an eight-year period. The "trainees" were selected from area agencies, specifically chosen on criteria consistent with the description of an associate-degree-level indigenous paraprofessional.

Role playing, written analyses of case scenarios, field supervisor ratings, questionnaires, interviews, and quizzes were part of the training program. These paraprofessionals were also instructed on the medical, psychological, and social aspects of aging.

Santos et al. (1983) noted increases in knowledge and skills and changes from negative to positive attitudes as a result of the training. Similar programs could prove beneficial to nursing homes, where attitudes and skills in caring for the elderly are of critical importance.

How might a skills-training program that addresses these two areas be implemented in a nursing home? We recommend skills training focused on behavioral approaches to the management of the three types of problem behaviors exhibited by nursing home residents highlighted earlier in the book: disorientation, depression, and agitation. Behavioral approaches to working with mental health problems in nursing homes have been noted for their preventative as well as their remedial impact. Behavioral approaches to problems of aging provide positive, adaptive, "life-long-learning" options, and suggest concrete actions to caregivers for teaching and reinforcing resident self-maintenance and optimal functioning.[17]

A skills-training intervention that follows the principles of programmed instruction and parallels those of adult education is recommended. Those principles include (1) clear outcome objectives stated behaviorally; (2) straightforward pre- and postintervention tests; (3) scripts to include small steps, frequent practice, varied exercises, opportunity for application to one's life and feedback/confirmation of learning; and (4) materials (written and supplementary) that respect the adult-learning principles of autonomy, appeal, feedback, immediacy, modeling, and practice.[18] A programmed format is recommended because of its user flexibility, its economy for training in small nursing homes, and its consistency. The effectiveness of programmed instruction has been found to be equal to or better than other methods of instruction.

## SUMMARY

In this chapter, we suggested a strategy for putting a mental health paraprofessional role for primary caregivers into operation. This strategy is a combination of job-enrichment and skills-training interventions. We attempted to provide information that would enhance the probability of successfully implementing this strategy within the nursing home setting. This was done by moving from the theoretical background through practical suggestions with the nursing home setting specifically in mind. These interventions need to be theoretically based, in order to provide direction, but flexible, in recognizing that no two settings are identical and, therefore, no two interventions will be identical.

## NOTES

1. The term *job enrichment* is used to refer to activities that involve alterations of jobs with the intent of improving both productivity and the quality of employee job experiences. For this purpose the term will not be distinguished from closely related terms, such as *job design, job enlargement,* or *work redesign.* See Strauss (1974) for a discussion of the specific connotations of each of these terms.

2. For a discussion of the relationship between attitudes and behavior see Bem (1970).

3. For a partial listing of these rules see Campion and Thayer (1985).

4. Principles of the mechanistic job-design approach include task functionalization/specialization, specialization of materials, task simplification, skill simplification, repetition, pacing, idle time/capacity and motion economy. Detailed discussions of these principles can be found in Taylor (1911), Gilbreth (1911), Ireson and Grant (1971), Maynard (1971), Barnes (1980), and Konz (1979).

Principles of the biological job-design approach include seating, tool design, endurance, strength, anthropometry, static effort, muscular adequacy and stress concentration. This approach derives from the work of Tichauer (1978), Astrand and Rodahl (1977), and Davis and Miller (1971).

Principles of the perceptual-motor job-design approach include workplace lighting, displays, controls, warning devices, panel layout, information-processing requirements, memory requirements, boredom, and arousal. Relevant literature includes works by McCormick (1976), Woodson (1981), Van Cott and Kinkdale (1972), Grandjean (1980), and Rasmussen (1981).

5. See Nystrom (1981).

6. For a more detailed discussion of the problem of turnover in nursing homes see Kraus (1974), Pecarchik and Nelson (1973), Stryker (1981), Waxman, Carner, and Berkenstock (1984), Schwartz (1974).

7. Falcone (1985) is an example of this in the recent nursing home industry literature.

8. Discussions of the impact of job enrichment on turnover and absenteeism can be found in Kopelman (1985), Orpen (1979), Ford (1969), Locke, Sirota, and Wolfson (1976), and Paul, Robertson, and Herzberg (1969).

9. Kasteler et al. (1979) discuss the relationship between productivity and turnover in nursing in detail.

10. The degree of commitment necessary is discussed in Paul, Robertson, and Herzberg (1969), Tichy (1976), Ketchum (1984), and Locke, Sirota, and Wolfson (1976).

11. For a discussion of the relationship between growth-need strength and job enrichment, see Orpen (1979) and Kemp and Cook (1983).

12. Examples of this interest can be seen in Gordon (1982), Leader (1986), Hinkley (1986), Bowman (1986), and Lindeman (1984).

13. Consultation regarding job design requires a more substantial knowledge base than can be provided here. Knowledge of motivation, task structure, and other management issues as they relate to job redesign are important components. These concerns, as well as the job-redesign process are treated thoroughly in Hackman and Oldham (1980).

14. A complete discussion of the implications of scores on the JDS is found in Oldham, Hackman, and Pearce (1976).

15. The relative advantages of employee participation in job-redesign projects are discussed in Ford (1969), Paul, Robertson, and Herzberg (1969), and Glaser (1975).

16. The extended impact of job redesign is discussed in Lawler, Hackman, and Kaufman (1973) and Cordery and Wall (1985).

17. Behavioral approaches are discussed in detail in Dupree, O'Sullivan, and Patterson (1982), Dye (1985), and Richards and Thorpe (1978).

18. To review instructional research in this regard see Clark (1983), Gagne and Reiser (1982), Kraut (1976), and Nash, Muczyk, and Vettori (1971). For examples, see Burke (1981), Johnson and Johnson (1971), and Scott (1968).

# Afterword

Mental health consultation is an effort to use professional expertise most efficiently. It requires indirect intervention, in effect multiplying the impact of a single well-trained mental health professional through the efforts of those consulted with. The mental health-consultation process is complex enough when carried out in community settings. When consultation approaches are applied to the nursing home, the complexity becomes almost overwhelming.

This book has been designed as an introduction to the organized complexity of mental health consultation in nursing homes. We have covered a wide range of topics—from the federal health-care environment to individual psychological assessment, from family functioning to dimensions of job design. We did so, however, with two purposes in mind: First, we felt that both the consultant and the consulter need to appreciate the broader context of mental health consultation in the nursing home. As a friend of ours put it: "You have to know the game to play your part." Second, we designed this book as an introduction to the area rather than as an exhaustive discussion of a single topic. We have tried to provide leads to the larger literatures on specific issues of concern, realizing that our current efforts are illustrative of the range of approaches that are appropriate for the setting, rather than a definitive treatment of any particular approach.

In the area of individual assessment, for example, we have not provided a detailed discussion of psychiatric and psychological testing of older adults with dementia or delirium. Instead, we have chosen to provide a general framework for considering the assessment task—a framework that may be useful to a wider range of professionals and staff members in the nursing home setting. Similarly, in discussing organizational-development approaches, we have necessarily been selective, focusing our attention on behaviorally oriented consultations and on job-redesign strategies.

In making our choices of emphasis and exclusion, we have tried to keep several audiences in mind. For nursing home administrators, we have tried to provide both a framework for considering mental health consultation as well as some sense of the possible benefits from including consultants in the work of the nursing home community. For mental health practitioners, we have tried to point out the relevance of their skills for the nursing home setting. Consulting and diagnostic approaches used in the community are directly applicable in the nursing home. For staff members who are responsible for mental health functions, we have tried to highlight the types of assistance potentially available from consultation.

The quality of institutional care is already on the public agenda, mainly because of the recent Institute of Medicine report and its attendant publicity (1986). The costs of institutional care are also emerging as an important public concern, mainly because of recent congressional debate over the scope and coverage of catastrophic health-care insurance. These developments in the public life of our nation may make it possible for mental health consultation to be included as an essential element in the expected range of nursing home services. Through this volume, we hope to help prepare consultants to assist in the growing task of adapting the nursing home community to meet the mental health needs of its community members better.

# References

## INTRODUCTION

Gatz, M.; Smyer, M. A.; and Lawton, M. P. 1980. The mental health system and the older adult. In *Aging in the 1980s: Selected contemporary issues in the psychology of aging,* ed. L. W. Poon. Washington, D.C.: American Psychological Association.

Glasscote, R. M., and Biegel, A. 1976. *Old folks at homes.* Joint information service of the American Psychiatric Association and the National Association for Mental Health.

Institute of Medicine. 1986. *Improving the quality of care in nursing homes.* Washington, D.C.: National Academy Press.

Levine, M. 1981. *The history and politics of community mental health.* New York: Oxford University Press.

Lindeman, C. 1985. Manpower in nursing homes: Implications for research. In *Mental illness in nursing homes: Agenda for research,* ed. M. S. Harper and B. Lebowitz. Rockville, Md.: NIMH, U.S. Department of Health and Human Services.

## CHAPTER 1

Bloom, A. W. 1983. *My experience with health care delivery systems for the elderly.* Unpublished manuscript prepared for the W. K. Kellogg Foundation National Fellows Program.

Branch, L., and Jette, A. 1982. A prospective study of long-term care institutionalization among the aged. *American Journal of Public Health* 72: 1373–1379.

Cohen, M. A.; Tell, E. J.; and Wallack, S. S. 1986. Client-related risk factors of nursing home entry among elderly adults. *Journal of Gerontology* 41 (6): 785–792.

Crose, R.; Duffy, M.; Warren, J.; and Franklin, B. 1987. Project OASIS: Volunteer mental health praprofessionals serving nursing home residents. *Gerontologist* 27: 359–362.

Dunlop, B. D. 1976. Need for and utilization of long-term care among elderly Americans. *Journal of Chronic Diseases* 29: 75–87.

Frankfather, D. L.; Smith, M. J.; and Caro, F. G. 1981. *Family care of the elderly.* Lexington, Mass.: Lexington Books.

Goffman, E. 1961. *Asylums: Essays on the social situation of mental patients and other inmates.* Garden City, N.Y.: Doubleday.

Goffman, E. 1968. Characteristics of total institutions. In *The mental patient: Studies in the sociology of deviance,* ed. S. P. Spitzer and N. K. Denzin. New York: McGraw-Hill.

Gottesman, L. E., and Bourestom, N. C. 1974. Why nursing homes do what they do. *Gerontologist* 14: 501–506.

Greenberg, J., and Ginn, A. 1979. A multivariate analysis of the predictors of long-term care placement. *Home Health Care Services Quarterly* 1: 75–99.

Gubrium, J. F. 1974. On multiple realities in a nursing home. In *Late life: Communities and environmental policy,* ed. J. F. Gubrium. Springfield, Ill.: Charles C. Thomas.

———. 1975. *Living and dying at Murray Manor.* New York: St. Martin's Press.

Gurland, B. J. 1980. The assessment of the mental health status of older adults. In *Handbook of mental health and aging,* ed. J. E. Birren and R. B. Sloane. Englewood Cliffs, N.J.: Prentice-Hall.

Haber, P. A. L. 1987. Nursing homes. In *The encyclopedia of aging,* ed. G. L. Maddox. New York: Spring.

Health Care Financing Administration (HCFA). 1981. *Long-term care: Background and future directions.* HCFA Publication No. 81-20047. Washington, D.C.: U.S. Department of Health and Human Services.

Johnson, C. L., and Grant, L. A. 1985. *The nursing home in American society.* Baltimore, Md.: Johns Hopkins University Press.

Kastenbaum, R., and Candy, S. E. 1973. The 4% fallacy: A methodological and empirical critique of extended care facility population statistics. *International Journal of Aging and Human Development* 4: 15–21.

Knight, B. 1986. *Psychotherapy with older adults.* Beverly Hills, Calif.: Sage Publications.

Liang, J., and Tu, E. J. C. 1986. Estimating lifetime risk of nursing home residency: A further note. *Gerontologist* 26: 560–563.

Litwak, E. 1985. *Helping the elderly.* New York: Guilford Press.

Maddox, G. 1975. Families as context and resource in chronic illness. In *Long-term care: A handbook for researchers, planners, and providers,* ed. S. Sherwood. Holliswood, N.Y.: Spectrum/Wiley.

McConnel, C. E. 1984. A note on the lifetime risk of nursing home residency. *Gerontologist* 24: 193–198.

National Center for Health Statistics. 1979. *National nursing home survey: 1977, summary for the United States.* Hyattsville, Md.: U.S. DHEW.

Palmore, E. 1976. Total chance of being institutionalized among the aged. *Gerontologist* 16: 504–507.

Shanas, E. 1979. Social myth as hypothesis: The case of family relations of old people. *Gerontologist* 19: 3–9.

Smallegan, M. 1985. There was nothing else to do: Needs for care before nursing home admission. *Gerontologist* 25: 364–369.

Swift, C. F., and Cooper, S. 1986. Settings, consultees, and clients. In *Handbook of mental health consultation,* ed. F. V. Mannino, E. J. Trickett, M. F. Shore, M. G. Kidder, and G. Levin. Department of Health and Human Services, Publication No. (ADM) 86-1446. Washington, D.C.

Tobin, S., and Kulys, R. 1980. Older persons and their responsible others. *Social Work* 25 (2): 138–145.

Troll, L. E.; Miller, S. J.; and Atchley, R. C. 1979. *Families in later life.* Belmont, Calif.: Wadsworth Publishing.

U.S. Department of Commerce. Bureau of the Census. 1978. *1976 survey of institutionalized persons: A study of persons receiving long term care.* Washington, D.C.: Government Printing Office.

Wack, J., and Rodin, J. 1978. Nursing homes for the aged: The human consequences of legislation-shaped environments. *Journal of Social Issues* 34 (4): 6–21.

Warren, R. L. 1963. *The community in America.* Chicago: Rand McNally.

## CHAPTER 2

Avorn, J. L. 1986. Medicine, health and the geriatric transformation. *Daedalus* 115 (1): 211–225.

Baldwin, C. Y. and Bishop, C. E. 1984. Return to nursing home investment: Issues for public policy. *Health Care Financing Review* 5: 43–52.

Blumenthal, D.; Schlesinger, M.; Drumheller, P. D.; and the Harvard Medicare Project. 1986. The future of Medicare. *New England Journal of Medicine* 314 (11): 722–728.

Callahan, D. 1986. Adequate health care and an aging society: are they morally compatible? *Daedalus* 115 (1): 247–267.

Cole, T. R. 1987. Class, culture, and coercion: A historical look at longterm care. *Geriatrics* 11 (4): 9–15.

Davis, K. 1986. Aging and the health-care system: Economic and structural issues. *Daedalus* 115 (1): 227–246.

Fries, B. E., and Cooney, L. M. 1985. Resource utilization groups: A patient classification system for long-term care. *Medical Care* 23 (2): 110–122.

Gaylin, W.; Glasser, I.; Marcus, S.; and Rothman, D. 1978. *Doing good.* New York: Pantheon Books.

Greene, V., and Monahan, D. 1981. Structural and operational factors affecting quality of patient care in nursing homes. *Public Policy* 29: 399–415.

Harrington, C.; Estes, C. L.; Lee, P. R.; and Newcomer, R. J. 1986. Effects of state Medicaid policies on the aged. *Gerontologist* 26: 437–443.

Hing, E. 1987. Use of nursing homes by the elderly: Preliminary data from the 1985 National Nursing Home Survey. *Advance Data* 135 (May 14): 1–12.

Institute of Medicine. 1986. *Improving the quality of care in nursing homes.* Washington, D.C.: National Academy Press.

Jones, A. A. 1984. Prospective payment: Curbing Medicare costs at patient's expense? *Generations,* fall: 19–21.

Kerschner, P. A. 1987. Personal communication with the authors. Dr. Kerschner is president of the National Foundation for Long Term Health Care.

LaViolette, S. 1983. Nursing home chains scramble for more private-paying patients. *Modern Health Care* 13: 110–138.

Lyles, Y. M. 1986. Impact of Medicare diagnosis-related groups (DRGs) on nursing homes in the Portland, Oregon Metropolitan Area. *Journal of the American Geriatrics Society* 34: 573–578.

McArthur, R. F. 1970. The historical evolution from almshouse to ECF: A three-part discussion. *Nursing Homes* 19 (April): 26–27; (June): 26–27; (August): 14–15.

Mechanic, D. 1987. Challenges in long-term care policy. *Health Affairs* 6 (2): 22–34.

*Modern Healthcare.* 1987. Financial digest, July 31, 88–89.

*Nation's Health.* 1987. HHS, Congress seeks nursing home reform. American Public Health Association. August, 5.

Office of Technology Assessment. 1983. *Diagnosis related groups (DRGs) and the Medicare program: Implications for medical technology—A technical memorandum.* OTA-TM-H-17. Washington, D.C.: Government Printing Office.

———. 1987. *Losing a million minds: Confronting the tragedy of Alzheimer's disease and other dementias.* Washington, D.C.: Government Printing Office.

Palmer, H. C. 1985. Studies of nursing home costs. In *Long term care: Perspectives from research and demonstrations,* ed. R. J. Vogel and H. C. Palmer. Rockville, Md.: Aspen.

Pear, R. 1987. Crisis is predicted in care of elderly. *New York Times,* September 13, A1, A43.

Pincus, J. D. 1986. Public relations: prescription for an ailing public image. *Journal of Long Term Care Administration* 14: 3–6.

Rabin, D. L., and Stockton, P. 1987. *Long-term care for the elderly: A factbook.* New York: Oxford University Press.

Scanlon, W. J. 1980. A theory of the nursing home market. *Inquiry* 17: 25–41.

Shaughnessy, P.; Schlenker, R.; Harley, B.; Shanks, N. H.; Tricario, G.; Perry, V.; Kurowski, B.; and Woodson, A. 1980. *Long term care reimbursement and regulation: A study of cost, casemix and quality.* Working Paper No. 4, University of Colorado, Center for Health Services Research.

Smallwood, D. E.; Simon, H. J.; and Brody, B. L. 1987. Questioning long-term care IRAs. *Health Care* 6 (2): 132–143.

Siebel, R. V. 1986. Health care policies: Industry incentives. *Journal of Long Term Care Administration* 14: 7–11. Epigraph from p. 10.

Strahan, G. 1987. Nursing home characteristics: Preliminary data from the 1985 national nursing home survey. *Advance Data* 131 (March 27): 1–12.

Sulvetta, M. S., and Holohan, J. 1986. Cost and case-mix differences between hospital-based and freestanding nursing homes. *Health Care Financing Review* 7: 75–84.

Thorburn, P., and Meiners, M. R. 1986. Nursing home patient outcomes: the results of an incentive reimbursement experiment. Long Term Care Studies Program Research Report, DHHS Publication No. (PHS) 86-3400. National Center for Health Services Research and Technology Assessment.

Ullman, S. G. 1985. The impact of quality on cost in the provision of long-term care. *Inquiry* 22: 293–302.

U.S. General Accounting Office. 1986. *Post-hospital care: Efforts to evaluate Medicare prospective payments are insufficient.* GAO/PEMD-86-10. Washington, D.C.: Government Printing Office.

U.S. General Accounting Office. 1987. *Medicare: Preliminary strategies for assessing quality of care.* GAO/PEMD-87-15. Washington, D.C.: Government Printing Office.

U.S. Senate. Special Committee on Aging. 1987. *Developments in Aging: 1986.* Vols. 1–3. Washington, D.C.: Government Printing Office.

Uyeda, M. K.; De Leon, P. H.; Perloff, R.; and Kraut, A. G. 1986. Financing mental health services: A comparison of two federal programs. *American Behavioral Scientist* 30 (2): 90–110.

Vladeck, B. C. 1980. *Unloving care: The nursing home tragedy.* New York: Basic Books. Epigraph from p. 3.

Vogel, R. J. 1985. The industrial organization of the nursing home industry. In *Long term care: Perspectives from research and demonstrations,* ed. R. J. Vogel and H. C. Palmer. Rockville, Md.: Aspen.

Wack, J., and Rodin, J. 1978. Nursing homes for the aged: The human consequences of legislation-shaped environments. *Journal of Social Issues* 34 (4): 6–21.

Wiener, J.; Ehrenworth, D. A.; and Spence, D. A. 1987. Private long-term care insurance: Cost, coverage, and restrictions. *Gerontologist* 27: 487–493.

## CHAPTER 3

Birkel, R.; Lerner, R. M.; and Smyer, M. A. In preparation. Applied developmental psychology as an implementation of the life-span view of human development. *Journal of Applied Developmental Psychology.*

Birren, J. E., and Sloane, R. B., eds. 1980. *Handbook of mental health and aging.* Englewood Cliffs, N.J.: Prentice-Hall.

Bloom, B. 1975. *Community mental health: A general introduction.* Monterey, Calif.: Brooks/Cole.

Busse, E. W., and Blazer, D. G., eds. 1980. *Handbook of geriatric psychiatry.* New York: Van Nostrand Reinhold.

Caplan, G. 1964. *Principles of preventive psychiatry.* New York: Basic Books.

———. 1970. *The theory and practice of mental health consultation.* New York: Basic Books.

Conoley, J. C. 1986. Contributions of psychology to mental health consultation. In *Handbook of mental health consultation,* ed. F. V. Mannino, E. J. Trickett, M. F. Shore, M. G. Kidder, and G. Levin. Washington, D.C.: Department of Health and Human Services, Publication No. (ADM) 86-1446. Washington, D.C.

Fullan, M.; Miles, M.; and Taylor, G. 1980. Organization development in schools: The state of the art. *Review of Educational Research* 12: 121–183.

Goldmeier, J., and Mannino, F. V. 1986. The role of social work in consultation. In *Handbook of mental health consultation,* ed. F. V. Mannino, E. J. Trickett, M. F. Shore, M. G. Kidder, and G. Levin. Department of Health and Human Services, Publication No. (ADM) 86-1446. Washington, D.C.

Gutheil, T. G. 1984. The problem of resistance in the nursing home consultation. *Social Casework* 65 (1): 40–44.

Howard, L. A. 1986. Nursing and mental health consultation: A public health-community perspective. In *Handbook of mental health consultation,* ed. F. V. Mannino, E. J. Trickett, M. F. Shore, M. G. Kidder, and G. Levin. Department of Health and Human Services, Publication No. (ADM) 86-1446. Washington, D.C.

Jellineck, T., and Tennstedt, S. L. 1980. Prevention of chronicity in the nursing home. *Psychiatric Annals* 10 (9): 37–44.

Kelly, J. G. 1986. The mental health disciplines and their approaches to consultation: A commentary. In *Handbook of mental health consultation,* ed. F. V. Mannino, E. J. Trickett, M. F. Shore, M. G. Kidder, and G. Levin. Department of Health and Human Services, Publication No. (ADM) 86-1446. Washington, D.C.

Keys, C. B. 1986. Organization development: An approach to mental health consultation. In *Handbook of mental health consultation,* ed. F. V. Mannino, E. J. Trickett, M. F. Shore, M. G. Kidder, and G. Levin. Department of Health and Human Services, Publication No. (ADM) 86-1446. Washington, D.C.

Knight, B. 1986. *Psychotherapy with older adults.* Beverly Hills, Calif. Sage Publications.

Levin, G.; Trickett, E. J.; and Kidder, M. G. 1986. The themes, promise, and challenges of mental health consultation. In *Handbook of mental health consultation,* ed. F. V. Mannino, E. J. Trickett, M. F. Shore, M. G. Kidder, and G. Levin. Department of Health and Human Services, Publication No. (ADM) 86-1446. Washington, D.C.

Mannino, F. V.; Trickett, E. J.; Shore, M. F.; Kidder, M. G.; and Levin, G., eds. 1986. *Handbook of mental health consultation.* Department of Health and Human Services, Publication No. (ADM) 86-1446. Washington, D.C.

Maruyama, M. 1983. Cross-cultural perspectives on social and community change. In *Handbook of social intervention,* ed. E. Seidman. Beverly Hills, Calif.: Sage Publications.

Petry, S., and Gutheil, T. G. 1979. The hidden psychology of nursing home consultation. *The Transnational Mental Health Research Newsletter* 21 (1): 6–9.

Robinson, L. 1986. Nursing and mental health consultation: Psychiatric liaison perspective. In *Handbook of mental health consultation,* ed. F. V. Mannino, E. J. Trickett, M. F. Shore, M. G. Kidder, and G. Levin. Department of Health and Human Services, Publication No. (ADM) 86-1446. Washington, D.C.

Santos, J. F., and VandenBos, G. R., eds. 1982. *Psychology and the older adult: Challenges for training in the 1980s.* Washington, D.C.: American Psychological Association.

Sbordone, R. S., and Sterman, L. T. 1983. The psychologist as a consultant in a nursing home: Effect on staff morale and turnover. *Professional Psychology: Research and Practice* 14(2): 240–250.

Schwab, J. J. 1986. The psychiatrist's roles and functions in the 1980s. In *Handbook of mental health consultation,* ed. F. V. Mannino, E. J. Trickett, M. F. Shore, M. G. Kidder, and G. Levin. Department of Health and Human Services, Publication No. (ADM) 86-1446. Washington, D.C.

Smith, K. K., and Corse, S. J. 1986. The process of consultation: Critical issues. In *Handbook of mental health consultation,* ed. F. V. Mannino, E. J. Trickett, M. F. Shore, M. G. Kidder, and G. Levin. Department of Health and Human Services, Publication No. (ADM) 86-1446. Washington, D.C.

Smyer, M. A.; Gatz, M.; and Pruchno, R. A. 1987. Community psychology and aging. In *Community psychology: Theoretical and empirical approaches,* 2nd ed., ed. M. S. Gibbs, G. R. Lachenmeyer, and J. Sigal. New York: Gardner Press.

Stockdill, J. W. 1986. Foreword. In *Handbook of mental health consultation,* ed. F. V. Mannino, E. J. Trickett, M. F. Shore, M. G. Kidder, and G. Levin. Department of Health and Human Services, Publication No. (ADM) 86-1446. Washington, D.C.

Tobin, S. S.; Ellor, J. W.; and Anderson-Rorg, S. M. 1986. *Enabling the elderly: Religious institutions within the community service system.* Albany, N.Y.: SUNY Press.

Vernberg, E. M., and Reppucci, N. D. 1986. Behavioral consultation. In *Handbook of mental health consultation,* ed. F. V. Mannino, E. J. Trickett, M. F. Shore, M. G. Kidder, and G. Levin. Department of Health and Human Services, Publication No. (ADM) 86-1446. Washington, D.C.

Verwoerdt, A. 1981. *Clinical geropsychiatry.* 2nd ed. Baltimore: Williams and Wilkins.

Zeisel, J. 1981. *Inquiry by design: Tools for environment-behavior research.* Monterey, Calif.: Brooks/Cole.

## CHAPTER 4

American Psychiatric Association. 1980. *Diagnostic and statistical manual of mental disorders* (DSM-III). 3rd ed. Washington, D.C.: American Psychiatric Association.

———. Ad hoc committee on the chronic mental patient. 1978. *The chronic mental patient.* Washington, D.C.: American Psychiatric Association.

Blazer, D. 1980. The epidemiology of mental illness in late life. In *Handbook of geriatric psychiatry,* ed. E. W. Busse and D. G. Blazer. New York: Van Nostrand Reinhold.

Butler, R. N., and Lewis, M. I. 1982. *Aging and mental health.* 3rd ed. St. Louis: C.V. Mosby.

Davies, A. M. 1985. Epidemiology and the challenge of aging. *International Journal of Epidemiology* 14 (1): 9–19.

Department of Health and Human Services. 1980. *Care of the mentally ill in nursing homes.* Publication No. (ADM) 81-1077. Addendum to national plan for the chronically mentally ill. Washington, D.C.

Dohrenwend, B. P., and Dohrenwend, B. S. 1982. Perspectives on the past and future of psychiatric epidemiology (the 1981 Rema Lapouse lecture). *American Journal of Public Health* 72: 1271–1279.

Dohrenwend, B. P.; Dohrenwend, B. S.; and Gould, M. S. 1980. *Mental illness in the United States: Epidemiological estimates.* New York: Praeger.

Eaton, W. W.; Holzer, C. E.; Von Korff, M.; Anthony, J. C.; Helzer, J. E.; and George, L. 1984. The design of the epidemiologic catchment area surveys: The control and measurement of error. *Archives of General Psychiatry* 41 (10): 942–948.

Eaton, W. W.; Reiger, D. A.; Locke, B. Z.; and Taube, C. A. 1981. The epidemiologic catchment area program of the National Institute of Mental Health. *Public Health Report* 96: 319–325.

Folstein, M. F.; Folstein, S. E.; and McHugh, P. R. 1975. Mini mental state: A practical method for grading the cognitive state of patients for the clinician. *Journal of Psychiatric Research* 12: 189–198.

Gatz, M.; Smyer, M. A.; Garfein, A.; and Seward, M. In press. Essentials of assessment in nursing homes. In *Mental health services in nursing homes,* ed. M. S. Harper. Baltimore, Md.: Williams and Wilkins.

Gatz, M.; Smyer, M. A.; and Lawton, M. P. 1980. The mental health system and the older adult. In *Aging in the 1980s: Selected contemporary issues in the psychology of aging,* ed. L. W. Poon. Washington, D.C.: American Psychological Association.

German, P. S. 1987. Personal communication with the author. May.

German, P. S.; Shapiro, S.; and Kramer, M. 1986. Nursing home study of the eastern Baltimore epidemiological catchment area study. In *Mental illness in nursing homes: Agenda for research,* ed. M. S. Harper and B. D. Lebowitz. Rockville, Md.: National Institute of Mental Health.

Glass, R. I. 1986. New prospects for epidemiologic investigations. *Science* 234: 951–955.

Goldfarb, A. 1962. Prevalence of psychiatric disorders in metropolitan old age and nursing homes. *Journal of American Geriatric Society* 10: 77–84.

Gottesman, L. E. 1977. Clinical psychology and aging: A role model. In *Geropsychology,* ed. D. Gentry. Cambridge, Mass.: Ballinger.

Honigfeld, G., and Klett, C. J. 1965. Nurses' Observation Scale for Inpatient Evaluation: A new scale for measuring improvement in chronic schizophrenia. *Journal of Clinical Psychology* 21: 65–71.

Kahn, R. L. 1975. The mental health system and the future aged. *Gerontologist* 15: 24–31.

Kay, D. W. K., and Bergmann, K. 1980. Epidemiology of mental disorders among the aged in the community. In *Handbook of mental health and aging,* ed. J. E. Birren and R. B. Sloane. Englewood Cliffs, N.J.: Prentice-Hall.

Kermis, M. D. 1986. The epidemiology of mental disorders in the elderly: A response to the Senate/AARP report. *Gerontologist* 26: 482–487.

Kramer, M. 1986. Trends of institutionalization and prevalence of mental disorders in nursing homes. In *Mental illness in nursing homes: Agenda for research,* eds. M. S. Harper and B. D. Lebowitz. Rockville, Md.: National Institute of Mental Health.

La Rue, A.; Dessonville, C.; and Jarvik, L. F. 1985. Aging and mental disorders. In *Handbook of the psychology of aging,* 2nd ed., ed. J. E. Birren and K. W. Schaie. New York: Van Nostrand Reinhold.

Levine, M. 1981. *The history and politics of community mental health.* New York: Oxford University Press.

Liptzin, B. 1986. Major mental disorders/problems in nursing homes: Implications for research and public policy. In *Mental illness in nursing homes: Agenda for research,* ed. M. S. Harper and B. D. Lebowitz. Rockville, Md.: National Institute of Mental Health.

MacMahon, B., and Pugh, T. F. 1970. *Epidemiology: Principles and methods.* Boston: Little, Brown.

National Center for Health Statistics. 1979. *National nursing home survey: 1977 summary for the United States.* Hyattsville, Md.: U.S. DHEW.

———. 1983. *An overview of the 1980 national master facility inventory survey of nursing and related care homes,* by A. Sirrocco. Vital and Health Statistics, No. 91.; Department of Health and Human Services, Publication No. (PHS) 83-1250.

National Institute of Aging (NIA) Task Force. 1980. Senility reconsidered: Treatment possibilities for mental impairment in the elderly. *Journal of the American Medical Association* 244 (3): 259–263.

President's Commission on Mental Health, The (PCMH). 1978a. *Task panel reports submitted to the President's Commission on Mental Health.* Vol. 4. Washington, D.C.: Government Printing Office.

———. 1978b. *Report to the president.* Vol. 1. Washington, D.C.: Government Printing Office.

Regier, D. A.; Goldberg, I. D.; and Taube, C. A. 1978. The de facto U.S. mental health services system: A public health perspective. *Archives of General Psychiatry* 35: 685–693.

Regier, D. A.; Myers, J. K.; Kramer, M.; Robins, L. N.; Blazer, D. G.; and Hough, R. L. 1984. The NIMH epidemiologic catchment area program: Historical context, major objectives, and study population characteristics. *Archives of General Psychiatry* 41: 934–941.

Robins, L. N. 1978. Psychiatric epidemiology. *Archives of General Psychiatry* 31: 697–702.

Robins, L. N.; Helzer, J. E.; Croughan, J.; and Ratcliff, K. S. 1981. National Institute of Mental Health diagnostic interview schedule: Its history, characteristics, and validity. *Archives of General Psychiatry* 38: 381–389.

Robins, L. N.; Helzer, J. E.; Ratcliff, K. S.; and Seyfried, W. 1982. Validity of the diagnostic interview schedule version II: DSM-III diagnoses. *Psychological Medicine* 12: 855–870.

Rovner, B. W.; Kafonek, S.; Filipp, L.; Lucas, M. J.; and Folstein, M. F. 1986. Prevalence of mental illness in a community nursing home. *American Journal of Psychiatry* 143 (11): 1446–1449.

Sabin, T. D.; Vitug, A. J.; and Mark, V. H. 1982. Are nursing home diagnoses and treatment inadequate? *Journal of the American Medical Association* 248 (3): 321–322.

Sartorius, N. 1982. Epidemiology and mental health policy. In *Public mental health: Perspectives and prospects,* ed. M. D. Wagenfeld, P. V. Lemkau, and B. Justice. Beverly Hills, Calif.: Sage Publications.

Seidman, E. 1983. Introduction. In *Handbook of social intervention,* ed. E. Seidman. Beverly Hills, Calif.: Sage Publications.

Sherwood, S., and Mor, V. 1980. Mental health institutions and the elderly. *Handbook of mental health and aging,* ed. J. E. Birren and R. B. Sloane. Englewood Cliffs, N.J.: Prentice-Hall.

Smith, K. K., and Corse, S. J. 1986. The process of consultation: Critical issues. In *Handbook of mental health consultation,* ed. F. V. Mannino, E. J. Trickett,

M. F. Shore, M. G. Kidder, and G. Levin. Department of Health and Human Services, Publication No. (ADM) 86-1446. Washington, D.C.

Smyer, M. A.; Cohn, M. D.; Droogas, A.; Garfein, A.; and Hermansen, S. 1985. Mental health training in nursing homes: A view from administrators and aides. Paper presented at the annual meeting of the Association for Gerontology in Higher Education, Washington, D.C.

Spitzer, R. L.; Endicott, J.; and Robins, E. 1978. Research diagnostic criteria: Rationale and reliability. *Archives of General Psychiatry* 35: 773–782.

Swift, C. F., and Cooper, S. 1986. Settings, consultees, and clients. In *Mental health consultation handbook,* ed. F. V. Mannino, E. J. Trickett, M. F. Shore, M. G. Kidder, and G. Levin. Department of Health and Human Services, Publication No. (ADM) 86-1446. Washington, D.C.

U.S. Senate. Subcommittee on Long-Term Care, Special Committee on Aging. 1976. *The role of nursing homes in caring for discharged mental patients (and the birth of a for-profit boarding home industry).* Supporting paper no. 7. Washington, D.C.: Government Printing Office.

Weissman, M. M.; Myers, J. K.; Tischler, G. L.; Holzer, C. E., III; Leaf, P. J.; and Orvaschel, H. 1985. Psychiatric disorders (DSM-III) and cognitive impairment among the elderly in a U.S. urban community. *Acta Psychiatrica Scandinavia* 71 (4): 366–379.

White, L. 1987. Epidemiology. In *The encyclopedia of aging,* ed. G. L. Maddox. New York: Springer.

## CHAPTER 5

Albert, M. S. 1981. Geriatric neuropsychology. *Journal of Consulting and Clinical Psychology* 49: 835–850.

Beck, A. T.; Ward, C. H.; Mock, J.; and Erbaugh, J. 1961. An inventory for measuring depression. *Archives of General Psychology* 4: 53–63.

Bellak, L., and Bellak, S. S. 1973. *Manual for the Senior Apperception Technique.* Larchmont, N.Y.: CPS.

Blumenthal, D.; Schlesinger, M.; Drumheller, P. D.; and The Harvard Medicare Project. 1986. The future of Medicare. *New England Journal of Medicine* 314 (11): 722–728.

Brink, T. L., ed. 1986. *Clinical gerontology: A guide to assessment and intervention.* New York: Haworth Press.

Busse, E. W., and Blazer, D. G., eds. 1980. *Handbook of geriatric psychiatry.* New York: Van Nostrand Reinhold.

Butler, R. N., and Lewis, M. I. 1982. *Aging and mental health,* 3d ed. St. Louis: C. V. Mosby.

Cohen, G. D. 1987. Alzheimer's disease. In *The encyclopedia of aging,* ed. G. L. Maddox. New York: Springer.

Colligan, R. C.; Osborne, D.; Swenson, W. M.; and Offord, K. P. 1984. The aging MMPI: Development of contemporary norms. *Mayo Clinic Proceedings* 59: 377–390.

Crook, T.; Ferris, S.; and Bartus, R., eds. 1983. *Assessment in geriatric psychopharmacology.* New Canaan, Conn.: Mark Powley Associates.

Cummings, J. L., and Benson, D. F. 1983. *Dementia: A clinical approach.* Boston: Butterworth.

Danish, S. J.; D'Augelli, A. R.; and Hauer, A. L. 1979. *Helping skills: A life development training program.* New York: Human Services Press.

Edinberg, M. A. 1985. *Mental health practice with the elderly.* Englewood Cliffs, N.J.: Prentice-Hall.

Fillenbaum, G. G., and Smyer, M. A. 1981. The development, validity, and reliability of the OARS multidimensional functional assessment questionnaire. *Journal of Gerontology* 36 (4): 428–434.

Finch, C. E., and Schneider, E. L., eds. 1985. *Handbook of the biology of aging.* New York: Van Nostrand Reinhold.

Folstein, W. F.; Folstein, S. E.; and McHugh, P. R. 1975. "Mini-Mental State": A practical method for grading the cognitive state of patients for the clinician. *Journal of Psychiatric Research* 12: 189–198.

Gallagher, D.; Thompson, L. W.; and Levy, S. M. 1980. Clinical psychological assessment of older adults. In *Aging in the 1980s: Selected contemporary issues in the psychology of aging,* ed. L. W. Poon. Washington, D.C.: American Psychological Association.

Gatz, M.; Smyer, M. A.; Garfein, A.; and Seward, M. In press. Essentials of assessment in nursing homes. In *Mental health services in nursing homes,* ed. M. S. Harper. Baltimore, Md.: Williams and Wilkins.

Gilhooly, M. L. M., Zarit, S. H., and Birren, J. E., eds. 1986. *The dementias: Policy and management.* Englewood Cliffs, N.J.: Prentice-Hall.

Golden, C. J. 1981. A standardized version of Luria's neuropsychological tests. In *Handbook of clinical neuropsychology,* ed. S. Filskov and T. J. Boll. New York: Wiley-Interscience.

Gurland, B. J. 1980. The assessment of mental health status of older adults. In *Handbook of mental health and aging,* ed. J. E. Birren and R. B. Sloane. Englewood Cliffs, N.J.: Prentice-Hall.

Hathaway, S. R., and McKinley, J. C. 1951. *The Minnesota multiphasic personality inventory manual.* Rev. ed. New York: Psychological Corporation.

Helmes, E.; Csapo, K. G.; and Short, J. A. 1987. Standardization and validation of the Multidimensional Observation Scale for Elderly Subjects (M.O.S.E.S.). *Journal of Gerontology* 42 (4): 395-405.

Hersch, E. L., Csapo, K. G., and Palmer, R. B. 1978. Development of the London Psychogeriatric Rating Scale. *London Psychiatric Hospital Research Bulletin* 1: 3–21.

Honigfeld, G., and Klett, C. J. 1965. Nurses' Observation Scale for Inpatient Evaluation: A new scale for measuring improvement in chronic schizophrenia. *Journal of Clinical Psychology* 21: 65–71.

Hussian, R. A. 1986. Severe behavioral problems. In *Geropsychological assessment and treatment,* ed. L. Teri and P. M. Lewinsohn. New York: Springer.

Institute of Medicine. 1986. *Improving the quality of care in nursing homes.* Washington, D.C.: National Academy Press.

Jazwiecki, T., and Press, S. 1986. Federal reimbursement for long-term care of the mentally ill. In *Mental illness in nursing homes: Agenda for research,* ed. M. S. Harper and B. D. Lebowitz. Rockville, Md.: National Institute of Mental Health.

Kahn, R. L. 1975. The mental health system and the future aged. *Gerontologist* 15 (1): 24–31.

Kahn, R. L.; Goldfarb, A. I.; Pollack, M.; and Peck, A. 1960. Brief objective measures for the determination of mental status in the aged. *American Journal of Psychiatry* 117: 326–328.

Kahn, R. L., and Miller, N. E. 1978. Assessment of altered brain function in the aged. In *The clinical psychology of aging,* ed. M. Storandt, I. C. Siegler, and M. F. Elias. New York: Plenum Press.

Kane, R. A., and Kane, R. L. 1981. *Assessing the elderly: A practical guide to measurement.* Lexington, Mass.: Lexington Books.

Katz, S.; Ford, A. B.; Moskowitz, R. W.; Jackson, B. A.; and Jaffee, M. W. 1963. Studies of illness in the aged. The index of ADL: A standardized measure of biological and social function. *Journal of the American Medical Association* 185: 914–919.

Knight, B. 1986. *Psychotherapy with older adults.* Beverly Hills, Calif.: Sage Publications.

Lawton, M. P., and Storandt, M. 1984. Clinical and functional approaches to the assessment of older people. In *Advances in psychological assessment,* ed. P. McReynolds and G. J. Chelune, vol. 6. San Francisco: Jossey-Bass.

Lawton, M. P.; Whelihan, W. M.; and Belsky, J. K. 1980. Personality tests and their use with older adults. In *Handbook of mental health and aging,* ed. J. E. Birren and R. B. Sloane. Englewood Cliffs, N.J.: Prentice-Hall.

Lezak, M. D. 1987. Norms for growing older. *Developmental Neuropsychology* 3 (1): 1–12.

Lindeman, C. 1986. Manpower in nursing homes: Implications for research. In *Mental illness in nursing homes: Agenda for research,* ed. M. S. Harper and B. D. Lebowitz. Rockville, Md.: National Institute of Mental Health.

Lubin, B., and Rinck, C. M. 1986. Assessment of mood and affect in the elderly: The Depression Adjective Check List and the Multiple Affect Adjective Check List. In *Clinical Gerontology: A guide to assessment and intervention,* ed. T. L. Brink. New York: Haworth Press.

Margolis, R. B., and Scialfa, C. T. 1984. Age differences in Wechsler Memory Scale performance. *Journal of Clinical Psychology* 40: 1442–1449.

Mattis, S. 1976. Mental status examination for organic mental syndrome in the elderly patient. In *Geriatric psychiatry,* ed. L. Bellak and T. B. Karasu. New York: Grune and Stratton.

Miller, E. 1980. Cognitive assessment of the older adult. In *Handbook of mental health and aging,* ed. J. E. Birren and R. B. Sloane. Englewood Cliffs, N.J.: Prentice-Hall.

Murray, H. A. 1943. *Thematic apperception test.* Cambridge: Harvard University Press.

Nesselroade, J. R., and Ford, D. H. 1985. P-technique comes of age: Multivariate, replicated, single-subject designs for research on older adults. *Research on aging* 7 (1): 46–80.

Overall, J. E., and Gomez-Mont, F. 1974. The MMPI-168 for psychiatric screening. *Educational and Psychological Measurement* 34: 315–319.

Overall, J. E., and Gorham, D. R. 1962. The Brief Psychiatric Rating Scale. *Psychological Reports* 10: 799–812.

Pearson, J. S.; Swenson, W. M.; and Rome, H. 1965. Age and sex differences related to MMPI response frequency in 25,000 medical patients. *American Journal of Psychiatry* 121: 988–995.

Pfeiffer, E. 1968. *Disordered behavior: Basic concepts in clinical psychiatry.* New York: Oxford University Press.

———, ed. 1975. *Multidimensional functional assessment: The OARS methodology.* Durham, N.C.: Center for the Study of Aging and Human Development, Duke University.

———. 1980. The psychosocial evaluation of the elderly patient. In *Handbook of geriatric psychiatry,* ed. E. W. Busse and D. G. Blazer. New York: Van Nostrand Reinhold.

Poon, L. W. 1986. *Handbook for clinical memory assessment of older adults.* Washington, D.C.: American Psychological Association.

Rabins, P. V., and Mace, N. L. 1986. Some ethical issues in dementia care. In *Clinical gerontology: A guide to assessment and intervention,* ed. T. L. Brink. New York: Haworth Press.

Radloff, L. S., and Teri, L. 1986. Use of the Center for Epidemiological Studies—Depression scale with older adults. In *Clinical gerontology: A guide to assessment and intervention,* ed. T. L. Brink. New York: Haworth Press.

Reichlin, R. E. 1984. Current perspectives on Rorschach performance among older adults. *Journal of Personality Assessment* 47: 562–582.

Rorschach, H. 1942. *Psychodiagnostics: A diagnostic test based on perception* 4th ed. New York: Grune and Stratton.

Rubenstein, L. 1983. The clinical effectiveness of multidimensional geriatric assessment. In *Handbook of mental health and aging,* ed. J. E. Birren and R. B. Sloane. Englewood Cliffs, N.J.: Prentice-Hall.

Santos, J., and VandenBos, G. R., eds. 1982. *Psychology and the older adult: Challenges for training in the 1980s.* Washington, D.C.: American Psychological Association.

Savage, R. D., and Britton, P. G. 1968. The factorial structure of the WAIS in an aged sample. *Journal of Gerontology* 23 (2): 183–186.

Schaie, K. W. 1984. Historical time and cohort effects. In *Life-span developmental psychology: Historical and generational effects,* ed. K. A. McCluskey and H. W. Reese. New York: Academic Press.

Schaie, K. W., and Schaie, J. P. 1977. Clinical assessment and aging. In *Handbook of the psychology of aging,* ed. J. E. Birren and K. W. Schaie. New York: Van Nostrand Reinhold.

Schaie, K. W., and Stone, V. 1982. Psychological assessment. In *Annual review of gerontology and geriatrics,* ed. C. Eisdorfer, vol. 3. New York: Springer.

Schulz, R. 1980. Aging and control. In *Human helplessness: Theory and applications,* ed. J. Barber and M. E. P. Seligman. New York: Academic Press.

Seligman, M. E. P. 1975. *Helplessness: On depression, development, and death.* San Francisco: W. H. Freeman.

Seligman, M. E. P., and Elder, G. H. 1986. Learned helplessness and life-span development. In *Human development and the life course: Multidisciplinary perspectives,* ed. A. Sorenson, F. Weinert, and L. Sherrod. Hillsdale, N.J.: Erlbaum.

Smyer, M. A. 1980. The differential usage of services by impaired elderly. *Journal of Gerontology* 35 (2): 249–255.

Storandt, M. 1977. Graduate education in gerontological psychology: Results of a survey. *Educational Gerontology* 2: 141–146.

U.S. General Accounting Office (USGAO). 1977. *Report to the Congress: The well-being of older people in Cleveland, Ohio.* Document No. HRD-77-70. Washington, D.C.

Verwoerdt, A. 1981. *Clinical geropsychiatry,* 2d ed. Baltimore: Williams and Wilkins.

Wechsler, D. 1945. A standardized memory scale for clinical use. *Journal of Psychology* 19: 87–95.

———. 1955. *Wechsler adult intelligence scale manual.* New York: Psychological Corporation.

Williams, T. F. 1983. Comprehensive functional assessment: An overview. *Journal of the American Geriatrics Society* 31 (11): 637–641.

Yesavage, J. A.; Brink, T. L.; Lum, O.; Huang, O.; Adey, M. B.; Leirer, V. O. 1983. Development and validation of a geriatric depression rating scale: A preliminary report. *Journal of Psychiatric Research* 17: 37–49.

Zarit, S. H. 1980. *Aging and mental disorders: psychological approaches to assessment and treatment.* New York: Macmillan.

Zarit, S. H., and Anthony, C. R. 1985. Interventions with dementia patients and their families. In *The dementias: Policy and management,* ed. M. L. M. Gilhooly, S. H. Zarit, and J. E. Birren. Englewood-Cliffs, N.J.: Prentice-Hall.

Zarit, S. H.; Eiler, J.; and Hassinger, M. 1985. Clinical assessment. In *Handbook of the psychology of aging,* ed. J. E. Birren and K. W. Schaie, 2d ed. New York: Van Nostrand Reinhold.

Zarit, S. H.; Orr, N. K.; and Zarit, J. M. 1985. *The hidden victims of Alzheimer's disease: Families under stress.* New York: New York University Press.

## CHAPTER 6

Angel, J. E. 1987. *Physicians' desk reference.* 41st ed. Oradell, N.J.: Medical Economics Company.

Banziger, G., and Rousch, S. 1983. Nursing homes for the birds: A control-relevant intervention with bird feeders. *Gerontologist* 23: 527–531.

Beck, P. 1982. Two successful interventions in nursing homes: The therapeutic effects of cognitive activity. *Gerontologist* 22: 378–383.

Blazer, D. G. 1982. *Depression in late life.* St. Louis: C. V. Mosby.

Brink, T. L. 1979. *Geriatric psychotherapy.* New York: Human Sciences Press. Epigraph is from p. 145.

Burnside, I. M. 1978. *Working with the elderly: Group process and techniques.* North Scituate, Mass.: Duxbury Press.

———. 1980. Symptomatic behaviors in the elderly. In *Handbook of mental health and aging,* ed. J. E. Birren and R. B. Sloane. Englewood Cliffs, N.J.: Prentice-Hall.

Busch, C. D. 1984. Common themes in group psychotherapy with older adult nursing home residents: A review of selected literature. *Clinical Gerontologist* 2 (3): 25–38.

Carman, M. B., and Nordin, S. R. 1984. Psychodrama: A therapeutic modality for the elderly in nursing homes. *Clinical Gerontologist* 3 (1): 15–24.

Craighead, W. E.; Kazdin, A. E.; and Mahoney, M. J. 1981. *Behavior modification: Principles, issues, and applications.* Boston: Houghton Mifflin.

Gaitz, C. M., and Varner, R. V. 1980. Preventive aspects of mental illness in late life. In *Handbook of mental health and aging,* ed. J. E. Birren and R. B. Sloane. Englewood Cliffs, N.J.: Prentice-Hall.

Goldfried, M. R. 1982. Behavioral assessment: An overview. In *International handbook of behavior modification and therapy,* ed. A. S. Bellack and A. E. Kazdin. New York: Plenum Press.

Goodstein, R. K. 1982. Individual psychotherapy and the elderly. *Psychotherapy: Theory, Research, and Practice* 19 (4): 412–418.

Gotesman, K. G. 1980. Behavioral and dynamic psychotherapy with the elderly. In *Handbook of mental health and aging,* ed. J. E. Birren and R. B. Sloane. Englewood Cliffs, N.J.: Prentice-Hall.

Guy, D. W., and Morice, H. O. 1985. A comparative analysis of behavior management in the nursing home. *Clinical Gerontologist* 4 (2): 11–17.

Hicks, R., Funkenstein, H. H., Davis, J. M., and Dysken, M. W. 1980. Geriatric psychopharmacology. In *Handbook of mental health and aging,* ed. J. E. Birren and R. B. Sloane. Englewood Cliffs, N.J.: Prentice-Hall.

Hussian, R. A. 1981. *Geriatric psychology: A behavioral perspective.* New York: Van Nostrand Reinhold.

Hussian, R. A., and Davis, R. L. 1985. *Responsive care: Behavioral interventions with elderly persons.* Champaign, Ill.: Research Press.

Johnson, D. R. 1985. Expressive group psychotherapy with the elderly: A drama therapy approach. *International Journal of Group Psychotherapy* 35 (1): 109–127.

Keisler, D. J. 1971. Experimental designs in psychotherapy research. In *Handbook of psychotherapy and behavior change,* ed. A. E. Bergin and S. L. Garfield. New York: Wiley.

Knight, B. 1986. *Psychotherapy with older adults.* Beverly Hills, Calif.: Sage Publications.

Korchin, S. J. 1976. *Modern clinical psychology.* New York: Basic Books.

Langer, E. J., and Rodin, J. 1979. Environmental determinants of memory improvement in late adulthood. *Journal of Personality and Social Psychology* 37 (11): 2003–2013.

Patterson, R. L. 1982. *Overcoming deficits of aging: A behavioral approach.* New York: Plenum Press.

Rodin, J., and Langer, E. J. 1977. Long-term effects of a control-relevant intervention with the institutionalized aged. *Journal of Personality and Social Psychology* 35 (12): 897–902.

Rosenstein, J. C., and Swenson, E. W. 1980. Behavioral therapy approaches to therapy with the elderly. In *Non-traditional therapy and counseling with the aging,* ed. S. S. Sargent. New York: Springer.

Spayd, J. A. 1987. *The paradox of role assignment: An observation of the role of nursing assistants in Pennsylvania long-term care facilities.* Master's thesis, Columbia Pacific University, San Rafael, Calif.

Sundberg, N. D.; Taplin, J. R.; and Tyler, L. E. 1983. *Introduction to clinical psychology: Perspectives, issues, and contributions to human service.* Englewood Cliffs, N.J.: Prentice-Hall.

Wattis, J., and Church, M. 1986. *Practical psychiatry of old age.* New York: New York University Press.

Weinstein, W. S., and Khanna, P. 1986. *Depression in the elderly.* New York: Philosophical Library.

Whanger, A. D. 1980. Treatment within the institution. In *Handbook of geriatric psychiatry,* ed. E. W. Busse and D. G. Blazer. New York: Van Nostrand Reinhold.

Whelihan, W. M. 1978. Psychotherapy with elderly clients: A behavioral approach. *Proceedings of the Annual Convention of the American Psychological Association,* 1978: 2–12.

Williamson, P. N., and Ascione, F. R. 1983. Behavioral treatment of the elderly: Implications for theory and therapy. *Behavior Modification* 7 (4): 583–610.

Zarit, S. H. 1980. *Aging and mental disorders: Psychological approaches to assessment and treatment.* New York: Free Press.

———. 1987. Personal communication.

Zevon, H. A.; Karuza, J.; and Brickman, P. 1982. Responsbility and the elderly: Applications to psychotherapy. *Psychotherapy: Theory, Research, and Practice* 19 (4): 405–411.

## CHAPTER 7

American Psychiatric Association. 1980. *Diagnostic and statistical manual of mental disorders* (DSM-III). 3rd ed. Washington, D.C.: American Psychiatric Association.

Barnes, J. A. 1974. Effects of reality orientation classroom on memory loss, confusion, and disorientation in geriatric patients. *Gerontologist* 14: 138–142.

Beck, A. T. 1973. *The diagnosis and management of depression.* Philadelphia: University of Pennsylvania Press.

Blazer, D. G. 1982. *Depression in late life.* St. Louis: C. V. Mosby.

Brickel, C. M. 1984. The clinical use of pets with aged. *Clinical Gerontologist* 2 (4): 72–75.

Brook, P., Degun, G.; and Miller, M. 1975. Reality Orientation, a therapy for psychogeriatric patients: A controlled study. *British Journal of Psychiatry* 127: 42–45.

Burnside, I. M. 1978. *Working with the elderly: Group process and techniques.* North Scituate, Mass.: Duxbury Press.

———. 1980. Symptomatic behaviors in the elderly. In *Handbook of mental health and aging,* ed. J. E. Birren and R. B. Sloane. Englewood Cliffs, N.J.: Prentice-Hall.

Carman, M. B., and Nordin, S. R. 1984. Psychodrama: A therapeutic modality for the elderly in nursing homes. *Clinical Gerontologist* 3 (1): 15–24.

Citrin, R. S., and Dixon, D. N. 1977. Reality orientation: A milieu therapy used in an institution for the aged. *Gerontologist* 17: 39–43.

Cohen, G. D. 1987. Alzheimer's disease. In *The encyclopedia of aging,* ed. G. L. Maddox. New York: Springer.

Cohen-Mansfield, J. 1986. Agitated behaviors in the elderly: II. Preliminary results in the cognitively deteriorated. *Journal of the American Geriatrics Society* 34: 722–727.

Cohen-Mansfield, J., and Billig, N. 1986. Agitated behaviors in the elderly: I. A conceptual review. *Journal of the American Geriatrics Society* 34: 711–721.

Eyde, D. R., and Rich, J. A. 1983. *Psychological distress in aging: A family management model.* Rockville, Md.: Aspen.

Folsom, J. C. 1968. Reality orientation for the elderly mental patient. *Journal of Geriatric Psychiatry* 1: 291–307.

Fozard, J. L. 1980. The time for remembering. In *Aging in the 1980s,* ed. L. W. Poon. Washington, D.C.: American Psychological Association.

Fry, P. S. 1984. Cognitive training and cognitive-behavioral variables in the treatment of depression in the elderly. *Clinical Gerontologist* 3 (1): 25–45.

Gallagher, D. 1979. Behavior group therapy with the elderly. Paper presented at the meeting of the American Psychological Association, New York.

Gallagher, D. E., and Thompson, L. W. 1983. Effectiveness of psychotherapy for both endogenous and nonendogenous depression in older adult outpatients. *Journal of Gerontology* 38 (6): 707–712.

Gatz, M., and Warren, C. 1986. *Electroconvulsive therapy and the elderly: Contemporary trends.* Unpublished manuscript, University of Southern California, Ethel Percy Andrus Center and Social Science Research Institute.

Goddard, P., and Carstensen, L. L. 1986. Behavioral treatment of chronic depression in an elderly nursing home resident. *Clinical Gerontologist* 4 (4): 13–20.

Goodstein, R. K. 1982. Individual psychotherapy and the elderly. *Psychotherapy: Theory, Research, and Practice* 19 (4): 412–418.

Haight, B. K., and Bahr, R. T. 1984. The therapeutic role of the life review in the elderly. *Academic Psychology Bulletin* 6 (3): 287–299.

Haley, W. 1983. Behavioral self-management: An application to a case of agitation in an elderly chronic psychiatric patient. *Clinical Gerontologist* 1 (3): 45–52.

Harris, C. S., and Ivory, P. B. 1976. An outcome evaluation of reality orientation therapy with geriatric patients in a state mental hospital. *Gerontologist* 16: 496–503.

Hart, J., and Fleming, R. 1985. An experimental evaluation of a modified reality orientation therapy. *Clinical Gerontologist* 3 (4): 34–45.

Hogstel, M. 1979. Use of reality orientation with aging confused patients. *Nursing Research* 28 (3): 161–165.

Hussian, R. A. 1981. *Geriatric psychology: A behavioral perspective.* New York: Van Nostrand Reinhold.

Hussian, R. A., and Davis, R. L. 1985. *Responsive care: Behavioral interventions with elderly persons.* Champaign, Ill.: Research Press.

Ingersoll, B., and Silverman, A. 1978. Comparative group psychology for the aged. *Gerontologist* 18: 201–206.

Johnson, D. R. 1985. Expressive group psychotherapy with the elderly: A drama therapy approach. *International Journal of Group Psychotherapy* 35 (1): 109–127.

Kaye, V. G. 1985. An innovative treatment modality for elderly residents of a nursing home. *Clinical Gerontologist* 3 (4): 45–51.

Langer, E. J., and Rodin, J. 1979. Environmental determinants of memory improvement in late adulthood. *Journal of Personality and Social Psychology* 37 (11): 2003–2013.

Lehmann, H. E. 1982. Affective disorders in the aged. *Psychiatric Clinics of North America* 5 (1): 27–44.

Lewinsohn, P. M. 1974. Clinical and theoretical aspects of depression. In *Innovative treatment methods in psychopathology,* ed, K. S. Calhoun, H. E. Adams, and K. Mitchell. New York: Wiley.

Mishara, B. L. 1978. Geriatric patients who improve in token economy and general milieu treatment programs: A multivariate analysis. *Journal of Consulting and Clinical Psychology* 46 (6): 1340–1348.

Patterson, R. L., and Teigen, J. R. 1973. Conditioning and post-hospital generalization of non-delusional responses in a chronic psychotic patient. *Journal of Applied Behavioral Analysis* 6: 65–70.

Powell-Proctor, L., and Miller, E. 1982. Reality orientation: A critical appraisal. *British Journal of Psychiatry* 140: 457–463.

Salzman, C., and Shader, R. I. 1978. Depression in the elderly. I. Relationship between depression, psychological defense mechanism, and physical illness. *Journal of the American Geriatric Society* 26: 253–260.

Schwenk, M. A. 1979. Reality orientation for the institutionalized aged: Does it help? *Gerontologist* 19 (4): 373–377.

Spar, J. E. 1982. Dementia in the aged. *Psychiatric Clinics of North America* 5 (1): 67–86.

Steuer, J. 1982. Psychotherapy for depressed elders. In *Depression in late-life,* ed. D. Blazer. St. Louis: C. V. Mosby.

Strauss, D., and Solomon, K. 1983. Psychopharmacologic intervention for depression in the elderly. *Clinical Gerontologist* 2 (1): 3–29.

Sundberg, N. D.; Taplin, J. R.; and Tyler, L. E. 1983. *Introduction to clinical psychology: Perspectives, issues, and contributions to human service.* Englewood Cliffs, N.J.: Prentice-Hall.

Taulbee, L. R. 1976. Reality orientation and the aged. In *Nursing and the aged,* ed. I. Burnside. Hightstown, N.J.: McGraw-Hill.

———. 1978. Reality orientation: A therapeutic group activity for elderly persons. In *Working with the elderly: Group process and technique,* ed. I. Burnside. North Scituate, Mass.: Duxbury Press.

Thompson, L. W., and Gallagher, D. 1984. Efficacy of psychotherapy in the treatment of late-life depression. *Advances in Behavior Research and Therapy* 6 (2): 127–139.

VA Hospital, Tuscaloosa. 1984. *Guide for reality orientation.* Tuscaloosa: VA Hospital.

Vezina, J., and Bourque, P. 1984. The relationship between cognitive structure and symptoms of depression in the elderly. *Cognitive Therapy and Research* 8 (1): 29–36.

Waller, M., and Griffen, M. 1984. Group therapy for depressed elders. *Geriatric Nursing* 5 (7): 309–311.

Wattis, J., and Church, M. 1986. *Practical psychiatry of old age.* New York: New York University Press.

Weinstein, W. S., and Khanna, P. 1986. *Depression in the elderly.* New York: Philosophical Library.

Wetzel, J. W. 1980. Interventions with the depressed elderly in institutions. *Social Casework: The Journal of Contemporary Social Work,* April: 234–239.

Wetzler, M. A., and Feil, N. 1979. *Validation therapy with disoriented elders who use fantasy. Manual.* Cleveland: Edward Feil Productions.

Whelihan, W. M. 1978. Psychotherapy with elderly clients: A behavioral approach. *Proceedings of the Annual Convention of the American Psychological Association,* 1978: 2–12.

Williamson, P. N., and Ascione, F. R. 1983. Behavioral treatment of the elderly: Implications for theory and therapy. *Behavior Modification* 7 (4): 583–610.

Zarit, J. M.; Zarit, S. H.; and Rosenberg, S. 1987. *A special treatment unit for Alzheimer's disease: Development and implementation.* Unpublished manuscript.

Zarit, S. H. 1987. Personal communication.

Zemore, R., and Eames, N. 1979. Psychic and somatic symptoms of depression among young adults, institutionalized aged, and noninstitutionalized aged. *Journal of Gerontology* 34 (5): 716–722.

Zepelin, H., and Wade, S. 1975. *A study of the effectiveness of reality orientation classes.* Paper presented at the 28th annual meeting of the Gerontological Society, Louisville.

Zepelin, H.; Wolfe, C. S.; and Kleinplatz, F. 1977. *Evaluation of a year long reality orientation program.* Paper presented at the 30th annual meeting of the Gerontological Society, San Francisco.

## CHAPTER 8

Aizenberg, R., and Treas, J. 1985. The family in late life: Psychosocial and demographic considerations. In *Handbook of the psychology of aging,* ed. J. E. Birren and K. W. Schaie. New York: Van Nostrand Reinhold.

Arling, G., and McAuley, W. J. 1983. The feasibility of public payments for caregiving. *Gerontologist* 23: 300–306.

Bengtson, V. L., and Treas, J. 1980. The changing context of mental health and aging. In *Handbook of mental health and aging,* ed. J. E. Birren and R. J. Sloane. Englewood Cliffs, N.J.: Prentice-Hall.

Blieszner, R., and Mancini, J. A. 1987. Enduring ties: Older adults' parental role and responsibilities. *Family Relations* 36: 176–180.

Bowers, B. J. 1987. Reconceptualizing intergenerational caregiving: A grounded theory analysis of middle aged women caring for their aging parents. *Advances in Nursing Science* 9: 20–31.

Brody E. 1985. Parent care as a normative family stress. *Gerontologist* 25: 19–29.

Cantor, M. 1983. Strain among caregivers: A study of experience in the United States. *Gerontologist* 23: 597–604.

Cantor, M., and Little, V. 1985. Aging and social care. In *Handbook of aging and the social sciences,* ed. R. H. Binstock and E. Shanas. New York: Van Nostrand Reinhold.

Cicirelli, V. G. 1983. A comparison of helping behavior to elderly parents of adult children with intact and disrupted marriages. *Gerontologist* 23: 619–625.

Cohen, S., and Gans, B. 1978. *The other generation gap.* Chicago: Follet.

Duvall, E. M. 1971. *Family development.* 4th ed. Philadelphia: Lippincott.

Furse, D. M. 1983. Who are the real nursing home consumers? *American Health Care Association Journal* 1 (6): 51–54.

Greene, V. L., and Monahan, D. J. 1982. The impact of visitation on patient well-being in nursing homes. *Gerontologist* 22: 418–423.

Hagestad, G. O. 1986. The family: Women and grandparents as kin-keepers. In *Our aging society: Paradox and promise,* ed. A. Pifer and L. Bronte. New York: W. W. Norton.

———. 1981. Problems and promises in the social psychology of intergenerational relations. In *Aging: Stability and change in the family,* ed. R. Fogel, E. Hatfield, S. Kiesler, and J. March. New York: Academic Press.

Hing, E. 1987. Use of nursing homes by the elderly: Preliminary data from the 1985 National Nursing Home Survey. *Advance Data* 135 (May 14).

Hook, W. F., Sobal, J., and Oak, J. C. 1982. Frequency of visitation in nursing homes: Patterns of contact across boundaries of total institutions. *Gerontologist* 22: 424–428.

Hooyman, N., Gonyea, J., and Montgomery, R. 1985. The impact of in-home services termination on family caregivers. *Gerontologist* 25: 141–145.

Horowitz, A. 1985. Family caregiving to the frail elderly. In *Annual Review of Gerontology and Geriatrics,* ed. C. Eisdorfer, M. P. Lawton, and G. L. Maddox. New York: Springer.

Janis, I. L., and Mann, L. 1977. Emergency decision making—theoretical analysis of responses to disaster warnings. *Journal of Human Stress* 3 (2): 35.

Johnson, C. L. 1983. Dyadic family relations and social support. *Gerontologist* 23: 377–383.

Johnson, C. L., and Catalano, D. J. 1981. Childless elderly and their family supports. *Gerontologist* 21: 610–618.

———. 1983. A longitudinal study of family supports to impaired elderly. *Gerontologist* 23: 612–618.

Johnson, M. A., and Van Meter, M. J. 1985a. Family decision making, long-term care for the elderly, and the role of religious organizations: Part I: Issues and the challenge. *Journal of Religion and Aging* 1 (3): 61–70.

———. 1985b. Family decision making, long-term care for the elderly: Part II: A review. *Journal of Religion and Aging* 1 (4): 59–73.

Johnson, M. A., and Werner, C. 1982. We had no choice: A study in family guilt feelings surrounding home care. *Journal of Gerontological Nursing* 8 (11): 641–654.

Kahan, J.; Kemp, B.; Staples, F. R.; and Brummel-Smith, K. 1985. Decreasing the burden in families caring for a relative with a dementing illness: A controlled study. *Journal of the American Geriatrics Society* 33 (6): 664–670.

Kingson, E. R.; Hirshorn, B. A.; and Cornman, J. M. 1986. *Ties that bind: The interdependence of generations.* Washington, D.C.: Seven Locks Press.

Litwak, E. 1985. *Helping the elderly: The complementary roles of informal networks and formal systems.* New York: Guilford Press.

Miller, B.; Linsk, N.; and Pflaum, R. 1986. *Family expectations of nursing home involvement.* Paper presented at the 39th annual meeting of the Gerontological Society of America, Chicago, Ill., November.

Montgomery, R. J. V. 1982. Impact of institutional care policies on family integration. *Gerontologist* 22: 54–58.

Montgomery, R. J. V.; Gonyea, J. G.; and Hooyman, N. R. 1985. Caregiving and the experience of subjective and objective burden. *Family Relations* 34: 19–26.

National Center for Health Statistics. 1979. *National nursing home survey: 1977, summary for the United States.* Hyattsville, Md.: U.S. DHEW.

Poulschock, S. W., and Deimling, G. T. 1984. Families caring for elders in residence: Issues in the measurement of burden. *Journal of Gerontology* 39 (2): 230–231.

Rakowski, W., and Clark, N. M. 1985. Future outlook, caregiving, and care-receiving in the family context. *Gerontologist* 25: 618–623.

Rubin, A., and Shuttlesworth, G. E. 1983. Engaging families as support resources in nursing home care: Ambiguity in the subdivision of tasks. *Gerontologist* 23: 632–636.

Seelbach, W. C. 1984. Filial responsibility and the care of aging family members. In *Independent aging: Family and social systems perspectives,* ed. W. H. Quinn and G. A. Hughston. Rockville, Md.: Aspen.

Shanas, E. 1979. Social myth as hypothesis: The case of the family relations of old people. *Gerontologist* 19: 3–9.

Shuttlesworth, G. E.; Rubin, A.; and Duffy, M. 1982. Families versus institutions: Incongruent role expectations in the nursing home. *Gerontologist* 22: 200–208.

Silverstone, B., and Hyman, H. K. 1983. *You and your aging parent.* New York: Pantheon Books.

Smith, K. F., and Bengtson, V. L. 1979. Positive consequences of institutionalization: Solidarity between elderly parents and their middle-aged children. *Gerontologist* 19: 438–447.

Smith, S. M. 1984. Family selection of long term care services: It's not just the facility that's important. *Health Marketing Quarterly* 1 (4): 101–113.

Smyer, M. A., and Cooney, T. M. 1987. *Family relations across adulthood: Implications for alimony and support decisions.* Paper presented at the National Symposium on Alimony and Child Support, sponsored by the American Bar Association Section of Family Law and the State Bar of Texas, Austin, Texas, April 24–25.

Soldo, B. J., and Myllyluoma, J. 1983. Caregivers who live with dependent elderly. *Gerontologist* 23: 605–611.

Steinman, L. A. 1979. Reactivated conflict with aging parents. In *Aging parents,* ed. P. K. Ragan. Los Angeles: Ethel Percy Andrus Gerontology Center.

Subcommittee on Human Services, of the Select Committee on Aging, House of Representatives. 1987. *Exploding the myths: Caregiving in America.* Washington, D.C. Government Printing Office.

Sussman, M. 1985. The family life of old people. *Handbook of aging and the social sciences,* ed. R. H. Binstock and E. Shanas. New York: Van Nostrand Reinhold.

Tobin, S. S., and Kulys, R. 1981. The family in the institutionalization of the elderly. *Journal of Social Issues* 37 (3): 145–157.

Troll, L. E.; Miller, S. J.; and Atchley, R. C. 1979. *Families in later life.* Belmont, Calif.: Wadsworth Publishing.

U.S. Department of Commerce. Bureau of the Census. 1978. *1976 survey of institutionalized persons: A study of persons receiving long-term care.* Washington, D.C.: Government Printing Office.

U.S. Senate. Special Committee on Aging. *Developments in Aging: 1985.* Vol. 3. Rept. 99-242. 99th Cong., 2nd sess. Pursuant to S. Res., Sec. 19, 2-28-85. Washington, D.C.: Government Printing Office.

York, J. L., and Caslyn, R. J. 1977. Family involvement in nursing homes. *Gerontologist* 17: 500–505.

Zarit, S. H. In press. Issues and directions in family intervention research. In *Alzheimer's disease treatment and family stress: Directions for research,* ed. E. Light and B. Lebowitz.

Zarit, S. H., and Zarit, J. M. 1982. Families under stress: Interventions for caregivers of senile dementia patients. *Psychotherapy: Theory, Research and Practice* 19 (4): 461–471.

Zarit, S. H.; Orr, N. K.; and Zarit, J. M. 1985. *The hidden victims of Alzheimer's disease: Families under stress.* New York: New York University Press.

## CHAPTER 9

Bandler, R.; Grinder, J.; and Satir, V. 1976. *Changing with families.* Palo Alto, Calif.: Science and Behavior Books.

Blieszner, R., and Mancini, J. A. 1987. Enduring ties: Older adults' parental role and responsibilities. *Family Relations* 36: 176–180.

Bowers, B. 1986. *Family involvement in nursing home care.* Paper presented at the 39th annual meeting of the Gerontological Society, Chicago, Ill., November.

Brager, G., and Holloway, S. 1978. *Changing human service organizations: Politics and practice.* New York: Free Press.

Braun, K. L., and Rose, C. L. 1987. Family perceptions of geriatric foster family and nursing home care. *Family Relations* 36: 321–327.

Breslin, L. 1978. Aging: A family dilemma. *Psychiatric Quarterly* 50: 55–58.

Buckholdt, D. R. 1983. The family conference: The social control of human development. *Journal of Family Issues* 4 (4): 613–632.

Buckwalter, K. C., and Hall, G. R. 1987. Families of the institutionalized older adult: A neglected resource. In *Aging, health and family,* ed. T. H. Brubaker. Newbury Park, Calif.: Sage Publications.

Clark, D. B.; Baker, B. L.; and Heifetz, L. J. 1982. Behavioral training for parents of mentally retarded children: Prediction of outcome. *American Journal of Mental Deficiency* 87: 14–19.

Dattilo, J., and Murphy, W. D. 1987. *Behavior Modification in Therapeutic Recreation.* State College, Pa.: Venture Publishing.

Eyde, D., and Rich, J. 1983. *Psychological distress in aging family management model.* Rockville, Md.: Aspen.

Furse, D. 1983. Who are the real nursing home consumers? *American Health Care Association Journal* 1 (6): 51–56.

Garner, J. D., and Mercer, S. D. 1980. Social work practice in long term care facilities: Implications of the current model. *Journal of Gerontological Social Work* 3 (2): 71–72.

Germaine, C. B., and Gitterman, A. 1980. *The life model of social work practice.* New York: Columbia University Press.

Goldmeier, J., and Mannino, F. V. 1986. The role of social work in consultation. In *Handbook of mental health consultation,* ed. F. V. Mannino, E. J. Trickett, M. F. Shore, M. G. Kidder, and G. Levin. Department of Health and Human Services, Publication No. (ADM) 86-1446. Washington, D.C.

Goodstein, L. 1978. *Consulting with human service systems.* Reading, Mass.: Addison-Wesley.

Greene, R. 1986. The functional-age model of intergenerational therapy. A social casework model. In *Clinical gerontology: A guide to assessment and intervention,* ed. T. L. Brink. New York: Haworth Press.

Guerney, B. 1987. *Relationship enhancement.* San Francisco: Jossey-Bass.

Hatch, R. C., and Franken, M. L. 1984. Concerns of children with parents in nursing homes. *Journal of Gerontological Social Work* 7 (3): 9–30.

Hausman, C. P. 1979. Short-term counseling groups for people with elderly parents. *Gerontologist* 19: 102–107.

Herr, J. H., and Weakland, J. J. 1979. *Counseling older adults.* New York: Springer.

Hook, W. F.; Sobal, J.; and Oak, J. C. 1982. Frequency of visitation in nursing homes: Patterns of contact across boundaries of total institutions. *Gerontologist* 22: 424–428.

Horsman, M. N., and Echtenacher, B. 1981. Working with the family council. *American Health Care Association Journal* 1981 (November): 20–22.

Hussian, R. A., and Davis, R. L. 1985. *Responsive care: Behavioral interventions with elderly persons.* Champaign, Ill.: Research Press.

Kramer, C., and Kramer, J. 1976. *Basic principles of long-term care.* Springfield, Ill.: Charles C. Thomas.

Kreiger, D. 1981. *Foundations for holistic health nursing practices: The Renaissance nurse.* Philadelphia: Lippincott.

Lewis, K. 1980. Services for families of the institutionalized aged. *Aging,* no. 309–310: 14–19.

Linn, M. W., and Gurel, L. 1969. Wives' attitudes toward nursing homes. *Journal of Gerontology* 24 (3): 368–372.

Manaster, A. 1967. The family group therapy program at Park View Home for the Aged. *Journal of the American Geriatrics Society* 15 (3): 302–306.

McCubbins, H. I.; McCubbins, M. A.; and Cauble, E. 1979. *Coping health inventory for parents.* St. Paul, Minn.: University of Minnesota.

Mercer, S., and Garner, J. D. 1981. Social work consultation in long term care facilities. *Health and Social Work* 6 (May): 5–13.

Moos, R.; Insel, P. M.; and Humphrey, B. 1974. *Family work and group environment scales manual.* Palo Alto, Calif.: consulting Psychologists.

National Center for Health Statistics. 1979. *National Nursing Home Survey: 1977, Summary for the United States.* Hyattsville, Md.: U.S. DHEW.

Numeroff, R. 1983. Building and maintaining bridges: Meeting the psychological needs of nursing home residents and their families. *Clinical Gerontologist* 1 (4): 53–67.

Pratt, C.; Schmall, V.; Wright, S.; and Hare, J. 1987. The forgotten client, family caregivers to institutionalized dementia patients. In *Aging, health, and family,* ed. T. H. Brubaker. Newbury Park, Calif.: Sage Publications.

Qualls, S. H. 1987. Problems in families of older adults. In *Cognitive-behavioral therapy with families,* ed. N. Epstein, S. Schlesinger, and W. Dryden. New York: Brunner-Mazel.

Reid, W. J., and Epstein, L. 1977. *Task-centered practice.* New York: Columbia University Press.

Reisman, B. 1986. Adjusting to a residential facility for older persons: A child's perspective. *Journal of Gerontological Social Work* 9 (2): 91–100.

Reppucci, N. D., and Saunders, J. T. 1983. Focal issues for institutional change. *Professional Psychology: Research and Practice* 14: 514–528.

Riehl, J. P., and Roy, C. 1974. *Conceptual models for nursing practice.* New York: Appleton Century.

Roberts, R., and Northern, H. 1976. *Theories of social group work.* New York: Columbia University Press.

Rubin, A., and Shuttlesworth, G. E. 1983. Engaging families as support resources in nursing home care. Ambiguity in the subdivision of tasks. *Gerontologist* 23: 632–636.

Safford, F. 1980. A program for families of the mentally impaired elderly. *Gerontologist* 20: 656–660.

Satir, V. 1967. *Conjoint family therapy.* Palo Alto, Calif.: Science and Behavior Books.

Shuttlesworth, G. E.; Rubin, A.; and Duffy, M. 1982. Families versus institutions: Incongruent role expectations in the nursing home. *Gerontologist* 22: 200–208.

Silverstone, B., and Burack-Weiss, A. 1983. *Social work practice with frail elderly and their families: The auxillary function model.* Springfield, Ill.:Charles C. Thomas.

Silverstone, B., and Hyman, H. K. 1976. *You and your aging parent.* New York: Pantheon Books.

Smith, K. F., and Bengtson, V. L. 1979. Positive consequences of institutionalization: Solidarity between elderly parents and their middle-aged children. *Gerontologist* 19: 438–447.

Smoyak, S. 1975. *The psychiatric nurse as a family therapist.* New York: Wiley.

Smyer, M. A., and Frysinger, M. 1985. Mental health interventions in the nursing home community. In *Annual review of geriatrics and gerontology,* ed. M. P. Lawton and G. Maddox, vol. 5. New York: Springer.

Solomon, R. 1983. Serving families of institutionalized aged: The four crises. In *Gerontological social work practice in long-term care,* ed. S. Getzel and M. J. Mellor. New York: Haworth Press.

Stamm, I. 1972. Family therapy. In *Casework: A psychosocial therapy,* ed. E. A. Carter and M. McGoldrick. New York: Random House.

Tobin, S. S., and Kulys, R. 1981. The family in the institutionalization of the elderly. *Journal of Gerontological Social Work* 3: 3–16.

Vernberg, E. M., and Reppucci, N. D. 1986. Behavioral consultation. In *Handbook of mental health consultation,* ed. F. V. Mannino, E. J. Trickett, M. F. Shore, M. G. Kidder, and G. Levin. Department of Health and Human Services, Publication No. (ADM) 86-1446. Washington, D.C.

Wentzel, M. 1979. *The emotional effects of institutionalization upon the family.* Denton: North Texas State University, Center for Studies of Aging.

Zarit, S. H.; Orr, N. K.; and Zarit, J. M. 1985. *The hidden victims of Alzheimer's disease: Families under stress.* New York: New York University Press.

## CHAPTER 10

Alley, S.; Blanton, J.; Feldman, R. E.; Hunter, G. D.; and Rolfson, M. 1979. *Case studies of mental health paraprofessionals: Twelve effective programs.* New York: Human Sciences Press.

Austin, M. J. 1978. *Professionals and paraprofessionals.* New York: Human Sciences Press.

Baltes, M. M., and Reisenzein, R. 1986. The social world in long-term care institutions: Psychosocial control towards dependency? In *The psychology of control and aging,* ed. M. M. Baltes and P. B. Baltes. Hillsdale, N.J.: Erlbaum.

Brannon, D.; Smyer, M.; Cohn, M.; Borchardt, L.; Garfein, A.; Jay, G.; Landry, J.; Malonebeach, E.; and Walls, C. 1986. Caregiving as Work: An analysis of aide and LPN job characteristics in nursing homes. Paper presented at the 39th Annual Scientific Meeting, The Gerontological Society of America, October.

Charns, M. P., and Schaefer, M. J. 1983. *Health care organizations: A model for management.* Englewood Cliffs, N.J.: Prentice-Hall.

Durlak, J. A. 1979. Comparative effectiveness of paraprofessionals and professional helpers. *Psychological Bulletin* 86: 80–92.

Ellsworth, R. B. 1968. *Nonprofessionals in psychiatric rehabilitation.* New York: Appleton-Century-Crofts.

Gartner, A. 1979. The effectiveness of paraprofessionals in service delivery. In *Paraprofessionals in mental health: Theory and practice,* ed. S. Alley, J. Blanton, and R. E. Feldman. New York: Human Sciences Press.

Hackman, J. R., and Oldham, G. R. 1980. *Work redesign.* Reading, Mass.: Addison-Wesley.

Hage, J. T., and Aiken, M. 1969. Routine technology, social structure and organizational goals. *Administrative Science Quarterly* 14 (3): 366–377.

Institute of Medicine. 1986. *Improving the quality of care in nursing homes.* Washington, D.C.: National Academy Press.

James, V. 1979. Paraprofessionals in mental health: A framework for the facts. In *Paraprofessionals in mental health: Theory and practice,* ed. S. Alley, J. Blanton, and R. E. Feldman. New York: Human Sciences Press.

Joiner, C.; Johnson, V.; Chapman, J. B.; and Corkrean, M. 1982. The motivating potential in nursing specialties. *The Journal of Nursing Administration* 12: 26–30.

Kahn, M. W. 1981. *Basic methods for mental health practitioners.* Cambridge, Mass.: Winthrop Publishers.

Karlsruher, A. E. 1974. The nonprofessional as a psychotherapeutic agent: A review of the empirical evidence pertaining to his effectiveness. *American Journal of Community Psychology* 2: 61–77.

Lawton, M. P., and Nahemow, L. 1973. Ecology and the aging process. In *The psychology of adult development and aging,* ed. C. Eisdorfer and M. P. Lawton. Washington, D.C.: American Psychological Association.

Levine, M.; Tulkin, S.; Intagliata, J.; Perry, J.; and Whitson, E. 1979. In *Paraprofessionals in mental health: Theory and practice,* ed. S. Alley, J. Blanton, and R. E. Feldman. New York: Human Sciences Press.

Litwak, E. 1985. *Helping the elderly: The complementary roles of informal networks and formal systems.* New York: Guilford Press.

March, J. G., and Simon, H. 1958. *Organizations.* New York: Wiley.

McPheeters, H. 1979. Training, supervision, and evaluation of paraprofessionals in mental health. In *Paraprofessionals in mental health: Theory and practice,* ed. S. Alley, J. Blanton, and R. E. Feldman. New York: Human Sciences Press.

Moffic, H. S.; Patterson, G. K.; Laval, R.; and Adams, G. L. 1984. Paraprofessionals and psychiatric teams: An updated review. *Hospital and Community Psychiatry* 35: 61–67.

Nash, K. B.; Lifton, N.; and Smith, S. E. 1978. Paraprofessionals and community mental health. *Community Mental Health Review* 3: 1–8.

National Center for Health Statistics. 1981. *Employees in nursing homes in the United States: 1977 National Nursing Home Survey.* DDHS Publication No. PHS 81-1820. Hyattsville, Md.: Department of Health and Human Services.

Nietzel, M. T., and Fisher, S. G. 1981. Effectiveness of professional and paraprofessional helpers: A comment on Durlak. *Psychological Bulletin* 89: 555–565.

Oldham, G. R.; Hackman, J. R.; and Stepina, L. P. 1979. Norms for the job diagnostic survey. *JSAS Catalog of Selected Documents in Psychology* 9: 14.

Patterson, R. L.; Dupree, L. W.; Eberly, D. A.; Jackson, G. M.; O'Sullivan, J. J.; Penner, L. A.; and Dee-Kelly, K. 1982. *Overcoming deficits of aging: A behavioral treatment approach.* New York: Plenum Press.

Perrow, C. B. 1967. A framework for the comparative analysis of organizations. *American Sociological Review* 32 (2): 194–208.

Reingold, J.; Grossman, H. D.; and Burros, N. 1987. Merit gram: A form of recognition in a long-term care setting. *Gerontologist* 27: 147–149.

Sheridan, J. E.; Fairchild, T. J.; and Kaas, M. 1983. Assessing job performance of nursing home staff. *Nursing Research* 32 (2): 102–107.

Smyer, M. A.; Cohn, M. D.; Hermansen, S.; Droogas, A. S.; Garfein, A. 1985. *Mental health training in nursing homes: A view from administrators and aides.* Paper presented at the annual meeting of the Association of Gerontology in Higher Education, Washington, D.C.

Smyer, M. A., and Frysinger, M. 1985. Mental health interventions in the nursing home community. In *Annual Review of Geriatrics and Gerontology,* ed. M. P. Lawton and G. Maddox, vol. 5. New York: Springer.

Sobey, F. 1970. *Nonprofessional revolution in mental health.* New York: Columbia University Press.

Spaulding, J. 1985. *A consumer perspective on quality care: The residents' point of view.* Washington, D.C.: National Citizens' Coalition for Nursing Home Reform.

Strahan, G. 1987. Nursing home characteristics: Preliminary data from the 1985 National Nursing Home Survey. *Advance Data* 13 (March 27): 1–12.

Tarail, M. 1979. The community mental health worker: The role and function of indigenous paraprofessionals in a comprehensive community mental health center. In *Paraprofessionals in mental health: Theory and practice,* ed. S. Alley, J. Blanton, and R. E. Feldman. New York: Human Sciences Press.

Wagenfeld, M. O., and Robin, S. S. 1981. Reality, rhetoric and the paraprofessional: A concluding note. In *Paraprofessionals in the human services,* ed. S. S. Robin and M. O. Wagenfeld. New York: Human Sciences Press.

Woodward, J. 1965. *Industrial organization: Theory and practice.* Oxford: Oxford University Press.

## CHAPTER 11

Astrand, P. O., and Rodahl, K. 1977. *Textbook of work physiology: Physiological bases of exercise.* 2nd ed. New York: McGraw-Hill.

Barnes, R. M. 1980. *Motivation and time study: Design and measurement of work.* New York: Wiley.

Bem, D. J. 1970. *Beliefs, attitudes and human affairs.* Belmont, Calif.: Brooks/Cole.

Bowman, M. 1986. Peer level leaders spark higher job performance. *Providers* 12 (3): 44–45.

Burke, E., Sr. 1981. Sensory changes in the elderly, a programmed unit. *American Journal of Nursing* 81 (10): 1851–1880.

Campion, M. A., and Thayer, P. W. 1985. Development and field evaluation of an interdisciplinary measure of job design. *Journal of Applied Psychology* 70:29–43.

Clark, R. A. 1983. Reconsider research from learning media. *Review of Educational Research* 53 (4): 445–459.

Cordery, J. L., and Wall, T. D. 1985. Work design and supervisory practice: A model. *Human Relations* 38 (5): 425–441.

Davis, L. E., and Miller, C. I. 1971. Human productivity and work design. In *Industrial engineering handbook,* ed. H. B. Maynard. New York: McGraw-Hill.

Dawes, P. L. 1981. The nurses' aide and the team approach in the nursing home. *Journal of Geriatric Psychiatry* 14 (2): 265–276.

Dupree, L. W.; O'Sullivan, M. S.; and Patterson, R. L. 1982. Problems relating to aging: Rationale for a behavioral approach. In *Overcoming deficits of aging: A behavioral approach,* ed. R. L. Patterson, et al. New York: Plenum Press.

Dye, C. J. 1985. Behavioral approaches for enhancing mental health in the nursing home. In *Mental illness in nursing homes: Agenda for research,* ed. M. S. Harper and B. Lebowitz. Rockville, Md.: NIMH, U.S. Department of Health and Human Services.

Falcone, A. R. 1985. Patient oriented management is key to balancing quality and cost. *American Health Care Association Journal* 11 (8): 3–6.

Ford, R. N. 1969. *Motivation through the work itself.* New York: American Management Association.

Frank, L. L., and Hackman, J. R. 1975. A failure of job enrichment: The case of the change that wasn't. *Journal of Applied Behavioral Science* 11: 413–436.

Gagne, R. M., and Reiser, R. A. 1982. Characteristics of media selection models. *Review of Educational Research* 52 (4): 199–212.

Gartner, A. 1981. Paraprofessionals: Past, present, and future. In *Paraprofessionals in the human services,* ed. S. S. Robin and M. O. Wagenfeld. New York: Human Sciences Press.

Gilbreth, F. B. 1911. *Motion study: A method for increasing the efficiency of the workman.* New York: Van Nostrand.

Glaser, E. M. 1975. *Improving the quality of worklife . . . and in the process, improving productivity.* Los Angeles: Human Interaction Research Institute.

Gordon, G. K. 1982. Developing a motivating environment. *Journal of Nursing Administration* 12 (12): 11–16.

Grandjean, E. 1980. *Fitting the task to the man: An ergonomic approach.* London: Taylor and Francis.

Hackman, J. R. 1976. Work design. In *Improving life at work: Behavioral science approaches to organizational change,* ed. J. R. Hackman and J. L. Suttle. Pacific Palisades, Calif.: Goodyear.

Hackman, J. R., and Oldham, G. R. 1976. Development of a job diagnostic survey. *Journal of Applied Psychology* 60: 159–170.

———. 1980. *Work Redesign.* Reading, Mass.: Addison-Wesley.

Hackman, J. R.; Oldham, G.; Janson, R.; and Purdy, K. 1975. A new strategy for job enrichment. *California Management Review* 17 (4): 57–71.

Herzberg, F. 1966. *Work and the nature of man.* Cleveland: World.

———. 1968. One more time: How do you motivate employees? *Harvard Business Review* 48 (1): 53–62.

Hinkley, N. E. 1986. Training assures edge on competition. *Provider* 12 (3): 28–32.

Ireson, W. G., and Grant, E. L., eds. 1971. *Handbook of industrial engineering and management.* Englewood Cliffs, N.J.: Prentice-Hall.

Johnson, R. B., and Johnson, S. R. 1971. *Assuring learning with self instructional packages.* Chapel Hill, N.C.: Self Instructional Packages.

Kasteler, J. M.; Ford, M. H.; White, M. A.; and Caruth, J. L. 1979. Personnel turnover: A major problem for nursing homes. *Nursing Homes* 28 (Jan.–Feb.): 20–25.

Kemp, N. J., and Cook, J. D. 1983. Job longevity and growth need strength as joint moderators of the task design–job satisfaction relationship. *Human Relations* 36 (10): 883–898.

Ketchum, L. 1984. How redesigned plants *really* work. *National Productivity Review* 3 (3): 246–254.

Konz, S. 1979. *Work design.* Columbus, Ohio: Grid.

Kopelman, R. E. 1985. Job redesign and productivity: A review of the evidence. *National Productivity Review* 4 (3): 237–255.

———. 1986. Objective feedback. In *Generalizing from laboratory to field settings,* ed. E. A. Locke. Lexington, Mass.: Lexington Books.

Kraus, E. A. 1974. Study reveals reasons for personnel turnover rates. *Modern Nursing Home* 11: 48–50.

Kraut, A. I. 1976. Developing managerial skills via modeling techniques: Some positive research findings—a symposium. *Personnel Psychology* 24: 397–418.

Kreitner, R.; Reif, W. E.; and Morris, M. 1977. Measuring the impact of feedback on the performance of mental health technicians. *Journal of Organizational Behavior Management* 1: 105–109.

Lawler, E. E.; Hackman, J. R.; and Kaufman, S. 1973. Effects of job redesign: A field experiment. *Journal of Applied Psychology* 3: 49–62.

Leader, M. E. 1986. Nursing assistants get boost in career and self-esteem. *Provider* 12 (3): 41–42.

Lindeman, H. 1984. Training makes nursing assistants "front line" professionals. *American Health Care Association Journal* 11 (7): 65–66.

Locke, E. A.; Sirota, D.; and Wolfson, A. D. 1976. An experimental case study of the successes and failures of job enrichment in a government agency. *Journal of Applied Psychology* 61 (6): 701–711.

Maynard, H. B. 1971. *Industrial engineering handbook.* New York: McGraw-Hill.

McCormick, E. J. 1976. *Human factors in engineering and design.* New York: McGraw-Hill.

Moffic, H. S.; Patterson, G. K.; Laval, R.; and Adams, G. L. 1984. Paraprofessionals and psychiatric teams: An updated review. *Hospital and Community Psychiatry* 35: 61–67.

Nash, A.; Muczyk, J. P.; and Vettori, F. L. 1971. The relative practical effectiveness of programmed instruction. *Personnel Psychology* 24: 397–418.

Nystrom, P. C. 1981. Designing jobs and assigning employees. In *Handbook of organizational design,* ed. P. C. Nystrom and W. Starbuck. New York: Oxford University Press.

Oldham, G. R.; Hackman, J. R.; and Pearce, J. L. 1976. Conditions under which employees respond positively to enriched work. *Journal of Applied Psychology* 61 (4): 395–403.

Orpen, C. 1979. The effects of job enrichment on employee satisfaction, motivation, involvement, and performance: A field experiment. *Human Relations* 32 (3): 189–217.

Paul, W. J.; Robertson, K. B.; and Herzberg, F. 1969. Job enrichment pays off. *Harvard Business Review* 47 (2): 61–78.

Pecarchik, R., and Nelson, B. H. 1973. Employee turnover in nursing homes. *American Journal of Nursing* 73 (2): 289–290.

Pommer, D. A., and Streedbeck, D. 1974. Motivating staff performance in an operant learning program for children. *Journal of Applied Behavior Analysis* 7 (2): 217–221.

Prue, D. M.; Krapfl, J. E.; Noah, J. C.; Cannon, S.; and Maley, R. F. 1980. Managing the treatment activities of state hospital staff. *Journal of Organizational Behavior Management* 2 (3): 165–181.

Quilitch, H. R. 1975. A comparison of three staff-management procedures. *Journal of Applied Behavior Analysis* 8 (1): 59–66.

Rasmussen, J. 1981. Models of mental strategies in process plant diagnosis. In *Human detection and diagnosis of system failures,* ed. J. Rasmussen and W. B. Rouse. New York: Plenum Press.

Richards, W. S., and Thorpe, G. L. 1978. Behavioral approaches to the problems of later life. In *The clinical psychology of aging,* ed. M. Storandt, I. C. Siegler, and M. F. Elias. New York: Plenum Press.

Santos, J. F.; Burdick, D. C.; Hubbard, R. W.; and Santos, M. A. 1983. Training in mental health outreach. In *Mental health and aging: Programs and evaluations,* ed. M. A. Smyer and M. Gatz. Beverly Hills, Calif.: Sage Publications.

Sbordone, R. J., and Sterman, L. T. 1983. The psychologist as a consultant in a nursing home: Effects on staff morale and turnover. *Professional Psychology: Research and Practice* 14 (2): 240–250.

Schwab, D. P., and Cummings, L. L. 1976. A theoretical analysis of the impact of task scope on employee performance. *Academy of Management Review* 1: 23–25.

Schwartz, A. N. 1974. Staff development and morale building in nursing homes. *Gerontologist* 14: 50–53.

Scott, L. 1968. *Programmed instruction and review for practical and vocational nurses: Foundations and fundamentals of nursing.* New York: Macmillan.

Seeborg, I. S. 1978. The influence of employee participation in job redesign. *The Journal of Applied Behavioral Science* 14 (1): 87–98.

Shook, G. L.; Johnson, C. M.; and Uhlman, W. F. 1978. The effect of response effort reduction, instructions, group and individual feedback, and reinforcement on staff performance. *Journal of Organizational Behavior Management* 1 (2): 206–215.

Sims, H. P.; Szilagyi, A. D.; and Keller, R. T. 1976. The measurement of job characteristics. *Academy of Management Journal* 19: 195–224.

Sirota, D., and Wolfson, A. 1972. Job enrichment: Surmounting the obstacles. *Personnel* 1972 (July–August): 9–19.

Strauss, G. 1974. Job satisfaction, motivation, and job redesign. In Organizational behavior: Research and issues, ed. G. Strauss, R. E. Miles, C. S. Snow, and A. S. Tannenbaum. Madison, Wis.: Industrial Relations Research Association.

Stryker, R. 1981. *How to reduce employee turnover in nursing homes.* Springfield, Ill.: Charles C. Thomas.

Taylor, F. W. 1911. *The principles of scientific management.* New York: Harper.

Tichauer, E. E. 1978. *The biological basis of ergonomics: Anatomy applied to the design of work situations.* New York: Wiley.

Tichy, N. M. 1976. When does work restructuring work: Organizational innovations at Volvo and GM. *Organizational Dynamics,* summer: 63–80.

Trist, E. L.; Higgin, G. W.; Murray, H.; and Pollock, A. B. 1963. *Organizational Choice.* London: Tavistock Institute of Human Relations.

Umstot, D. D.; Bell, C. H.; and Mitchell, T. R. 1976. Effects of job enrichment and task goals on satisfaction and productivity: Implications for job design. *Journal of Applied Psychology* 61 (4): 379–394.

Van Cott, H. P., and Kinkdale, R. G., eds. 1972. *Human engineering guide to equipment design.* Washington, D.C.: Government Printing Office.

Vladeck, B. 1980. *Unloving care: The nursing home tragedy.* New York: Basic Books. Epigraph is from pp. 19–20.

Waxman, H. M.; Carner, E. A.; and Berkenstock, G. 1984. Job turnover and job satisfaction among nursing home aides. *Gerontologist* 24: 503–509.

Whittset, D. A. 1971. Job enrichment, human resources and profitability. In *New perspectives in job enrichment,* ed. J. R. Maher. New York: Van Nostrand Reinhold.

Woodson, W. E. 1981. *Human factors design handbook.* New York: McGraw-Hill.

## AFTERWORD

Institute of Medicine. 1986. *Improving the quality of care in nursing homes.* Washington, D.C.: National Academy Press.

# Name Index

# Subject Index